Cases in
Health Services
Management

Cases in Health Services Management

FIFTH EDITION

edited by

Jonathon S. Rakich, Ph.D.
Indiana University Southeast

Beaufort B. Longest, Jr., Ph.D., FACHE
University of Pittsburgh

Kurt Darr, J.D., Sc.D., FACHE
The George Washington University

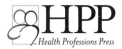
HPP
Health Professions Press

Baltimore • London • Sydney

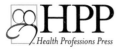

Health Professions Press, Inc.
Post Office Box 10624
Baltimore, MD 21285-0624

www.healthpropress.com

Typeset by Barton Matheson Willse & Worthington, Baltimore, Maryland.
Manufactured in the United States of America by Versa Press, Inc.,
East Peoria, Illinois.

This casebook can be used alone or in conjunction with other texts. To help instructors use the cases most effectively in the classroom, the editors have prepared an instructor's guide, *Instructor's Manual for Cases in Health Services Management*, available on CD-ROM or online from Health Professions Press (see Web site and address above or call 1-888-337-8808 or 1-410-337-9585). *Cases in Health Services Management* can also be used in conjunction with the textbook, *Managing Health Services Organizations and Systems*, also published by Health Professions Press.

The cases presented in this volume are based on the case authors' field research in a specific organization or are composite cases based on experiences with several organizations. In most instances, the names of organizations and individuals and identifying details have been changed. Cases are intended to stimulate discussion and analysis and are not meant to reflect positively or negatively on actual persons or organizations.

Library of Congress Cataloging-in-Publication Data.
Cases in health services management / edited by Jonathon S. Rakich, Beaufort B.
  Longest, Jr., Kurt Darr.—5th ed.
    p.   cm.
  Includes bibliographical references and index.
  ISBN 978-1-932529-59-3 (pbk.)
    1. Health services administration—United States—Case studies.   2. Health
facilities—United States—Administration—Case studies.   3. Hospitals—United
States—Administration—Case studies.   I. Rakich, Jonathon S.   II. Longest, Beaufort B. Jr.
III. Darr, Kurt.

    [DNLM: 1. Hospital Administration—United States.   2. Organizational Case
Studies—United States.   3. Total Quality Management—United States. WX 150 C338 2010]
    RA971.C34 2010
    362.10973—dc22   2010002241

British Library Cataloguing in Publication data are available from the British Library.

Contents

**PART I   PUBLIC POLICY AND THE ENVIRONMENT
OF HEALTH SERVICES DELIVERY**

    Alexandra Piriz and Kurt Darr

    Under the leadership of a new CEO, the efforts of a mid-
    Atlantic acute-care hospital system to develop a vertically inte-
    grated clinic health system result in allegations of antitrust,
    excessive healthcare costs, disruption of physician referral pat-
    terns, and use of harsh collection practices, all of which cause
    a negative reaction in the community.

    Gary E. Crum

    State health department managers must address financial, politi-
    cal, programmatic, and ethical issues in attempting to reduce
    health agency budgets, including the special challenges posed by
    agency employees who are primarily civil servants, and the need
    for legislative approval for reductions.

    Mary K. Feeney

    Flu vaccine shortages in 2004–2005 are caused by a major manu-
    facturer's problems with quality control. Federal and state efforts

to secure the vaccine raise public policy and resource-allocation issues. Three student role-play scenarios facilitate discussion.

David M. Currie and Mark Arundine

FDA approval of high-cost, drug-coated stents for angioplasty procedures as alternatives to uncoated stents and coronary bypass surgery raises issues of a trade-off between quality improvement and costs of medical treatment. Students will also examine the effect on stakeholders—patients, hospitals, and insurers.

Kimberly A. Rucker and Kurt Darr

A pharmaceutical manufacturer encounters significant negative stakeholder reaction to its introduction of a new medication for human immunodeficiency virus (HIV) despite having met expectations for clinical rigor and carefully assessing stakeholders and the external environment.

PART II   STRATEGIC MANAGEMENT

Michael J. King and Robert C. Myrtle

The CEO of a 350-bed hospital explores strategic alternatives to enhance its financial situation and reputation by asking the hospital's board of directors to approve a worksite wellness program. The program is to be marketed to area companies for the purpose of improving workers' health and decreasing employers' healthcare costs. Includes pro forma financial statements.

Jonathon S. Rakich and Alan S. Wong

The organization life cycle of a 96-bed hospital is traced from inception by community leaders, facility decline, and sale to a for-profit system, as well as regeneration with the city's acquisi-

tion and change to not-for-profit status. The CEO reflects on
strategies that returned the hospital to profitability and ponders
its future direction.

Anthony R. Kovner

A general acute-care, not-for-profit, 350-bed hospital in an economically depressed section of the city struggles with rising costs
and deteriorating quality of care. Two major issues are the need
for investment in facilities and technology as well as continuing
support for six off-site clinics partially funded by the city.

*Brent C. Pottenger, Douglas Archer, Stephen Cheung,
and Robert C. Myrtle*

The new CEO of a 30-bed, not-for-profit rural hospital faces a
turnaround situation to make the hospital profitable after 3 years
of losses. Problems include challenging payer mix, too many
full-time equivalent staff members per occupied bed, and difficulty recruiting physicians.

William E. Aaronson

A not-for-profit, faith-based continuing care retirement community seeks help with long-range planning. A consultant encounters resistance to change, questionable financial management
practices, and a lack of business acumen in the board of directors.

Randi Priluck

A not-for-profit home health agency explores strategies to
increase revenue through for-profit ventures without jeopardiz-
ing its charitable culture. The business planning group considers

an assisted-living facility, a private-pay home care program, and an eldercare services program to be marketed to building owners with a high percentage of elderly residents.

PART III   MANAGEMENT, MEDICAL STAFF, AND GOVERNING BODY

A nursing home chain of over 400 facilities has governance challenges in replacing the CEO who founded and built the company; board conflict complicates solving problems of poor financial performance and missed opportunities.

A fired CEO reflects on the board's lack of understanding of medical staff and individual physician relationships with the hospital. Confident that he had board support in a contract dispute with hospital-based radiologists seeking to build a competing off-site imaging center, he was surprised when he was fired; he failed to appreciate the power of the medical staff and the four physician board members.

Vice president for nursing services at a 285-bed for-profit hospital decides what action to take regarding her in-box, which includes e-mails, correspondence, phone messages, and challenges (e.g., two angry nurses, a wandering patient, staff shortages, increasing OR infections). Emphasizes priority setting, decision making, and delegation.

Management of a community hospital is unwilling to recognize and address the major problems in its radiology department, which is directed by a radiologist whose disruptive behavior and preoccupation with income and stock market speculation have diminished the quality of radiograph readings with tragic results.

The CEO has difficulty overcoming barriers and pitfalls in implementing TQM in a chain of seven nursing homes. The embroilment of the TQM initiative in negotiations with the union representing nurses threatens the initiative's future.

A tax district community hospital has major problems with its governance structure because of historical animosities among internal stakeholders, medical staff politics, weak and ambivalent senior management, and a disruptive member of the medical staff with ambitions to attain major power in the hospital.

PART IV   RESOURCE UTILIZATION AND CONTROL

The CFO assesses the financial feasibility of establishing a satellite health park consisting of an ophthalmic surgery center, a diagnostic facility, and a rehabilitation facility. Data on investment, cost, and projected revenue based on patient mix are provided for each proposed health park service. The CFO determines present value of cash flow and conducts payback analysis.

A community hospital experiences the negative financial impact of a city hospital's decision to divert medically indigent ER patients. Left unchecked, the practice will create a large deficit. Turning the patients away will also create the double bind of serious public relations problems for the hospital.

PART VI   ETHICS INCIDENTS

Kurt Darr

Ten mini–case studies cover the spectrum of administrative and clinical ethical issues, from conflicts of interest to dishonest contractors and from infection control to advance directives.

Administrative Ethics

Incident 1:   Borrowed Time
Incident 2:   Emergency Department Repeat Admissions: A Question of Resource Use
Incident 3:   The Administrative Institutional Ethics Committee
Incident 4:   Bits and Pieces
Incident 5:   A Potentially Shocking Revelation

Clinical Ethics

Incident 6:   Protecting the Community
Incident 7:   Decisions
Incident 8:   The Missing Needle Protector
Incident 9:   Demarketing to Avoid Bankruptcy
Incident 10:   Something Must Be Done, But What?

About the Editors

Jonathon S. Rakich, Ph.D., Professor of Management, School of Business, Indiana University Southeast, New Albany, Indiana 47150
Dr. Rakich received his master of business administration from the University of Michigan–Ann Arbor and his doctorate in business from Saint Louis University. His university instructional areas are strategic management at the undergraduate and graduate levels and health services administration. During his 42-year teaching career, Dr. Rakich has coauthored 3 books in 13 editions, 45 journal articles (including those in *Health Care Financing Review*, *Health Care Management Review*, *Hospital & Health Services Administration*, *Journal of Health & Society Policy*, and *Hospital Topics*), and more than 60 conference proceedings and professional papers.

Professor Rakich was awarded a postdoctoral federal faculty fellowship with the U.S. Department of Health and Human Services and has served on the board of trustees of a home health agency and health systems agency. During academic sabbaticals, he served an administrative residency at Summa Health System and conducted on-site research of the Canadian healthcare system. He holds membership in the Academy of Management, including in the Health Care Management and Business Policy divisions.

Professor Rakich is Distinguished Professor Emeritus of Management and Health Services Administration at the University of Akron, where he taught from 1972 to 1999. During that period he held administrative positions as Director of Graduate Programs in Business, Director of Executive Development Programs, and Coordinator of the MBA–Health Services Administration option program.

Beaufort B. Longest, Jr., Ph.D., FACHE, M. Allen Pond Professor and Director of the Health Policy Institute, Department of Health Policy and Management, Graduate School of Public Health, University of Pittsburgh, Pittsburgh, Pennsylvania 15261
Professor Longest holds a doctorate from Georgia State University. He is a fellow of the American College of Healthcare Executives and holds memberships in the Academy of Management, AcademyHealth, American Public Health Association, and the Association for Public Policy Analysis

and Management. He is an elected member of the Beta Gamma Sigma Honor Society in Business as well as in the Delta Omega Honor Society in Public Health.

Professor Longest's research has led to the publication of numerous peer-reviewed articles in respected national and international journals. He has authored or coauthored 10 books and 30 chapters in other books. His current research and scholarship address corporate citizenship, health policy making, and governance and management in healthcare settings. His work in these areas has been published in refereed journals and as chapters in books and has underpinned his most recent books, *Managing Health Services Organizations and Systems, Fifth Edition, Managing Health Programs and Projects,* and *Health Policymaking in the United States.*

Professor Longest consults with healthcare organizations and systems, universities, associations, and government agencies on health policy and management.

Kurt Darr, J.D., Sc.D., FACHE, Professor of Hospital Administration, Department of Health Services Management and Leadership, School of Public Health and Health Services, The George Washington University Medical Center, Washington, D.C. 20037
Dr. Darr holds a doctor of science from The Johns Hopkins University and a master of hospital administration and a juris doctor from the University of Minnesota.

Professor Darr completed an administrative residency at Rochester (Minnesota) Methodist Hospital and subsequently worked as an administrative associate at the Mayo Clinic. After being commissioned in the U.S. Navy, he served in administrative and educational assignments at St. Albans Naval Hospital and Bethesda Naval Hospital. He completed postdoctoral fellowships with the Department of Health and Human Services, the World Health Organization, and the Accrediting Commission on Education for Health Services Administration.

Professor Darr is a fellow of the American College of Healthcare Executives. He is admitted to practice before the Supreme Court of the state of Minnesota and the Court of Appeals of the District of Columbia. Dr. Darr is a mediator for the Civil Division of the Superior Court of the District of Columbia. He has served as a hearing officer for the American Arbitration Association.

Teaching and research focuses include health services management, administrative and clinical ethics, hospital organization and management, quality improvement, and application of the Deming method in health services. Professor Darr is the author and editor of books used in graduate health services administration programs and numerous articles on health services topics.

Professors Longest and Darr are coauthors of the textbook, *Managing Health Services Organizations and Systems, Fifth Edition* (2008), published by Health Professions Press.

Professors Rakich, Longest, and Darr have collaborated in authoring and editing books in the field of health services management for over 30 years.

Contributors

William E. Aaronson, PhD
Associate Professor of Healthcare
  Management
Temple University
409 Ritter Annex (006-00)
1810 North 13th Street
Philadelphia, PA 19122

Douglas Archer, MHA
State Capital Center
School of Policy, Planning, and
  Development
University of Southern California
Sacramento, CA 95811

Mark Arundine
c/o Richard Ivey School of
  Business
The University of Western
  Ontario
1151 Richmond Street North
London, Ontario N6A 3K7
CANADA

Bryan Boliard, MBA
Sykes College of Business
University of Tampa
401 West Kennedy Boulevard
Tampa, FL 33606

**Ronnie R. Boongaling, MS,
  MHA**
Practice Administrator
North Valley Dermatology
  Center
251 Cohasset Road, Second Floor
Chico, CA 95926

Stephen Cheung, MHA
State Capital Center
School of Policy, Planning, and
  Development
University of Southern California
Sacramento, CA 95811

George S. Cooley, MBA
President
Long Green Associates, Inc.
Post Office Box 15
Long Green, MD 21092

Gary E. Crum, PhD
Executive Director
SW Virginia Graduate Medical
  Education Consortium
The University of Virginia's
  College at Wise
One College Avenue
Wise, VA 24293

David M. Currie
c/o Richard Ivey School of
  Business
The University of Western
  Ontario
1151 Richmond Street North
London, Ontario N6A 3K7
CANADA

Kathryn H. Dansky, PhD
Associate Professor of Health
  Policy and Administration
Department of Health Policy
  and Administration

The Pennsylvania State
 University
114-H Henderson Building
University Park, PA 16802

Kurt Darr, JD, ScD
Professor
Department of Health Services
 Management and Leadership
School of Public Health and
 Health Services
The George Washington
 University
2175 K Street, N.W., Suite 320
Washington, DC 20037

Bonnie Eng-Suess, MHA
Contract and IPA Specialist
Central Health MSO, Inc.
1051 Parkview Drive, Suite 220
Covina, CA 91723

Bruce D. Evans, MBA
Professor of Management
Graduate School of Management
University of Dallas
Braniff Building, Room 260
1845 East Northgate
Irving, TX 75062

Mary K. Feeney, PhD
Assistant Professor
Department of Public
 Administration
University of Illinois at Chicago
412 S. Peoria St. (M/C 278)
Chicago, IL 60607

Elizabeth M. A. Grasby, PhD
c/o Richard Ivey School of
 Business
The University of Western
 Ontario
1151 Richmond Street North
London, Ontario N6A 3K7
CANADA

Amy J. Hillman
c/o Richard Ivey School of
 Business
The University of Western
 Ontario
1151 Richmond Street North
London, Ontario N6A 3K7
CANADA

Mike Jasperson, MBA, MSHA
Sykes College of Business
University of Tampa
401 West Kennedy Boulevard
Tampa, FL 33606

**Richard L. Johnson, FACHE,
 FAAHC, MBA**
Executive Vice President
Physician Management
 Resources, Inc.
Post Office Box 188
Clarendon Hills, IL 60514

Michael J. King, MHA, CPA
Chief Operating Officer
Doctors Medical Center of
 Modesto
1441 Florida Avenue
Modesto, CA 95350

Anthony R. Kovner, PhD
Professor of Public and Health
 Management
Robert F. Wagner Graduate
 School of Public Service
New York University
40 West 4th Street
600 Tisch Hall
New York, NY 10003

Cynthia Mahood Levin, MHSA
Sr. Director of Executive
 Programs & Service Quality
Guest Services
Stanford Hospital & Clinics
300 Pasteur Drive
Stanford, CA 94305

Curtis P. McLaughlin, DBA
Professor Emeritus of Health
  Policy and Administration
Kenan-Flagler School of Business
University of North
  Carolina–Chapel Hill
Chapel Hill, NC 27599

Robert C. Myrtle, DPA
Professor of Health Services
  Administration and
  Gerontology
School of Policy, Planning, and
  Development
University of Southern California
Lewis Hall 312
Los Angeles, CA 90089

John E. Paul
Clinical Associate Professor
Department of Health Policy and
  Management
1102B McGavran-Greenburg
  Hall C.B. #7411
University of North Carolina at
  Chapel Hill
Chapel Hill, NC 27599-7411

Alexandra Piriz
Candidate for the Master of
  Health Services Administration
Department of Health Services
  Management and Leadership
School of Public Health and
  Health Services
The George Washington
  University
Washington, DC 20052

Brent C. Pottenger, MHA
State Capital Center
School of Policy, Planning, and
  Development
University of Southern California
Sacramento, CA 95811

Randi Priluck, PhD
Assistant Professor of Marketing
Lubin School of Business
Pace University
One Pace Plaza W482
New York, NY 10038

Jonathon S. Rakich, PhD
Professor of Management
School of Business
Indiana University Southeast
4201 Grant Line Road
New Albany, IN 47150

Michael F. Rolph, MBA, CPA
Senior Vice President and Chief
  Financial Officer
First Health of the Carolinas
Post Office Box 3000
Pinehurst, NC 28374

Kent V. Rondeau, PhD
Associate Professor
School of Public Health
Faculty of Medicine and
  Dentistry
University of Alberta
13-103 Clinical Sciences Building
Edmonton, Alberta T6G 2G3
CANADA

Kimberly A. Rucker, MHSA
Segment Manager, Direct Pay
  Market
Marketing Strategy and Analysis
Kaiser Foundation Health Plan of
  the Mid-Atlantic States
Rockville, MD 20852

Marilyn Seymann
c/o Richard Ivey School of
  Business
The University of Western Ontario
1151 Richmond Street North
London, Ontario N6A 3K7
CANADA

Earl Simendinger, PhD
Professor of Management
Sykes College of Business
University of Tampa
Campus Box 148F
401 West Kennedy Boulevard
Tampa, FL 33606

Jason Stornelli
c/o Richard Ivey School of
   Business
The University of Western Ontario
1151 Richmond Street North
London, Ontario N6A 3K7
CANADA

William E. Stratton, PhD
Professor of Management
College of Business
Idaho State University
Campus Box 8020
Pocatello, ID 83209

Cara Thomason, MHA, MSG
Dementia Care Coordinator
Park Terrace Senior Living
21952 Buena Suerte
Rancho Santa Margarita, CA 92688

Rosalie Wachsmuth, MHA, MSG
Program Manager
Aging and Disability Services
   Administration
State of Washington
9315 58th Avenue Court S.W.
#R-204
Lakewood, WA 98499

Mary Anne Watson, PhD
Associate Professor of
   Management
Sykes College of Business
University of Tampa
Campus Box 122F
401 West Kennedy Boulevard
Tampa, FL 33606

Gary R. Wells, PhD
Professor of Finance
College of Business
Idaho State University
Campus Box 8020
Pocatello, ID 83209

Michael Wiltfong

Alan S. Wong, PhD
Professor of Finance
School of Business
Indiana University Southeast
4201 Grant Line Road
New Albany, IN 47150

Preface

Like its predecessors, the fifth edition of *Cases in Health Services Management* describes management problems and issues in a variety of healthcare settings. The primary criterion used for selecting the cases was that each had to be rich in applied lessons. The result is a comprehensive set of health services management cases in one volume, 36% of them new. Selection was tempered by the editors' 90 years of combined experience teaching with the case method.

The cases in this edition are of various lengths and complexities and are grouped into six parts. Of the 28 cases, 10 are new. One carryover case, Hartland Memorial Hospital, has been completely revised. Cases that have stood the test of time are retained in this edition. Almost half of the cases feature settings outside acute care hospitals, including long-term care facilities, health networks, a continuing care retirement community, an emergency department, a hospital burn unit, a pharmaceutical company, a city health department, a home health agency, and a software company. Part I is new and focuses on public policy and the environment of health services delivery.

Acute care hospital cases include a range of sizes, types, ownerships, and geographic locations, including rural and inner-city settings. One hospital case is set in a multi-institutional system; another applies the principles of continuous quality improvement. An in-box exercise set in a hospital simulates the time pressures and importance of prioritizing issues that confront managers.

Depending on depth of analysis and the amount of time available for out-of-class preparation, most cases can be addressed adequately in one or two class hours. A few cases are short and present single issues. Most, however, are integrative and complex, and involve multiple problems and issues. Analyses will require applying several discrete disciplines and knowledge areas. Users must synthesize and apply knowledge, skills, and experience from the social-behavioral sciences; administrative and clinical ethics; individual, social, and environmental determinants of health; management and administration (e.g., strategic planning and policy formulation, marketing, organizational and administrative relationships, problem solving, resource allocation and utilization, control, financial management, human resources management); and health services organization, financing, and delivery.

The primary audience for this book is students in health services management programs. Cases are especially effective in integrating the curriculum, and many students will use this book in a capstone course. Case analysis bridges theory and practice. In this regard, new and experienced managers will find the cases informative as they hone analytical and problem-solving skills. These cases can also be used in continuing professional development seminars for practicing managers. (A broad definition of managers is appropriate here because department heads and mid- and senior-level managers perform similar generic management activities.)

By their nature, cases present events, situations, problems, and issues. It is the dynamics of the analysis, especially the group discussion, that make the case method such a powerful and rich tool for learning. Therefore, users are urged to review the Introduction, which describes the case method and case analysis.

The cases included in this volume are intended to stimulate class discussion and analysis. In most instances, the names of organizations and individuals are disguised. In all instances authors of the cases have prepared well-written, factual situations that are based on field research in a specific organization, or a composite case based on experience with several organizations. None of these cases is meant to reflect positively or negatively on actual persons or organizations, or to depict either effective or ineffective handling of administrative situations.

The 28 cases and 10 ethics incidents are organized in six parts:

Part I: Public Policy and the Environment of Health Services Delivery (five cases)

Part II: Strategic Management (six cases)

Part III: Management, Medical Staff, and Governing Body (six cases)

Part IV: Resource Utilization and Control (five cases)

Part V: Human Resource Management and Organizational Dynamics (six cases)

Part VI: Includes 10 ethics incidents that sensitize and educate students about the administrative and clinical issues that managers confront.

The synopsis of each case in the table of contents identifies the organizational setting, dominant themes, and issues.

As experiential learning in health services management education has given way to more discipline-based didactic education, and as younger, less-experienced students have entered graduate programs, cases that apply didactic work have taken on increased importance. This collection of cases, combined with a solid academic grounding in health services and management disciplines, will be of great aid in preparing students for situations they are certain to encounter as health services managers.

The core task of teaching others to manage effectively in the health services field is to provide the insight to identify and define problems and the judgment to apply the skills and methods needed to solve them. With instructor or seminar-leader guidance, cases such as those in this volume can make an important contribution to that end.

TEXTBOOK SUPPLEMENT AND INSTRUCTOR'S MANUAL

A useful supplement for students and instructors using the case method is *Managing Health Services Organizations and Systems, Fifth Edition*, published by Health Professions Press. This textbook will ground students in the healthcare system and give them the management knowledge necessary for case analysis. Chapter 6, "Managerial Problem Solving and Decision Making," is especially helpful in preparing to use the case method.

An Instructor's Manual, available on CD-ROM from Health Professions Press, accompanies *Cases in Health Services Management, Fifth Edition*. It contains the teaching notes that have been prepared by the authors of the cases. It is available without charge to instructors who adopt the casebook.

The Instructor's Manual also contains follow-up case supplements to the following four cases in the casebook:

1. Governance Challenges at Good Hands Healthcare (B, C, and D)— follow up to case #12

2. Hartland Memorial Hospital (Part 2: Organizational Diagnosis and Social-Networking Exercise)—follow up to case #14

3. West Florida Regional Medical Center (B)—follow up to case #21

4. Hospital Software Solutions (B)—follow up to case #24.

Instructors who use the follow-up cases are invited to reproduce them for classroom use.

Acknowledgments

The editors wish to acknowledge the generous contribution of the authors whose cases are included in this book. They are listed alphabetically beginning on page xix. We thank them for allowing us to use their cases. In addition, thanks are owed to the book and journal publishers who granted permission to reprint the cases to which they hold the copyright.

We are indebted to the staff of Health Professions Press for their help in producing the book, specifically Mary Magnus, director of publications; Cecilia González, book production editor and production manager; and Kristi Maxwell, marketing and sales manager. We recognize and thank staff members at our universities who assisted us: Cheryl Young, Linda Kalcevic, and Alexandra Piriz.

Finally, we thank our respective deans and chairs for nurturing an organizational environment that made our work possible.

Introduction

For decades the case method has played an essential role in the study of law, medicine, and business. It has become an established part of education in healthcare management programs and similar types of educational activities. The cases in this volume were selected for use in healthcare management education because they describe problems and situations that have been faced by managers in the past and provide meaningful learning opportunities for the managers of tomorrow. The cases facilitate the following:

- Assist students to develop the assessment, analytical, and conceptual skills necessary for effective problem solving and decision making

- Support students as they synthesize and integrate theory and its application

- Encourage dynamic and interactive discussion among students that challenges their experience and values

- Allow students to quickly acquire knowledge and insights.

Traditional didactic education provides background and foundation in disciplines and methodologies relevant to health services management. For many students, fellowships, residencies, internships, and similar types of field experience supplement didactic learning. Case studies blend didactic and experience-based learning; both are enhanced in the process.

This Introduction (1) describes the types of cases, (2) lists benefits of the case method, (3) discusses the roles of students and instructors in using cases, and (4) outlines a methodology for case analysis.

TYPES OF CASES

Cases are situation-specific descriptions of management issues and problems that students are asked to identify and evaluate. By definition, cases describe past events. The cases reflect contemporary situations, issues, and problems that managers confront. Thus, cases can impart valuable lessons and insights relatively unfettered by temporal change. The lessons learned analyzing and evaluating cases have enduring value and are applicable throughout a career.

Some cases are comprehensive and integrative and involve a variety of functional areas and a range of issues and problems that affect the whole organization. Others are more narrowly focused. All of the cases in this book permit students to:

- Operationally define the issue(s) or problem(s) that are present

- Identify facts and distinguish them from assertions, opinions, and hearsay

- Separate facts important to solving the problem from facts that are unimportant

- Distinguish relevant facts from irrelevant facts

- Make assumptions that are supported by facts, when necessary

- Apply appropriate management disciplines and methodologies

- Take the role of managers or external consultants when considering alternatives, offering recommendations, and planning implementation.

In sum, case studies and the case method offer a disciplined approach to problem solving and will provide a rich learning experience.

BENEFITS OF THE CASE METHOD

The case method offers numerous benefits. None is more important than giving students the opportunity to develop and sharpen their analytical skills and thought processes. The essence of case analysis is assessment and problem solving. Thus, cases enable students to hone skills in situation assessment, problem diagnosis and definition, alternative solution evaluation and selection, and development of plans to implement solutions and evaluate them. Because students must articulate and defend their recommendations, logic and communication skills are enhanced as well.

The case method also requires students to synthesize and integrate knowledge. Compartmentalized subject areas and underlying disciplines, such as organizational behavior, accounting, economics, marketing, finance, and law, must be linked, blended, and applied in a holistic way during case analysis. Cases require that students apply management theory to actual settings. Case study is an opportunity to practice being a manager—it puts the students at the scene of the events depicted and requires application of classroom theory. Case study exposes students to various organizational settings and managerial problems and provides a vehicle to introduce and discuss complementary subject matter relevant to the case, but not included in it.

Finally, cases are an opportunity for students to learn and practice group interactive skills. The case method is used in group forums. In either a structured or unstructured fashion, all participants discuss the case, present their analyses, and critique the analyses of others. The flow of facts, opinions, perceptions, and values results in productive student learning, including learning to work effectively within a group.

ROLES OF INSTRUCTORS AND STUDENTS

In using the case method, instructors depart from the usual role of lecturer and become discussion leaders and facilitators. The instructor's task in the case method is to encourage students to think independently and to formulate and defend their analyses. The burden of learning is properly on the students. Learning takes place most effectively in the case method if students use the opportunity provided by analysis and discussion to sharpen their skills.

Instructors are essential to the case method and contribute in several ways: selecting cases and the order in which they are assigned; providing a classroom environment that permits students to gain maximum benefit from the case analysis and interactive discussions; and giving direction to class discussion—expanding or contracting it, or changing the direction and focus, as appropriate. To effectively facilitate the use of the case method, instructors must be thoroughly knowledgeable about the case— virtually to the point of having memorized its key elements. Only then can instructors correct misunderstandings and misperceptions, as well as provide information and facts that students may have missed or misunderstood. Instructors may also define and address collateral issues. Instructors can provide direction in the analyses by using the Socratic method to pose key questions. Following discussion, the instructor should critique the group's work by commenting on class discussion, the analytical process, elements ignored or over- or underemphasized, and the quality of recommendations. Such critiques improve learning and the ability of students to use effectively the case analysis method.

Instructors may use several criteria to evaluate student performance:

- Mastery of the facts in the case—as well as of facts acquired by the student from other sources—and their use(s)

- Application of discipline-specific and analytical methodologies

- Soundness of assumptions, as supported by facts, and the logic of a student's reasoning

- Accuracy of identifying problems and the clarity and precision with which they are articulated

- Consistency and compatibility of analysis, recommendations, and whether the solution will solve the problem

- Quality of alternative solutions to the problem(s) identified and the comprehensiveness of decision criteria by which alternative solutions are judged

- Means to implement and evaluate application of the solution

- Degree to which the solution(s) and implementation are feasible and relevant to the issue(s) involved and whether they consider internal and external forces.

Pedagogically, instructors may choose an unstructured or structured approach to using the case method. In the unstructured approach, the instructor assigns a case. Students read and prepare an analysis of the case for class discussion. The instructor initiates discussion by asking open-ended questions of the class in general, or to specific students: What is the problem in the case? What contextual aspects should be considered? What facts are there? Which facts are important, unimportant? If you were the decision maker, what would you do? Why? How would you implement your recommendation(s)?

The structured approach is more formal and requires that each student prepare a written report using a specific format or outline. The instructor initiates discussion by asking one or two members of the class to present their case analysis. Alternatively, the instructor assigns the case to groups of students. Each group prepares a written analysis of the case. One group presents its analysis to the class and this is the basis for discussion.

The pedagogic technique an instructor uses will be influenced by factors such as personal preference; class size and length of the class period; and academic mix and previous experience of students, including their familiarity with the case method and their grounding in the underlying disciplines. Over time, the instructor's approach may change from structured to unstructured depending on the learning objectives, the degree to which the instructor introduces corollary subject matter through lectures or through controlled and directed discussion, and the progress students make in adapting to the case method.

Whatever the approach, two attributes of case study sometimes surprise students. First, it is impossible for case writers to include all of the relevant facts and circumstances of a situation. This means that cases are incomplete. These gaps can be partially filled by making assumptions that are supported by the facts that are available. This situation is typical for managers, who almost never have all of the facts that they would like to have before making a decision.

Second, it is not uncommon that the problems identified in cases have no right or wrong answers. This attribute makes case study dynamic, interesting, integrating, and powerful. Initially, students may be frustrated because answers to the problems in a case are elusive. Greater experience with case study will show them, however, that small differences in situation assessment, assumptions, or problem definition can lead to very different conclusions and recommendations.

The role of students in case study is demanding. Because they bear the responsibility of learning, this is as it should be. An often anxiety-laden aspect of using the case method is that students must present their analyses and recommendations in the classroom and have their peers and the instructor challenge their work. If class discussion is to be productive, students must be well prepared and be active participants. Effective participation means contributing substance, not merely talking or restating points already made.

PROCEDURES FOR CASE ANALYSIS

There are several effective case analysis models. Instructors may have developed their own. Most instructors require that students assume they are part of the organization or setting of the case, take the perspective of the manager(s), and apply a systematic analytical approach.

Typically, students begin their analysis by assessing the facts of a case and organizing them by category. Categories may include organizational objectives; expectations about performance held by internal and external stakeholders; past and present results of operations; internal organizational strengths and weaknesses; external influences, such as regulations or the actions of competitors; and similar relevant factors. In some cases, each category may be important. For others, only some categories are important. Regardless, the initial task is to gather and organize facts. When completed, the problem statement can be formulated.

The problem statement is the starting point for the analysis. The case may have one problem or several, and they may be explicit or implicit. Correctly stating the problem is a crucial aspect of the case method, and it is also a skill essential to effective management. It can be a difficult task, but the skill can be developed and is facilitated by experience with case analysis. Success depends on thoroughly and effectively assessing the facts in the case.

Care must be taken to distinguish the symptoms of a problem from its root causes. Exhibits and figures in a case must be thoroughly assessed. Data should be analyzed—to the point of performing calculations—so that the case and its problems can be better understood.

Making assumptions that are relevant to the problem statement follows. There are three types of assumptions: structural, personal (about the problem solver), and problem-centered. Facts must be available to support assumptions, which are inferences drawn from facts using deductive or inductive reasoning. Assumptions allow the problem solver to extend and enhance what is known.

The next step in case analysis is formulating alternatives that can solve the problem(s). Facts that delimit or distinguish obviously infeasible alternatives from those that can be considered further are particularly useful. Facility expansion, for example, may be infeasible if assessment of the current financial situation shows that capital funds are unavailable or that the organization's market area will not sustain the growth. Quantitative and financial analytical methods should be used to compare alternatives, as appropriate.

After feasible solutions have been developed, the analyst must evaluate them. Evaluating alternative solutions requires applying decision criteria that judge relative merit and effectiveness in solving the problem. Arraying the decision criteria and solutions in a matrix is especially effective in understanding the relationships. Appropriate questions to guide the process include the following:

- Are the alternatives consistent with the organization's philosophy, culture, and mission?

- Which alternative provides the greatest benefits?

- What are the relative costs of each alternative?

- Are internal capabilities to implement alternatives equal?

- Will external influences constrain or support implementation of the alternatives differently?

The answers to these and similar questions will determine which solution is selected.

Once a solution is chosen, implementation must be planned and undertaken. After implementation, the effectiveness of the solution must be evaluated. Implementation should include the means, methods, and staff who will perform the evaluation. The question to be answered is "How will we know that the problem has been solved?" For some cases, implementation is the primary focus, whereas for others evaluating alternative solutions and choosing one is the focus. Implementation is addressed more generally in the cases in this volume. Regardless of the emphasis in a case, attention must be given to implementation and evaluation of the solution. This makes case analysis more realistic, which is, after all, the central reason for using the case method.

OTHER RESOURCES IN USING THE CASE METHOD

A generic model for using case analysis is as follows:

1. Students should identify the role that they will play in the process of analysis.

2. State the problem to be solved: "In what ways can I (we) . . . ?"

3. Summarize, organize, and number the facts that are *relevant* to the problem statement.

4. Draw inferences (make assumptions) relevant to the problem statement, including the following:

   a. Structural assumptions (context, resources, constraints, laws, regulations)

   b. Personal assumptions about the problem solver (biases, risk taker, risk averse, escalating commitment, anchoring)

   c. Problem-centered assumptions (urgency, time frame, importance, degree of risk)

5. Link the inferences (assumptions) to the facts by citing the numbers of the facts that are supportive.

6. Identify tentative solutions.

7. Use general, broad-based criteria to perform initial screening of tentative alternative solutions.

8. Develop a decision matrix to compare and apply specific decision criteria to select the solution that will be implemented.

9. State in general terms how *and* by whom the solution will be implemented.

10. Identify how *and* by whom the solution, once implemented, can be evaluated.

Additional information about problem solving and application of the case method can be found in Chapter 6, "Managerial Problem Solving and Decision Making," of *Managing Health Services Organizations and Systems, Fifth Edition*, published by Health Professions Press.

PART I

Public Policy and the Environment of Health Services Delivery

1

Carilion Clinic

Alexandra Piriz

Kurt Darr
The George Washington University, Washington, D.C.

BACKGROUND: CITY OF ROANOKE

Nestled in the Commonwealth of Virginia, between Salem and Vinton, is the city of Roanoke. The city last recorded almost 95,000 residents; its metropolitan area population is just over 293,000.[1, 2] Bisected by the Roanoke River and surrounded by the Blue Ridge Mountain Parkway, Roanoke is the commercial and cultural hub of western Virginia and southern West Virginia.

The community that became Roanoke was established in 1852. Early economic development of Roanoke resulted from its importance as the junction point for the Shenandoah Valley Railroad and the Norfolk and Western Railway. These lines were essential to transport coal from mines in western Virginia and West Virginia.[3, 4] Within Roanoke's contemporary service area are a regional airport, shopping malls, corporate headquarters, and distribution centers for several national companies, among them Advanced Auto Parts.[1, 2]

CARILION CLINIC

Employing almost 13% of Roanoke's total population is Carilion Clinic (formerly Carilion Health System), which includes 12 different facilities within 20 miles of the city's center. The "Clinic" has a children's hospital and several breast care and lactation centers as well as acute care hospitals and a physician group practice. The Carilion Clinic employs over 500 physicians in a multispecialty group practice that is active in 10 not-for-profit hospitals within a 150-mile radius.[5] The system admits over 1 million patients annually.[5] In 2008, the eight main hospitals were licensed for 1,215 beds.[5] This does not include infant or inpatient rehabilitation beds at the cornerstone facility, Carilion Roanoke Memorial Hospital.[5]

The Clinic's additional joint ventures and other related companies include the following nonexhaustive list:

Roanoke Ambulatory Surgery Center (50% ownership)

New River Valley Surgery Center (50% ownership)

Carilion Clinic Physicians, LLC (real estate holding company)

Carilion Labs, LLC

Carilion Emergency Services, Inc.

Carilion Behavioral Health, Inc.

Led by Edward Murphy, M.D., since 1998, Carilion Health System has become Carilion Clinic, a vertically integrated system of 10 hospitals that includes graduate and undergraduate medical education programs, a group practice of over 500 physicians, and other ventures. The organization has net operating revenue of over $1.2 billion, with assets of $1.1 billion in 2007.[6, 7] Dr. Murphy's compensation totaled almost $2.3 million in 2007. Nancy Agee, the Clinic's chief operating officer, earned the next highest amount at less than $800,000, a more than $1.5 million difference.[8]

CONTROVERSY IN ROANOKE

Despite its philanthropic mission and positive effect on the growth of Roanoke, Carilion Clinic has not always enjoyed a positive relationship with its community. (Carilion Clinic's mission, vision, and values statements can be found in Appendix 1.)

In May 1988, the U.S. Justice Department's Antitrust Division sought to prevent the merger of the two hospitals located in Roanoke: Memorial Roanoke Hospital and Community Hospital of Roanoke Valley. These two hospitals later became known as Carilion Health System. The suit attempted to block the merger due to the likely monopoly it would create in the area. Less than one year after the suit was filed, the U.S. Court of Appeals (Fourth Circuit) found for the defendants:

. . . the merger between defendant hospitals would not constitute an unreasonable restraint of trade under the Sherman Act § 1. The merger would strengthen the competition between the hospitals in the area because defendant hospitals could offer more competitive prices and services.[9]

In the two separate appeals that followed, the courts found for the defendants. These decisions allowed for the major expansion of what has become Carilion Clinic.

IN A MARKET: WHAT CONSTITUTES A MONOPOLY?

A monopoly occurs when one or more persons or a company dominate an economic market. This market domination results in the potential to exploit or suppress those in the market or those trying to enter it (supplier, provider, or consumer).[10]

During the 19th century, the U.S. government began prosecuting monopolies under the common law as "market interference offenses" in an effort to block suppliers from raising prices. Companies were often found buying all of the supplies of a certain material or product in a particular area, a practice now referred to as "cornering the market."

In 1887, Congress increased its efforts and passed the Interstate Commerce Act in response to railway companies' monopolistic practices in small, local markets.[10] This legislation protected small farmers who were being charged excessive rates to transport their goods. Congress continued to address the issue of monopolistic practices by passing the Sherman Antitrust Act of 1890, which limited the anticompetitive practices of businesses. The act blocked the transfer of stock shares to trustees in exchange for a certificate entitling them to a share of earnings.[10] The Sherman Act became the basis for the Clayton Antitrust Act of 1914, the Federal Trade Commission Act of 1914, and the Robinson-Patman Act of 1936, which replaced the Clayton Act.[10]

Antitrust or competition laws address three main issues:

1. Prohibit agreements or practices that restrict free trade and competition among business entities.

2. Ban abusive behavior by a firm dominating a market, or anticompetitive practices that tend to lead to such a dominant position.

3. Supervise the mergers and acquisitions of large corporations, including some joint ventures.[11]

The Herfindahl-Hirschman Index helps implement these laws by providing a method to determine market "density" or the concentration of the market. (The index is found in Appendix 2.) Antitrust laws and methods of calculating market density, such as the Herfindahl-Hirschman Index, are imperfect and can leave gaps that are later exploited.[12]

VERTICAL INTEGRATION: THE MAYO CLINIC

The Mayo Clinic is the leading model for vertical integration in the delivery of healthcare in the United States. Founded in 1863 in Rochester, Minnesota, the Mayo Clinic began as the medical practice of William Worrall Mayo, M.D., and his two sons, who were also physicians. It grew to include a comprehensive array of specialties.[13] This expansion allowed the Mayo Clinic to develop different levels of care across the health services continuum. Eventually it became a fully integrated health system.[13] Notably, Mayo physicians are salaried at competitive market levels, and they control the management structure.

Headquartered in Rochester, Minnesota, and with satellite clinics and hospitals in Jacksonville, Florida, and Scottsdale, Arizona, the Mayo Clinic has continued to provide excellence and dedication in the delivery of care through a constant (and often, self-admittedly, stubborn) commitment to its core values. Among those values are the needs of the patient come first, integration of teamwork, efficiency, and a mission over profit mentality.[14]

The Mayo Clinic is internationally recognized for quality and excellence in the delivery of care. *U.S. News and World Report* has ranked it as a Best Hospital in its annual evaluation for 19 consecutive years and several times identified it as an Honor Roll hospital, making it one of the 19 elite hospitals so recognized.[15]

Its management team's efforts and successes have also been noticed. In 2008, *Management Lessons from Mayo Clinic* by Leonard L. Berry, a service industry authority, and Kent D. Seltman, Mayo Clinic's marketing administrator, was published.[15] The book is a revealing look at the business concepts that have produced stellar clinical results, efficiency, and patient satisfaction.[16]

FORESHADOWING A MAYO CLINIC CLONE

Before Dr. Murphy took the helm of Carilion Health System, the organization's actions had stirred significant but manageable controversy due to the antitrust case of 1988. Following the court's decision that the merger was legal and posed no threat of monopoly, the hospital resumed its quiet existence in the community.

Upon his arrival, Dr. Murphy began to vertically integrate the organization, and he presented a formal plan in Fall 2006. The resulting actions on the part of Carilion Health System, among them the purchase of existing practices and the closure of others, has placed Carilion at the forefront of a battle involving local physicians, community members, and, in August 2008, the national media.

WHO IS EDWARD MURPHY, M.D.?

What does it take to get ranked 23rd in the Top 100 Most Powerful People in Healthcare?[17] Or 4th in the Top 50 Most Powerful Physicians?[17] What do you have to do to be paid $2.27 million in one year ($1.37 million in salary and $901,206 in benefits [2007])?[6] For Dr. Murphy, you grow a two-hospital health system into a vertically integrated health system anchored by a 500-physician specialty group practice that includes 10 not-for-profit hospitals, undergraduate and graduate medical programs, a large array of tertiary referral services, and a multistate laboratory service.[7]

Dr. Murphy earned his B.S. from the University of Albany and his medical degree (with honors) from Harvard University Medical School.[7] Although he has never practiced medicine, Dr. Murphy has worked as a clinical professor at the University of Albany, School of Public Health, and as an adjunct assistant professor at Rensselaer Polytechnic Institute School of Management.[7] Before his departure from New York state, he was also a member of the New York State Hospital Review and Planning Council and served on its executive committee as the vice chair of the Fiscal Policy Council.[7]

From 1989–1991, Dr. Murphy served as vice president of clinical services at Leonard Hospital, a 143-bed facility north of Albany, New York.[18] In 1991, he was promoted to president and CEO of Leonard Hospital until its merger with St. Mary Hospital to form Seton Health System in 1994. Dr. Murphy became president and CEO of the newly formed health system and stayed with Seton until 1998, when he relocated to Roanoke to head Carilion Health System.[7, 17]

Dr. Murphy's other roles in the Roanoke community are as a board member of Healthcare Professionals Insurance Company and Trust, Luna Innovations, Inc., and HomeTown Bank. He is past chair of the Art Museum of Western Virginia. He also serves in an influential position with the Council on Virginia's Future, which works to proactively frame the growth and progress of the state, including its businesses, population, and health of the population.[7]

VERTICAL INTEGRATION: BECOMING A "CLINIC"

Dr. Murphy has been clear about his intentions for the future of Carilion Health System. In an August 2006 interview, he stated, "Right now . . . our core business is hospital services. In the new model, the core business will be physician services; the hospital will become ancillary." [19] In an interview in 2007 for *Health Leaders Magazine*, Dr. Murphy explained, "I've been enamored of this model of healthcare delivery for a long time . . ." [19]

In Fall 2006, Dr. Murphy, his staff, and the leadership board of Carilion Health System officially announced their intention to create a new approach to Carilion's management that was to be characterized by teamwork and salaried physicians and other caregivers focused on patient care across the spectrum of care.[20] Dr. Murphy explained,

> The essence of the clinic model is that hospitals stop becoming inde-
> pendent businesses and start becoming ancillary services to the physician
> practice . . . If hospitals eventually want to provide better and more cost-
> effective healthcare it's a necessary shift.[20]

The transformation was scheduled to take place over 7 years with an 18-month-long phase in of the name Carilion Clinic and phase out of the name Carilion Health System, which had been adopted in the early 1990s. The plans for Carilion Health System also included a 50–50 partnership with Virginia Tech University in Blacksburg, Virginia, to establish a private not-for-profit clinical research institute and new medical school. Further, over the next five years (2007–2012) Carilion Clinic was to add 4–5 additional fellowship positions to support its work.[20]

A year after the formal announcement, Carilion Health System and Virginia Tech University released a joint statement announcing the creation of a new medical school in Virginia as "a jointly operated private medical school, located in downtown Roanoke, adjacent to Carilion Roanoke Memorial Hospital." [21] Its much-anticipated groundbreaking was scheduled for early 2008.[21] On July 20, 2009, Virginia's State Council for Higher Education approved the Virginia Tech Carilion School of Medicine (VTCSM) for operation as a postsecondary institution.[22] This approval gave the VTCSM degree-granting authority and made it eligible for scholarship and grant funding and will be followed by an application for approval from the State Association of Colleges in Fall 2009.[20, 22] The VTCSM is scheduled to matriculate its inaugural class in Fall 2010.[23]

WALL STREET JOURNAL EXPOSÉ

Generally speaking, an organization would be pleased if the *Wall Street Journal (WSJ)* published an article about the organization. That is, of course, unless the story started a firestorm that led to separate citizen and physician coalitions working against you and raised the specter of a word from Carilion's pre-history: *monopoly.*

Published on the front page of the *WSJ* on August 28, 2008, was a piece titled "Nonprofit Hospitals Flex Pricing Power. In Roanoke, Va., Carilion's Fees Exceed Those of Competitors: The $4,727 Colonoscopy." (The complete article is found in Appendix 3.) Written by John Carreyrou, the article explores Carilion's history, including the 1989 antitrust case, its expanding "market clout," and positive strides toward its goal of vertical integration, with the suggestion that some of the means used were questionable.[24] Painting a less-than-rosy picture for millions of *WSJ* readers throughout the world, Carreyrou exposed a little-known secret in Roanoke, Virginia—its skyrocketing healthcare costs, affected in part by, and possibly even led by, Carilion Clinic.[24]

Carilion denied any allegations of monopolistic practices or exploitative pricing and claimed it faces robust competition from Lewis-Gale Medical Center located in nearby Salem, Virginia.[25] (The Carilion Clinic press release is located in Appendix 4, and general information about Lewis-Gale Medical Center is found in Appendix 5.) Carilion Clinic defended its pricing practices, stating that it needs to subsidize costly services such as emergency departments and the uncompensated care of the uninsured throughout its operations.[25]

Unsettling was Carreyrou's examination of Carilion's practice of suing former patients for unpaid medical bills. Once a court judgment is obtained, Carilion places a lien against the patient's home. A lien on real property puts a "cloud" on the title, which prevents the owner from conveying the property with a clear title until the lien has been satisfied. Responding in the *WSJ*, Dr. Murphy stated,

> Carilion only sues patients and places liens on their homes if it believes they have the ability to pay. . . . If you're asking me if it's right in a right-and-wrong sense, it's not. . . . But Carilion cannot be blamed for the country's "broken" healthcare system.[24]

Dr. Murphy seems to acknowledge that although Carilion's efforts to protect its financial interests meet legal requirements, they are morally flawed. This position appears to be inconsistent with its mission that "Patient Care Comes First." And perhaps this is only one of several contradictions at Carilion.

WHERE WERE THE LOCAL MEDIA?

As reported by Carreyrou, Carilion made several complaints to the editors of the *Roanoke Times* regarding reporter Jeff Sturgeon's coverage of the system and its activities. Shortly after these complaints were made, mainly in response to a May 2008 piece by Sturgeon that focused on Carilion's practice of awarding business deals to its board members (totaling over $19 million in one case), Carilion pulled much of its advertising from the *Roanoke Times*. At about the same time, Sturgeon, who was the paper's longtime health issues writer, was reassigned. (The article is reprinted in Appendix 6.)

But even with Sturgeon's removal, Carilion continued to be front-page news in the *Roanoke Times* through the reporting of Sarah Bruyn Jones, who has covered the community's reaction to the *WSJ* article and the impetus that it brought to the local coalitions. Some of her articles include: "Carilion Critics Draw Hundreds to Meeting" (September 2008); "Fed Agency Looks into Carilion Purchase" (September 2008); "Carilion Footprint Expands in Deal" (August 2008); and "Carilion to Buy Cardiology Practice" (August 2008). Jones's reporting continues to put Carilion's practices in the forefront of the minds of Roanoke's citizens, but as was noted by Carreyrou, Carilion's growth seems unstoppable; resistance is not taken well.

THE BACKLASH

The attention and close examination that resulted from the August 2008 *WSJ* article resulted in a backlash from the community and fueled physicians' efforts to address what they claim are specific concerns. Concerns include anticompetitive behavior, unfair pricing, and a desire for open referrals for patients who come from outside Carilion's health network.[26]

Citizen and physician coalitions have often met in hotel conference centers and community centers to discuss the "unfair practices and behaviors" of Carilion Clinic. One coalition, the Citizens Coalition for Responsible Healthcare, has sponsored a petition that reads,

> To Dr. Murphy and the Carilion Health System Board of Directors:
>
> Please reconsider your Carilion Clinic plans. I want to keep my right to choose my doctor, even if he or she is an independent physician. Please rethink spending $100 million of my community's money on a Clinic model that could ruin our hospitals! Monopolies are never good for healthcare.[27]

The coalition's Web site (www.responsiblehealthcare.org) offers copies of the *WSJ* article, video recordings of their meetings, information about a new forum program, and a membership form for those who wish to participate in their efforts.[27]

The citizen coalitions maintain that their intentions are to bring focus to what they deem the negative impact of Carilion's transformation into a physician-led clinic that will increase costs and drive out many local physicians.[26] Dr. Murphy's plan would bring into Carilion Clinic as many physicians as possible, and each of them would have a salaried position. The concerns of the citizen coalitions stem from the scope of the effort, which has resulted in the closure or sale of many physician practices. Physicians assert that they cannot compete. Further, Carilion's system of internal referrals, coupled with the purchase of existing practices, has given many physicians with specialty practices only two choices: pack up and leave, or stay and fight.[26]

Despite the controversy, Carilion's plans show no signs of slowing, and they have stayed the course outlined in Fall 2006.

CARILION'S RESPONSE

On August 28, 2008, less than 24 hours after publication of Carreyrou's *WSJ* article, Carilion launched a counterattack. Statements published in newspapers and posted on Carilion's Web site and press releases given to the media attacked the allegations and stated that most of the article's conclusions were misleading and misinformed.

Carilion stated that as evidenced by the Virginia Hospital and Healthcare Association (of which it is a member) PricePoint Web site, it is not only comparable to surrounding hospitals, but also generally has lower prices than its closest competitor, Lewis-Gale Medical Center in neighboring Salem.[25] In support of their position on pricing, Carilion stated, ". . . medical care in hospitals is more expensive . . . having staff and technology at the ready has its costs."[25] Also mentioned was the Carilion Clinic's Life-Guard helicopter, which is an additional subsidized service.[25]

Carilion provided $42 million in charity care in 2007 and an additional $25 million in free care (bad debt that was written off), thus illustrating its dedication and support of Roanoke and surrounding communities.[25] Carilion also supports research and education, which are substantial resource commitments and should be recognized as additional significant costs to the organization and subsidized services to the community.[25]

In explaining the practice of suing patients, Carilion claimed that efforts are made to qualify patients for public programs after they are admitted to its facilities. Further, Carilion stated that only "a small fraction of the nearly 2 million" patient billings it has each year go to court.[25]

Court filings are a final resort, and we try to be flexible. If the judgment includes a lien on an individual's property, we do not foreclose on the lien. The lien is satisfied if and when the property is sold.[25]

In response to concerns about the Clinic's internal referral practice, Carilion stated that referrals are sent internally from Carilion physician to Carilion physician with the intention of sending patients to better, more-qualified physicians who have "earned" the referral. Further, Carilion stated that this "earn, not force" mentality contributes to the ultimate goal of well-coordinated care and service, which is the first choice of patients.[25]

The press release closed by describing a wasteful and poorly organized U.S. healthcare system that they hoped to improve with the vertically integrated clinic model of providing care.[25] The hope is that comprehensive, high-quality, and cost-effective care will put the patient first. The reader of the press release is reminded that what happened at Mayo could be replicated at Carilion.

CURRENT SITUATION IN ROANOKE (2009)

Almost three years after its public announcement, Carilion Health System is but a distant memory. Carilion Clinic has taken its place. At present there is a new medical school partnership and an ever-expanding physician practice with a long specialty list. However, Roanoke may not have seen anything yet.

Two decades after the original controversy surrounding a small-town hospital merger in Roanoke, Virginia, the landscape has changed, the population is growing, and healthcare costs are rising.[24] When the antitrust case began in 1988, Roanoke had among the lowest health insurance premium rates in Virginia; they are now among the highest.[28]

The 1989 antitrust decision was a harbinger of events that have occurred since in the Roanoke Valley. Carilion Clinic's problems with the Federal Trade Commission (FTC) continue. In mid-2009, the FTC brought an administrative complaint against Carilion to force divestiture of physician-owned neurology and orthopedic practices that it had acquired. In less than one month, Carilion reached an agreement with the FTC requiring that it divest the two specialty practices.[29, 30] Such actions by the FTC will have a chilling effect on Carilion Clinic's ability to become a comprehensive, vertically integrated healthcare provider.[29, 30]

QUESTIONS

1. Identify the problems that Carilion Clinic faces as it seeks to become a comprehensive, vertically integrated healthcare provider. Rank these problems in terms of difficulty of resolution for Carilion.

2. Develop arguments to support Carilion Clinic's efforts to become a comprehensive, vertically integrated healthcare system.

3. Identify reasons why competition is useful *and* why it is not useful in terms of healthcare cost, quality, and access.

4. Why could the Mayo Clinic develop a comprehensive, vertically integrated healthcare system and Carilion Clinic seemingly cannot?

5. Identify the advantages and disadvantages of developing specialty services internally to achieve vertical integration compared with obtaining the same services by acquiring existing providers.

ENDNOTES

1. http://www.roanoke.org "Roanoke Region of Virginia; Roanoke Regional Partnership." Updated 2009. Accessed July 1, 2009.
2. http://quickfacts.census.gov/qfd/index.html U.S. Census Bureau. Updated July 13, 2009. Accessed July 17, 2009.
3. http://www.dgif.virginia.gov Virginia Department of Game and Inland Fisheries. Accessed August 14, 2009.
4. Cramer, John. "Southeast's decline followed industrial shifts." http://www.roanoke.com Accessed August 14, 2009.
5. http://www.carilionclinic.org/Carilion/About+Us Updated 2009. Accessed June 22, 2009.
6. Bruyn Jones, Sarah. "Carilion CEO earned $2.27 million last fiscal year." *Roanoke Times*, September 10, 2008. Available at http://www.roanoke.com/business/wb/174762
7. http://www.vtc.vt.edu/about/leadership/ed_murphy.html Updated 2009. Accessed June 23, 2009.
8. 2006 Carilion Clinic Income Tax Form. Tax Year 10/1/2006–09/30/2007.
9. *United States of America v. Carilion Health System and Community Hospital of Roanoke Valley.* 707 F. Supp. 840.
10. http://legal-dictionary.thefreedictionary.com/Monopoly Accessed June 20, 2009.
11. http://www.oecd.org Organization for Economic Co-Operation and Development Updated 2009. Accessed July 1, 2009.
12. Wildermuth, John. "Will political donations keep Microsoft intact?" *San Francisco Chronicle*, July 1, 2001, p. A-1. Available at http://www.sfgate.com/cgi-bin/article.cgi?file=/c/a/2001/07/01/MN221539.DTL&type=printable

13. http://www.diavlos.gr/orto96/ortowww/historym.htm Updated April 12, 1997. Accessed June 21, 2009.
14. http://electronic-engagement.elliance.com/index.php/2009/01/11/brand-building-mayo-clinic-style/ Updated 2009. Accessed June 24, 2009.
15. http://www.mayoclinic.org/feature-articles/honor-roll-2008.html 2001–2009 Mayo Foundation for Medical Education and Research. Accessed July 6, 2009.
16. http://www.mhprofessional.com/product.php?isbn=0071590730&cat=106 Accessed July 6, 2009.
17. Lugar, Norma. "Up Close with Dr. Edward Murphy." *Roanoker Magazine*, January/February 2008. Available at http://www.theroanoker.com/features/ EdMurphy_jf08/index.cfm
18. http://www.hospital-data.com/hospitals/LEONARD-HOSPITAL-TROY. html Accessed July 6, 2009.
19. Nason, Deborah. "Charting a new course: Dr. Edward Murphy plans a trans-formation at Carilion Health System." *Virginia Business Magazine*, August 2006. Available at http://www.gatewayva.com/biz/virginiabusiness/lifestyle/ 0806_options/op_pro.shtml
20. Betbeze, Philip. "Keep 'em close." *Health Leaders*, June 2007. Available at http://www.healthleadersmedia.com/content/90253/topic/WS_HLM2_ MAG/Keep-Em-Close.html
21. http://www.vtnews.vt.edu/story.php?relyear=2007&itemno=5 Updated 2009. Accessed July 6, 2009.
22. http://www.vtc.vt.edu/about/newsroom/releases/2009-07-20schev certification.html Updated 2009. Accessed July 22, 2009.
23. http://www.vtc.vt.edu/about/newsroom/releases/2009-06-03preliminary accreditation.html Accessed July 22, 2009.
24. Carreyrou, John. "Nonprofit hospitals flex pricing power. In Roanoke, Va., Carilion's fees exceed those of competitors: The $4,727 colonoscopy." *Wall Street Journal*, August 28, 2008. Available at http://online.wsj.com/ article/SB121986172394776997.html?mod=2_1566_topbox
25. Statement from Carilion Clinic in response to *Wall Street Journal* article. Carilion Clinic, August 29, 2008. Available at http://www.carilionclinic.org/ Carilion/Statement+from+Carilion+Clinic+in+response+to+Wall+Street+ Journa
26. Bruyn Jones, Sarah. "Carilion critics draw hundreds to meeting: The citizen group says Carilion Clinic is driving up costs." *Roanoke Times*, September 10, 2008.
27. http://www.responsiblehealthcare.org/ Accessed June 20, 2009.
28. http://online.wsj.com/public/resources/documents/cigna_email080827.pdf Updated 2009. Accessed June 28, 2009.
29. Bruyn Jones, Sarah. "FTC questions buys by Carilion. The federal agency wants to undo the sale of two medical centers to maintain competition." *Roanoke Times*, July 28, 2009. Available at http://www.roanoke.com/business/ wb/213330
30. Zeiger, Anne. "Pressured by FTC, Carilion Clinic agrees to sell outpatient centers." Fiercehealthcare.com. August 9, 2009. Available at http://www. fiercehealthcare.com/story/carilion-clinic-agrees-sell-outpatient-centers/ 2009-08-09?utm_medium=rss&utm_source=rss&cmp-id=OTC-RSS-FH0

APPENDIX 1

Carilion Clinic

Mission, Values, and Vision

Carilion Clinic's goal is to provide the best possible outcome for every patient by working together to practice, teach, and discover better ways to heal. We do that through our Commitment to Care:

Patient Care Comes First   Carilion Clinic's defining value is patient care. We will design better ways to put our patients at the center of everything we do.

Timely Access to Care   Time is of the essence in the delivery of care. We will work to eliminate delays in the delivery of care so that our patients will receive the treatment they need, when they need it.

Teamwork and Efficiency   Coordination of care is essential to positive outcomes. We will work together to provide the most accurate diagnoses and deliver the most appropriate treatments for our patients.

Measurable Quality   Healthcare is best measured by quality outcomes. We will do everything we can to continuously improve toward the most possible positive outcomes for our patients.

Continuous Learning   Medical education ensures our ability to care for future generations. We will train medical professionals in dynamic ways to attract and retain the most skilled staff to care for our patients.

Research and Discovery   Advances in medicine are critical to improving the care we provide. We will support clinical research to remain on the leading edge of medicine and make the latest treatments available to our patients.

Trust and Respect   A high level of trust is required for patients to face disease with dignity and courage. We will respect our patients as fellow human beings who need our compassion and deserve our care.

Transparency and Accountability   Patients have every right to expect open and honest answers from their healthcare provider. We will hold ourselves accountable to our patients and provide them access to the information they need to make informed decisions about their health.

Retrieved July 2, 2009, from http://www.carilionclinic.org/Carilion/Mission+Values+and+Vision (Updated 2009.)

APPENDIX 2

Herfindahl-Hirschman Index

"HHI" is the Herfindahl-Hirschman Index, a commonly accepted measure of market concentration. It is calculated by squaring the market share of each firm competing in the market and then summing the resulting numbers. For example, for a market consisting of four firms with shares of 30%, 30%, 20%, and 20%, the HHI is 2600 ($30^2 + 30^2 + 20^2 + 20^2 = 2600$).

The HHI takes into account the relative size and distribution of the firms in a market and approaches zero when a market consists of a large number of firms of relatively equal size. The HHI increases both as the number of firms in the market decreases and as the disparity in size between those firms increases.

Markets in which the HHI is between 1000 and 1800 points are considered to be moderately concentrated, and those in which the HHI is in excess of 1800 points are considered to be concentrated. Transactions that increase the HHI by more than 100 points in concentrated markets presumptively raise antitrust concerns under the Horizontal Merger Guidelines issued by the U.S. Department of Justice and the Federal Trade Commission.

Retrieved July 6, 2009, from http://www.usdoj.gov/atr/public/testimony/hhi.htm (Updated 2009.)

APPENDIX 3

Nonprofit Hospitals Flex Pricing Power

In Roanoke, Va., Carilion's Fees
Exceed Those of Competitors: The $4,727 Colonoscopy

By: John Carreyrou

ROANOKE, Va.—In 1989, the U.S. Department of Justice tried but failed to prevent a merger between nonprofit Carilion Health System and this former railroad town's other hospital. The merger, it warned in an unsuccessful antitrust lawsuit, would create a monopoly over medical care in the area.

Nearly two decades later, the cost of health care in the Roanoke Valley—a region in southwestern Virginia with a population of 300,000—is soaring. Health-insurance rates in Roanoke have gone from being the lowest in the state to the highest.

That's partly a reflection of Carilion's prices. Carilion charges $4,727 for a colonoscopy, 4 to 10 times what a local endoscopy center charges for the procedure. Carilion bills $1,606 for a neck CT scan, compared with the $675 charged by a local imaging center.

Carilion's market clout is manifest in other ways. With eight hospitals, 11,000 employees, and $1 billion in assets, the tax-exempt hospital system has become one of the dominant players in the Roanoke Valley's economy. Its dozens of subsidiaries include businesses ranging from athletic clubs to a venture-capital fund.

The power of nonprofit hospital systems like Carilion over their regional communities has increased in recent years as their incomes have surged. Critics charge this is creating untaxed local health-care monopolies that drive the costs of care higher for patients and businesses.

"It's a one-market town here in terms of health care," says Sam Lionberger, who owns a local construction firm. "Carilion has the leverage."

Carilion acknowledges its influence in the local community but says there is nothing untoward about it. The hospital says it doesn't have a monopoly over the Roanoke Valley health-care market because it faces robust competition from Lewis-Gale Medical Center, a hospital located in nearby Salem, Va., and owned by for-profit chain HCA Inc.

Carilion says it charges more for certain procedures because it has to subsidize operations such as an emergency department and treatment for the uninsured. Edward Murphy, Carilion's CEO, says the high cost of health care in Roanoke reflects the national increase in such costs, which he says is driven by overutilization of medical services. Carilion is converting to a clinic model, in which doctors are employees of the hospital system and work more closely together to coordinate care, in an effort to cut down on unnecessary tests and procedures, he says. "Fragmentation is the enemy of quality" and affordable care, Dr. Murphy says.

The Roanoke City General District Court in downtown Roanoke devotes one morning a week to Carilion cases—lawsuits the hospital files against patients who haven't paid bills.

However, the clinic project has provoked a backlash from a group of local independent doctors, who say it is designed to stifle competition.

Originally set up to serve the poor, nonprofit hospitals account for the majority of U.S. hospitals. They are exempt from taxes and are supposed to channel income they generate back into operations, while providing benefits to their communities. But they have come under fire from patient advocates and members of Congress for stinting on charity care even as they amass large cash hoards, build new facilities, and award big paychecks to their executives.

Fueled by large, untaxed investment gains, Carilion's profits have risen over the past five years, reaching $107 million last year. Over the same period, the total annual compensation of its chief executive, Dr. Murphy, nearly tripled to $2.07 million. His predecessor, Thomas Robertson, received a lump-sum pension from Carilion of $7.4 million in 2003, on top of more than $2 million in previous pension payouts.

Carilion says Dr. Murphy's compensation is in line with comparable health-care organizations and notes he doesn't receive car allowances, a spousal allowance, or club memberships. It says Mr. Robertson's pension accrued over a 32-year career at Carilion.

Carilion estimates it receives about $50 million a year in tax exemptions. It dispensed $42 million in charity care in 2007 and $30 million in 2006.

After the 1989 merger, Carilion continued to operate Roanoke's two hospitals separately. It later consolidated the hospital boards and in 2006, transferred most of Roanoke Community Hospital's staff and services to a renovated and enlarged Roanoke Memorial Hospital.

The moves eliminated any hospital competition in Roanoke proper, enabling Carilion to raise its prices and contributing to a spike in health-insurance rates in the region, one of the least affluent parts of the state, according to local doctors and health-insurance brokers.

The construction of a new medical campus around Roanoke Memorial Hospital began several years ago.

Alan Bayse, founder of a local benefits-consulting firm who has sold health insurance in the area for 30 years, says health-insurance rates in the Roanoke Valley used to be 20% lower than in Richmond, Virginia's capital, and the lowest in the state. Today, he says, they are the highest in the state and 25% higher than in Richmond, citing rate information from insurer Cigna Corp. Anthem, another health insurer, says its rates are 6% higher in Roanoke than in Richmond.

Mr. Lionberger, whose construction company has about 100 employees, says his health-care costs have risen 50% over the past three years, hampering his ability to compete with contractors from other parts of the state. "It's frustrating," he says.

While Carilion strengthened its power in the hospital market, Roanoke continued to be home to a community of independent doctors numbering in the hundreds.

Taking the Helm

In 2001, Dr. Murphy took the nonprofit hospital system's helm. Dr. Murphy, who has a medical degree from Harvard but doesn't practice medicine, says he was convinced that the cost and quality of care in Roanoke could be improved if doctors worked in a more centralized system. In June 2006, he announced a seven-year, $100 million plan to transform Carilion into a multispecialty clinic, like the Mayo Clinic.

Carilion began approaching private physician groups, offering to buy their practices and pay their salaries. Some accepted, but others balked. Some doctors who chose to remain independent say the number of patients referred to them by Carilion physicians plummeted. Carilion controls a large proportion of Roanoke's referrals because it employs a majority of doctors who make them, such as family practitioners, pediatricians, and emergency physicians.

Joseph Alhadeff, an orthopedic surgeon who is a member of a private practice called Roanoke Orthopedic Center, says the number of joint replacements he performed dropped off sharply after he stopped getting such referrals from Carilion doctors, prompting him to plan to relocate to Pennsylvania. "I spent seven years building up a practice and watched it evaporate in six months," he says.

Carilion spokesman Eric Earnhart says the hospital system didn't engage "in any activity to reduce or divert" referrals from Dr. Alhadeff. Mr. Earnhart adds that Carilion continues to refer numerous cases to Roanoke Orthopedic Center.

Geoffrey Harter, an ear, nose, and throat doctor at another Roanoke private practice, Jefferson Surgical Clinic, says Carilion-employed colleagues told him the hospital system asked them not to refer patients to doctors it didn't employ, calling such referrals "leakage." Keeping referrals within Carilion is lucrative for the hospital system because it ensures tests and procedures performed on patients take place at Carilion facilities.

Dr. Murphy says Carilion uses the term "leakage" in internal marketing discussions and that he would rather see its doctors refer patients to other Carilion doctors to optimize their care. But he says Carilion doesn't require its doctors to keep referrals in-house even though it would be legal to do so.

As tension between Carilion and Roanoke's independent doctors grew in 2006, a group of 200 doctors formed an organization called the Coalition for Responsible Healthcare to protest the Carilion Clinic plan. The group posted a petition on its Web site and put up billboards around Roanoke that read: "Carilion Clinic. Big Dream. Big Questions." The local newspaper, the *Roanoke Times*, covered the controversy in a series of articles written by its health-care reporter, Jeff Sturgeon.

A few months later, in March 2007, the *Roanoke Times* moved Mr. Sturgeon off the health-care beat after Carilion complained repeatedly about his coverage. Carilion says it communicated its displeasure to the paper's editors, but never asked that Mr. Sturgeon be reassigned. Carilion withdrew most of its advertising from the paper, but says it did that as part of a reallocation of its ad budget. "Any friction that exists between an organization like us and the media is entirely appropriate," Mr. Earnhart says.

Mr. Sturgeon, who now covers transportation, declined requests for comment. Carole Tarrant, the *Roanoke Times*'s editor, said: "We're covering Carilion like we always have and always will, and have no plans to change how we cover Carilion." She declined to elaborate.

New Campus

A large part of the clinic conversion's costs have involved the construction of a new medical campus around Roanoke Memorial Hospital that began several years earlier.

The lead contractor building the site is Swedish construction giant Skanska. But one of the project's biggest beneficiaries has been J.M. Turner & Co., which is owned by Carilion board member Jay Turner. Carilion says it paid J.M. Turner a total of $14.9 million in direct contracting work from 2004 to 2007.

Dr. Murphy says Carilion's board authorized "arm's length work" with J.M. Turner, but adds that "a case could be made that we shouldn't award work to J.M. Turner to avoid the appearance of impropriety."

Carilion also paid Skanska, the lead contractor, a total of $120.8 million from 2003 to 2007. Some of that money flowed back to J.M. Turner as subcontracting work, according to Skanska and J.M. Turner. The companies and Carilion declined to say how much.

In an email, Mr. Turner said he recuses himself from all Carilion board decisions that involve his company. He added that his firm passed on much of the $14.9 million in direct contracting work it received from Carilion to other subcontractors.

Mr. Turner isn't the only Carilion board member with a financial stake in the new medical campus. Another board member, Warner Dalhouse, has invested in a hotel being built on the campus to accommodate patients and their families. HomeTown Bank, a local bank Mr. Dalhouse founded and of which he was until recently chairman, is financing the hotel's construction. Dr. Murphy and Mr. Turner sit on HomeTown Bank's board.

Carilion and Mr. Dalhouse say he didn't make his $130,000 investment in the hotel until after Carilion sold the parcel to Texas developers in early 2006. "I wasn't dealing with Carilion. I was dealing with the new owners of that land who had paid fair market value for it," Mr. Dalhouse says.

Carilion says its transformation into a multispecialty clinic will eventually lower local health-care costs. But many patients say they have yet to see relief from Carilion medical bills.

The Roanoke City General District Court devotes one morning a week to cases filed by Carilion. In its fiscal year ended Sept. 30, Carilion says it sued 9,888 patients, garnished the wages of 5,478 people, and placed liens on 3,920 homes. Carilion says the people it takes to court have the means to pay their bills.

On a Thursday morning in June, a Carilion representative waited outside a courtroom to intercept the half-dozen patients who had responded to summonses to appear in court. She took them to a side room to work out payment plans. A judge later called out names of close to 100 patients who didn't show and, one-by-one, entered judgments against them.

One of the patients who came to court, a 32-year-old housewife named Christie Masellis, faced a $12,137.12 bill. She had gastric bypass surgery at a Carilion facility in 2005. After developing complications, she required two more surgeries. She says her insurer covered the first surgery but not the two follow-ups because it changed its coverage policy.

Mrs. Masellis has two children. Her husband, Mark, earns about $49,000 a year working for an auto-parts distributor. Mrs. Masellis says she inquired about qualifying for hospital financial assistance, but the Carilion representative told her she was no longer eligible for charity care because her account was past due. The representative agreed to put her account on hold until Sept. 30 but offered her no discount. The bill included $2,514.82 in interest charges Carilion added to the original debt of $9,622.30.

Carilion's Mr. Earnhart says Mrs. Masellis had already received more than $15,000 in charity-care discounts. The suit Carilion filed is "for the remainder of the bill," he says.

Mr. and Mrs. Masellis have begun the process of filing for personal bankruptcy. Mr. Masellis says the hospital bill was a big factor in the decision, though the couple has other debts, including a $68,000 mortgage.

When some patients don't pay their bills, Carilion places liens on their homes. Carilion says it doesn't track how many liens it has outstanding, but the close to 4,000 it filed in 2007 "is representative of a typical year," Mr. Earnhart says. Carilion doesn't foreclose on homes and only collects when properties are sold, he says.

Dr. Murphy says Carilion only sues patients and places liens on their homes if it believes they have the ability to pay. "If you're asking me if it's right in a right-and-wrong sense, it's not," he says. But Carilion can't be blamed for the country's "broken" health-care system, he says.

Published August 28, 2008. *The Wall Street Journal.* Available at
http://online.wsj.com/article/SB121986172394776997.html?mod=googlenews_wsj

APPENDIX 4

Carilion Clinic's Press Release in Response to the *Wall Street Journal* Article

Friday, Aug. 29, 2008

On Thursday, Aug. 28, the *Wall Street Journal* targeted Carilion Clinic in an article about not-for-profit healthcare providers. We would like to address some of the key issues raised by the *Journal*, and hopefully answer some of the questions you may have in relation to the article.

Insurance Rates and Costs   The article implies that Carilion is the reason that insurance premiums are rising in our part of the state. It is misleading to infer that Carilion is the cause when premiums—set by insurance companies—contain many factors outside our control. The hospital component of the premium is just 40 percent; other factors include drug costs, utilization by the population, insurance overhead, and insurance profits. About sixty percent of hospital utilization in this region occurs at Carilion facilities.

If you compare Carilion's hospital charges to Lewis-Gale Medical Center and to HCA Richmond hospitals, we are generally lower, as evidenced on the Virginia Hospital & Healthcare Association (VHHA) PricePoint consumer website (www.vapricepoint.org).

Yes, medical care in hospitals is more expensive than in outpatient settings. Having staff and technology at the ready has its cost. Also, it is no secret that care for the uninsured and for unprofitable services—such as the Carilion Life-Guard helicopter ambulance service and Emergency Room care—has to be subsidized. Carilion is the safety net for many people in our community who have no means to pay for services, and this burden is borne in part by paying patients.

Community Benefits   As stated in the article, we provided $42 million in charity care (at cost) in 2007 to qualifying patients. An additional $25 million in free care was written off as bad debt. The total amount far exceeds U.S. Senator Chuck Grassley's proposed 5 percent requirement for not-for-profit hospitals.

In addition, we support medical residency teaching programs, provide financial assistance to nursing education and allied health programs in the region, and give significant resources to area not-for-profit organizations such as the Roanoke Rescue Mission, Child Health Investment Partnership (CHIP), and Free Clinics. These are important investments in the community's health.

Collections We have a generous charity care policy, and we actively work to qualify the poor, uninsured, and underinsured for free and discounted care.

Part of our collection process does include filing court judgments against individuals who do not qualify for charity care and do not pay their bills. This represents a small fraction of the nearly 2 million patient visits that occur per year. It is only fair to patients who do pay their bills that we collect from those who are able to pay but choose not to. Court filings are a last resort, and we try to be flexible. If the judgment includes a lien on an individual's property, we do not foreclose on the lien. The lien is satisfied if and when the property is sold.

Referrals Our position all along has been to *earn*, not force, referrals to our physicians. It is our intent through well-coordinated, high-quality care and service to be the first choice of patients for their medical care.

Board Activities We have a conflict-of-interest policy to which our board members are held accountable. Jay Turner, President of J.M. Turner Construction, is not involved in contracting decisions and abstains from any vote that might involve work by his company, in keeping with the Board's policy. We have always voluntarily disclosed on our Form 990 filings the value of the work Mr. Turner's company contracts with Carilion.

Closing We share national concerns about the rising cost of healthcare. One reason we are re-organizing into a physician-led Clinic is to more effectively and efficiently provide medical care. It is estimated that 30 percent of all medical tests and procedures are unnecessary. Carilion Clinic is on a path to improve healthcare outcomes, to reduce medical waste, and to make a positive difference in the lives of our patients. We have a lot of important work to do to reach our vision of creating a healthier and more vibrant region.

Available at http://www.carilionclinic.org/Carilion/Statement+from+Carilion+Clinic+in+response+to+Wall+Street+Journa

APPENDIX 5

Lewis-Gale Medical Center

The Lewis-Gale Medical Center resulted from the 1996 merger of Lewis-Gale Hospital and Lewis-Gale Psychiatric Center. Currently, it is a 521-bed medical center. It serves as the hub of HCA (Hospital Corporation of America) Virginia Health System's southwestern region. HCA is composed of locally managed facilities that include 163 hospitals and 112 outpatient centers in 20 states and in England.

Lewis-Gale Medical Center is led by Victor E. Giovanetti, FACHE, President, Southwest Virginia region. Lewis-Gale includes specialty services such as neurosurgery, cardiac surgery, and cancer treatment. Its three hospitals are located in western Virginia: Alleghany Regional Hospital in Low Moor, Montgomery Regional Hospital in Blacksburg, and Pulaski Community Hospital in Pulaski. All three are west of Roanoke.

HCA Virginia (including Lewis-Gale Medical Center) is the state's fourth-largest private employer. Its workforce includes more than 13,500 direct employees, as well as contracted physicians.

In 2007, HCA Virginia provided $242 million in free charity care to low-income and uninsured patients. It also donated more than $1.3 million to nonprofit organizations and causes, and paid $27 million in taxes.

Retrieved July 28, 2009, from http://www.hcavirginia.com/ and http://www.lewis-gale.com/ (Respective copyrights 2009.)

APPENDIX 6

Carilion, Board Members Collaborate

A company whose chief is on
Carilion's board has received $19 million worth of work

By Jeff Sturgeon

Carilion Clinic awarded $19.3 million worth of construction work over a three-year period to the company of a builder who sits on its board of directors.

Roanoke-based J.M. Turner & Co., Inc., received $582,724, $9 million, and $9.7 million in 2006, 2005, and 2004, respectively. The company's chairman, chief executive officer, and co-owner is Jay Turner, a Carilion board member during each of those years. Turner said Carilion lets board members work for or sell products and services to the system, with oversight, and confirmed that his company provides needed health care construction services.

Carilion's hiring of the firm has not been his decision or a decision he influenced, he said, though he is pleased the company named after his father is a Carilion contractor.

Carilion said it values having business-minded individuals drawn from the community on its board.

"I'm not sure you could have a business-oriented board and not have somebody's company doing business at some level with Carilion in some way. You'd have to bring board members in from outside the state," Carilion spokesman Eric Earnhart said.

For protection, a conflict-of-interest policy exists whose aim, Earnhart said, is to ensure no board member benefits inappropriately from his or her position of power. Carilion spends roughly $1 billion annually in Southwest and Western Virginia.

"We have certainly abided by those rules, and I feel like our company provides a very valuable service," said Turner, 63.

Earnhart said all the work the Turner contracting firm received from Carilion was either competitively bid—meaning the company beat out other contractors for a project with a designated value—or awarded in a "design-build" environment in which only the project manager is chosen upfront after negotiations.

The money represents perhaps 10 percent of Carilion's construction spending during the three years under analysis and would have gone to J.M. Turner & Co. even if the company leader wasn't a board member, Earnhart said.

"We've had excellent experience with J.M. Turner & Co.," he said.

Although its board meetings are closed to the public, Carilion annually identifies board members and key personnel and their family members who have Carilion jobs or business relationships with the health system. Its bylaw also tells how much money the people or their companies received and why.

The law requires not-for-profit, tax-exempt organizations to put the information on a Form 990 that is a public record available from the Internal Revenue Service, the organization itself, and other sources.

Turner topped Carilion's payout lists that detail which system officials benefited financially for 2004 through 2006.

In other examples, Carilion said it bought $1,698 worth of furniture from Grand Home Furnishings, where former Carilion board Chairman George Cartledge is an executive, and paid salary and benefits of $33,297 in 2005 to the spouse of board member and physician James Nuckolls. Nuckolls' wife works at a Carilion-owned medical practice.

It is not publicly known how much business the Turner company received from Carilion last year. A report covering the final three months of 2006 and most of 2007 is due out in late summer or early fall.

Turner has played a role on many Carilion projects

The millions of dollars listed as going to J.M. Turner are not a surprise because the company, while not Carilion's exclusive builder by any means, has played key roles in many projects.

It is currently involved in erecting the large Carilion Clinic physician services building on South Jefferson Street at Reserve Avenue. It will have a role in a new Pearisburg hospital.

Jay Turner also received a fee of $23,000 for his board service from 2004–06, according to reports. Only Cartledge received more—$24,300—during that time.

Carilion uses other construction companies, too.

"Thor Inc. has performed a number of construction projects for Carilion over the last several years, and we have only positive things to say about our relationship with them as our client," company President Allen Whittle said by e-mail.

Despite the scrutiny given Jay Turner's board service, Earnhart said contracting decisions by and large fall to an internal construction team below board level.

As for compliance with the conflict-of-interest policy, Earnhart noted that the board chairman who presides over meetings is James Hartley, a former county prosecutor.

"The board does and always has run a tight ship," Earnhart said.

Turner said if contracting matters reach the board, he will abstain if his company is involved. He said he did abstain when the board hired J.M. Turner contracting to build a planned athletic club at Smith Mountain Lake. For unrelated reasons, the club was not built.

Several steps removed from the Carilion board, J.M. Turner is also picking up business as a subcontractor for a Swedish construction management firm that Carilion has used for various large construction jobs.

The company, Skanska USA Building in Parsippany, N.J., has chosen J.M. Turner to be part of its local construction team on a number of occasions. These payments, the amount of which is not publicly known, are not included in the $19 million Carilion said it paid Turner, according to Earnhart.

So in addition to the disclosed payments, J.M. Turner & Co. indirectly benefits from Carilion's building projects.

Flynn Auchey, an associate professor for Virginia Tech's Department of Building Construction, said companies needing construction services commonly rely on construction services providers with whom they have prior experience, and general contractors do the same with subcontractors.

"Once you find someone you can trust, when you are used to working with someone and communication is good, staying with the same contractors and subcontractors often makes sense," said Auchey, who is also an architect, engineer, and general contractor. "It's not unusual at all."

Concerns about potential conflicts of interest can be quieted, he said, if the client solicits bids from more than one contractor.

Scott Rivenbark, Skanska's on-site project executive in Roanoke, said J.M. Turner has earned all its work received from Skanska through pricing proposals, similar to bids. Skanska has sometimes invited other Southwest Virginia contractors to bid, though not all of the time, and has in some cases chosen other contractors, he said.

Skanska is not under any pressure from Carilion to use J.M. Turner, but "we do so in the best interests of the project when it does make sense," he said.

Duncan Adams and Chris Winston contributed to this report.

(Published May 31, 2008, *Roanoke Times*. Available at http://www.roanoke.com/business/wb/163971)

SUPPLEMENTAL MATERIAL

Lewis-Gale Medical Center: A Century of Care

Its roots in Roanoke, Lewis-Gale Medical Center
embraces technology to assure its growth beyond Salem

By Sarah Bruyn Jones

When Patsy Saville began her nursing career at Lewis-Gale Hospital, the building was in downtown Roanoke, the syringes were glass, and patients stayed for a long time.

"It was quite a different place," said Saville, 74. "It was a good place. A lot smaller, and everybody knew everybody. We didn't have as many departments, and the nurses floated on every floor."

Today the Salem-based hospital's name has changed to Lewis-Gale Medical Center, where there are many distinct medical departments, and as Saville put it, "the syringes are disposable—everything is disposable for safety."

Saville came to Lewis-Gale in 1952 to attend the hospital's nursing school. Back then the hospital was located at Luck Avenue and Third Street Southwest (currently a parking lot beside WSLS-TV).

Saville retired in 1998, but three months later she was back at the hospital working part time in the employee health department.

Saville's career spans more than half the lifetime of the hospital, which is celebrating its 100th anniversary this year.

"I've had people laugh at me and say, 'Were you here when Doctors Lewis and Gale were here?' " Saville said with a laugh. "I say, 'Almost, but not quite.' "

During the past century, Lewis-Gale has transformed from a 26-bed hospital in downtown Roanoke to the hub of a multihospital system in Salem with 386 staffed beds and the license to expand to as many as 521 in an emergency.

Scientific breakthroughs, developments in medical technology, and changes in how medicine is paid for have not only shaped the growth of Lewis-Gale but also the U.S. health care industry.

Over the years, Lewis-Gale has touted its state-of-the-art medical equipment as a way to best serve the community, from its first X-ray machine back in 1914 to the latest advances in electrophysiology and radiology.

"When you really sit down and you think about all these changes and the technology and how many more people have been helped . . . it really blows your mind when you stop and think about all the changes," Saville said.

Dr. John Rogers, a radiation oncologist at Blue Ridge Cancer Care, said the technology has driven his field and advanced the treatment of cancer.

"My field didn't even exist," Rogers said, when asked to reflect on Lewis-Gale's origins.

Even when radiology did begin to develop, it was something where the technology was available only at large, academic medical centers, he said.

"So to be to the point where the technology is in the community setting and patients do not have to travel to get these types of treatments is amazing," Rogers said, standing in the Lewis-Gale Regional Cancer Center. "I can't tell you how much the technology has driven our capabilities."

Technology defines history and future

Throughout 2009, Lewis-Gale will mark its 100th anniversary. Plans to display old photographs and to invite community leaders and the general public to celebratory events still are being formed.

The history of Lewis-Gale doesn't lie simply with old photographs and the countless stories of birth, illness, and death that have echoed through the halls. Instead, Lewis-Gale's history has mirrored the evolution of U.S. health care and the business of medicine.

For Victor Giovanetti, chief executive officer of Lewis-Gale, the future lies in the ability to blend the tradition of patient care with technological advancements and the complexities of health care finances.

"We are in the business of taking great care of patients," he said. "That is our business, and if you can't do that consistently and with care, then you shouldn't be in this business."

To do that, though, Giovanetti said it is imperative to embrace new technology, but be cognizant of the role expensive technology has played in driving up the cost of health care.

"We need to be on the cutting edge to be sure we provide the highest level of care available," he said. "Our patients expect us to have the latest and greatest."

The new technologies come with significant price tags. In September, Lewis-Gale completed a $2.4 million renovation of its electrophysiology lab, including purchasing new equipment to perform a new cardiac treatment procedure. Electrophysiology is the diagnosis and treatment of the heart's electrical activities.

In August, the hospital spent slightly less than $3 million to purchase a new digital stereotactic linear accelerator for administering precise, image-guided radiological treatments to tumors in cancer patients.

"It creates an opportunity for patients to get treatment in many cases where there were no more options," Rogers said of the new radiology equipment.

Plans to open an outpatient computerized tomography and magnetic resonance imaging center on Brambleton Avenue in the spring for an estimated $1.4 million are just one of many expansions on the horizon.

"In the next couple of years, we might see the need for expansion," Giovanetti said, declining to elaborate on specifics. "This is an important year not only because it's our 100th anniversary, but for our service line development and overall growth."

It's Lewis-Gale's commitment to medical technology advancements in electro-physiology that brought Dr. Stephan Vivian to the area in 2008 from his former practice in Ohio.

"The opportunity to have state-of-the-art equipment and develop an atrial fibrilla-tion program are what brought me here," Vivian said.

While the new lab and high-tech equipment can treat any number of different kinds of arrhythmias, or abnormal heartbeats, Vivian said he is specifically inter-ested in performing a relatively new treatment for atrial fibrillation, one of the most common types of arrhythmia.

The equipment allows the doctor to enter the heart using a catheter and apply electrical energy to the source of the heart's irregular beat. In the case of atrial fibrillation, this typically involves isolating the malfunctioning electrical signals from the four pulmonary veins.

Computer screens help map digital pictures of the heart and map the various electrical functions of the heart.

"In the past, we had medication to slow the rate, which helps a little bit but isn't a cure," he said.

While the new procedure isn't for everyone, Vivian said he expects the science and research to continue to focus on this type of procedure.

"In the years to come, both the understanding and technology will improve, and I suspect the success rates will get better and better," Vivian said. "This offers patients an option that they never had before."

Growing the business beyond Salem

Giovanetti has repeatedly said that Lewis-Gale experienced significant market growth in 2008 and expects that to continue into 2009.

Some of that growth has come as Lewis-Gale has positioned itself as an alter-native to Carilion Clinic, Southwest Virginia's largest hospital system.

With some local doctors concerned about changes to Carilion's business model, several physician practices have decided to switch their admissions from Carilion's flagship Roanoke Memorial Hospital to Lewis-Gale.

When asked about the biggest change to face Lewis-Gale during its history, Giovanetti didn't hesitate in pinpointing changes to how the federal government reimburses hospitals for the care of Medicare patients. The formation of the diagnosis-related group, or DRG, payment system created a dramatic shift in how hospitals operate, Giovanetti said.

A related significant change, Giovanetti said, is the escalating cost of health care that has come in part because of the technological advancements.

Higher costs and shrinking reimbursements have forced hospitals to be more efficient, he said. In a way, that drove the formation of HCA Southwest Virginia, where Lewis-Gale is the main hospital that supports several smaller regional hospitals in Pulaski, Alleghany, and Montgomery counties. Giovanetti also is president of HCA Southwest Virginia.

"We are a hub-and-spoke system," he said, saying the connectivity throughout the region has been a significant change to what began 100 years ago.

Amid the medical technology boom and business model changes, Saville said she hopes that nurses, doctors, and hospital administrators remember the past.

"I miss the old hospital sometimes," Saville said. "Those were the good old days."

(Available at http://www.roanoke.com/business/wb/192978)

2

State Health Department

Cutting Budgets in Times of Revenue Shortfall

Gary E. Crum
University of Virginia's College at Wise

He was elected on a no-tax-increase, humanitarian ticket, but Governor "Yersey" Yersinian was about to destroy some of the humanitarian capacity of public health agencies in this rural midwestern state.

Tax revenues projected for the fiscal year, which runs from July 1 to June 30, had come in $30 million short, and the fiscal year was nearly half over. If things continued, the second half of the year would double this shortfall and equal 7% of the state's annual budget.

The director of the state office of management and budget, Bernice Matthews, who had just told the governor the bad news, was sitting on the enclosed patio behind the governor's mansion, looking at a heavy snow falling outside the window. She was sipping a cup of warm tea with the governor's elderly chief of staff, Shep Conway.

Conway spoke first after hearing Matthews's unwelcome announcement of the shortfall. "Where in blazes are we going to find $60 million in the current budget, with only six months left?"

They all silently wished the question was rhetorical, but it was not.

"We can't raise taxes or government fees without going back on the promises we made only a little more than a year ago," Conway continued.

"Not even a sin tax on tobacco, or an increase in borrowing is politically feasible—we criticized both in the campaign against our predecessors."

"Well," the governor said, "we will just have to cut programs—but which ones? Should we cut every agency the same—across the board: public schools and higher education, national guard, state police, public health, welfare, state parks, Medicaid, transportation, tax bureau, the governor's office, legislative support services, and the like?"

"Cutting across the board is one option, and everyone is treated the same—no big losers, no targeted programs," Matthews said. "But don't we think there are some programs more worthy than others? Shouldn't we take the time to pick and choose?"

Discussion Questions

1. If you were governor, would you cut across the board or use some special criteria (suggest some good ones) to pick and choose?

2. Depending on what choice you make, what are the potential negative ramifications for your administration in terms of loss of political support in the legislature and at the local level, short- and long-term damage to important programs, reducing state civil service employee morale, and the like?

After an hour of discussion among the state's top elected official and two of his top political appointees, Governor Yersinian made his decision.

"In the final analysis," the governor said, "we cannot justify a truly across-the-board cut. The accounts are too complex and the political environment suggests clear favorites. We can start by having all state agencies do a plan for X dollars in cuts, asking for slightly bigger cuts than we really need, so we can refund some proposed cuts along the lines that I like."

STATE HEALTH DEPARTMENT GETS THE BAD NEWS

State Health Commissioner Curtis Healy returned from the governor's cabinet meeting the next day and called his top health department advisors in to hear the news. There were seven advisors: the four heads of his key public health service departments; his legal and political advisor, Audrey Pontifico; the director of Medicaid, Matt McDugal; and the health commissioner's chief of staff, Shirley Cohan (see Exhibit 1). They all arrived quickly, curious that an unscheduled policy meeting was called.

It did not take Commissioner Healy long to spell out the situation—they had to cut $2.3 million from the agency's budget, and they had one week to complete their plan and send it to the governor.

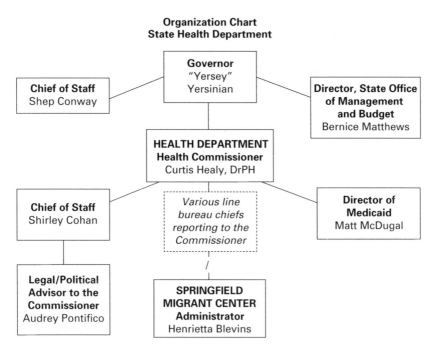

Organization Chart
State Health Department

Governor "Yersey" Yersinian

Chief of Staff — Shep Conway

Director, State Office of Management and Budget — Bernice Matthews

HEALTH DEPARTMENT Health Commissioner Curtis Healy, DrPH

Chief of Staff Shirley Cohan

Various line bureau chiefs reporting to the Commissioner

Director of Medicaid Matt McDugal

Legal/Political Advisor to the Commissioner Audrey Pontifico

SPRINGFIELD MIGRANT CENTER Administrator Henrietta Blevins

Exhibit 1. State Health Department, table of organization.

McDugal responded first, with an irritated voice: "Well, you and the governor know that Medicaid is a federal as well as a state program, and takes about 20% of the total state budget. It is a recipient 'entitlement' program—one with no budgeted ceiling. What is taken each year from state and federal coffers for medical care cannot be set ahead of time. Furthermore, in times of economic downturn, we have more, not fewer, people in need of and eligible for those financial-need-determined Medicaid services."

Cohan agreed: "And for every state dollar this state spends on its Medicaid services, we get two dollars from the feds: so, if we cut Medicaid by a million in state dollars, the healthcare providers in the state lose a total of three million."

"Don't get your pants in a bunch," Commissioner Healy said. "Bernice Matthews told us at the governor's cabinet meeting that Medicaid was not part of our problem. She is going to get greater cuts from reduced park service programs, reduced higher education programs, and cancellation of certain student loan programs. However, we will need to cancel the Medicaid dental payment and telemedicine reimbursement increases we were about to announce for the next fiscal year. Also, most departmental hiring and travel must be put on hold across all state agencies. That will save our department $300,000 this year from the start. That only leaves $2 million to go. Most agencies have it much worse."

The commissioner continued: "Another aspect of all this is that the legislature's approved capital budget—like for the new health department building on Vine Street—is off the table; it's not part of what we can cut. All the cuts have to come from the noncapital portions of state expenditures scheduled for this year."

Cohan added: "Let's look at the major categories for the budget for our agency and see where else we can find some fat. We will need $2 million cut from our non-Medicaid programs to get to the assigned mark, since we will get $300,000 from the travel cuts."

The public health commissioner handed out a table of departmental major expense budget categories (see Table 1) as he continued the conversation: "In talking briefly with Matthews after the cabinet meeting, she reviewed these budget categories and we discussed which ones would be easiest to cut. The biggest program on the sheet is the Special Supplemental Nutrition Program for Women, Infants, and Children (WIC [pronounced *wick*])." (Note: WIC is a large program funded in states by the United States Department of Agriculture [USDA]. Its task is to provide nutritious food for needy women and children.) Cohan added: "All but about $2 million is sent to grocery stores via redeemed negotiable vouchers women are given based on their nutritional status as well as that of their children."

"The budget we are reviewing," the commissioner said (Table 1, Column A), "is a rounded-off expense budget, and it includes all expenses, not just those related to income from state tax revenues. We need to pare it down to the state's portion. We do not want to cut program expenses, for instance, that are paid for by existing federal or foundation grants, rather than by state tax dollars."

As the conversation continued, McDugal summarized on a flip chart at the front of the room the many points that were made in the effort to find places to make cuts (listed in Table 1, Column B). For instance, in regard to WIC cuts, the public health department leaders were concentrating their attention on the $2 million in state tax–supported civil service costs, including salaries and fringe benefits such as state employee group health insurance, unemployment insurance, workers compensation insurance, vacation time banked, and the state's portion of pension allocations matching those of the employees. Not included were Social Security expenses; this state was one of the few approved in the distant past to have state employees be exempted from Social Security taxes (due to this fact, however, the state's retirees risk Social Security benefit cuts at retirement). Also included in the $2 million were the utilities, office

Table 1. State Health Department Budget Calculations

	Column A Current FY Projected Non-Medicaid Expenditures	Column B Portion of Column A Coming from State Tax Revenues	Column C Portion of Column B Not Yet Expended**	Column D Initial Cuts Proposed by Staff
Women, Infants, and Children (WIC) Program	$9,000,000	$2,000,000	$1,000,000	$175,000
Hospital and Nursing Home Inspection Program	$4,000,000	$500,000	$250,000	$90,000
Food Safety Inspections/Regulations	$3,000,000	$550,000	$275,000	$10,000
Health Education/Promotion Programs	$3,000,000	$3,000,000	$1,500,000	$300,000
Commissioner's Office, including Information Technology, Policy Planning, Intergovernmental Relations, Chief of Staff, Public Relations, Management Systems, etc.	$1,500,000	$1,415,000	$707,500	$250,000
Migrant Health Clinics	$4,000,000	$150,000	$75,000	$75,000
Maternal and Child Health Programs	$6,000,000	$0		
Family Planning	$2,000,000	$65,000	$32,500	?
Communicable Disease Control and Vital Records	$2,500,000	$2,500,000	$1,250,000	$30,000
Bioterrorism Control	$1,800,000	$0		
Primary Care (includes Rural Health, Minority Health, etc.)	$1,200,000	$1,200,000	$600,000	$30,000
Local Health Department Liaison Services (LHDs are run by county governments in this state)	$1,500,000	$1,500,000	$750,000	?
Special Programs				
Arthritis Prevention	$1,800,000	$1,800,000	$900,000	?
AIDS/Ryan White	$2,000,000	$0		
Oral Health	$500,000	$500,000	$250,000	$40,000
Breast and Cervical Cancer Diagnosis/Treatment	$2,300,000	$0		
Other Miscellaneous Programs	$560,000	$130,000*	$130,000	?
	$46,660,000	$15,310,000	$7,720,000	$1,000,000

* This $130,000 is all for a new program called the "First Lady's State Autism Project," for which no expenditures have yet been made.

** Either programs not started yet (see footnote above) or half of Column B: the approximate rounded-off amount remaining 6 months into the fiscal year.

furniture, equipment, and supplies state employees require as well as a detective agency hired for $100,000 a year to find fraud in the system. The remaining WIC budget (approximately $7 million) was USDA money that flows through the department as food vouchers for needy women and children.

The hospital and nursing home inspection program had an expenditure budget of $4 million, all but $500,000 of which was recovered each year by the fees charged to inspected facilities. The food safety inspection and regulation program had $550,000 in costs not supported by fees. The charge for an annual restaurant license in this state was based on the number of seats in a restaurant and may exceed $300, of which the state gets about half and the local health department gets the rest. Thus, only $550,000 is supported by state tax revenues.

The group discussed cutting the staff inspecting hospitals in the state by shortening the review process, reducing the size of inspection teams, or inspecting fewer hospitals each year (which means, however, that fewer fees will be received each year). Inspecting fewer hospitals is not as helpful for reaching the target of reducing the department's budget. The inspection fees could be raised on the health facilities, but it would be correctly considered the equivalent of a new tax.

After much additional discussion, the commissioner said, "Health education and promotion programs—that's $3 million—and my office are totally paid out of state tax revenues, except that my office's data staff is supported by a federal grant that brings in $85,000, which would not be in the state's interest to cut. Most of that $85,000 is to hire a new nosologist (an expert in classifying diseases and compiling disease statistics). Since this is an outside money source, and the salary and fringe benefits will be covered by a third party, the hiring of this person will not be prevented by the governor's hiring freeze, leaving $1,415,000 open for cuts out of the original $1.5 million."

McDugal took up the analysis at this point: "The migrant health clinics are supported mainly by private fees obtained from the patients and from payments within the department's own Medicaid program. Its remaining costs are pretty much solely in marketing outreach to the migrants, a program that costs $150,000 in state tax revenues each year. The benefit to cutting that program is that it may lower client loads, which will result in lower absorption of state tax dollars for Medicaid services. Here the lower Medicaid payments will not reduce the income of physicians, since all these migrant clinic physicians are salaried state employees. Thus, the cuts will be unlikely to generate public outcry.

"So, let's discuss some more of the programs that do not use any state tax revenues, but are supported by other funds. Cutting back these programs generates zero reductions in state expenditures," McDugal continued. "For example, maternal and child health (MCH) programs are 100% supported by federal Title V funds, and the family planning program is funded by federal Title X funds, except for a state program aimed at men, which is funded primarily by $65,000 in state tax revenues. Also, bioterrorism control, AIDS/Ryan White programs, and the breast and cervical cancer programs are completely funded by federal funds. On the other hand, we have programs that are good places maybe to find cuts because they are solely supported by state tax revenues: programs like communicable disease control and vital records, the primary care program, the local health department liaison effort, the arthritis prevention program, and the oral health program."

As the health department leaders continued talking, they noted that the $560,000 in "Other Miscellaneous Programs" (Table 1, bottom of Column A), with the exception of $130,000 for something called the "First Lady's State Autism Project," were small, local foundation–supported programs that use little or no state money.

"Well, once we adjust all the expense budget programs down to their portion of state tax revenue-supported actions, we are left with $15,310,000. So where can we find our $2 million in cuts?" the commissioner asked. "I need recommendations quickly."

After a larger staff meeting the next day, during which the commissioner was not present, the commissioner's political advisor, Audrey Pontifico, and his chief of staff, Shirley Cohan, discussed issues and proposals to take to the commissioner.

"Well, we've got to get $2 million in savings out of a vulnerable budget of $15,310,000" (Table 1, Column B), Cohan said.

"Yes," said Pontifico, "and we need to take it from an agency that is halfway through the fiscal year, so about half of every account has already been spent. The only program where 100% of the money remains to be spent this late in the fiscal year is the First Lady's State Autism Project, since it hasn't started yet. This means we have to take $2 million from a tax revenue budget remainder of less than $8 million. There is going to be a lot of blood on the floor."

In response to this comment about the fiscal year being half over, Cohan went to the flip chart McDugal had made the previous day, noted the remaining amounts in each account (Table 1, Column C), and totaled them as $7.72 million. She became more animated as she took up the conversation: "We're already under a hiring freeze for filling tax-supported positions, so we cannot use that toward the $2 million, but what about laying off some workers? Since we have a lot of highly educated people, the average salary and fringe benefit package for our agency is $70,000. We could get the total $2 million amount by laying off fewer than 30 people. In the private sector, where I was for 20 years before joining the governor's political appointees here last month, we would use layoffs to get rid of certain individuals we did not like, but who were too difficult to fire for various reasons—like people who had a long history of litigating against the company. Furthermore, we can do so with even fewer people laid off if we target the lawyers, physicians, and other highly paid workers."

Pontifico frowned as she responded slowly to this "private sector" solution: "The problem is that layoffs have heavy legal and financial barriers and complicated union procedures, not to mention the unemployment costs taken from the agency for the initial months, the payout of any compensatory or vacation time accrued, and the person-hours required to announce and implement a layoff under state government regulations. State civil servants also have special federal protections that they can appeal to if anything is not done just right. All of these protections can be traced back to a desire to solve the chaotic situation that was typical more than a hundred years ago in America: When a new governor or president was elected, almost all key government employees were fired so that the friends of the new official could be employed, a process known as the 'spoils (patronage) system.' The reality is that a layoff costs more in the first year or two than it will save, although it would be a help in more distant years, and the procedures are onerous.

"As for targeting professionals like physicians," Pontifico noted, "the important positions they fill often require expertise that cannot be handled by lower-level employees. For instance, you need a physician to handle statewide communicable disease outbreaks like the meningitis epidemic we had a few months ago in three of our colleges."

Pontifico continued speaking in a pensive tone: "And as for the targeting of undesired employees, the government is entirely different than the private sector. You can replace political appointees easily—they are 'at will' employees—but by law they are a small fraction of the total workforce. You cannot target specific civil servants for layoff due to budget cuts or reorganization, only specific *positions*. To target a specific person who is a poor performer, you would need to use disciplinary procedures over many months."

Pontifico finished her thought: "Termination of a position is complicated. Let's suppose that you have a civil servant named Fred in a Health Planner III job classification and maybe you secretly want to get Fred out of the organization without a lot of hearings and bother. You cancel his position on the organizational chart, but Fred does not get fired unless he has no seniority. If he has worked for the government, say, for 5 years, then he will be shifted over to another Health Planner III position on the organizational chart (assuming there is one) and 'bump' another Health Planner III with less seniority—let's say that person is named Helen. Helen maybe has 4½ years' employment with the state government and will bump someone hired 2 years ago named Jake, who is a Health Planner III, perhaps in another state agency entirely—and so on. Eventually several people may bump around and have to learn new jobs, and the person who is actually laid off is some newly hired employee named Yolanda, who everyone likes."

"So forget layoffs—what actual programs can be cut back, and what political problems do we risk?" Cohan asked.

"Well, let's look at the remaining tax-supported programs on the list and their characteristics and political aspects," Pontifico suggested. "Let's start with the WIC program. If we cancel plans for some new furniture for the new building on Vine Street, we can probably save a total of $150,000.

"We could also cut some of the WIC marketing programs encouraging more women to apply," Pontifico added, "but we have promised the USDA those programs will be continued and they are really pushing that. We might get some sympathy if we tell them about the state tax revenue problems, but the most we might expect is temporarily reducing some of our promised advertising by about $25,000."

"Well, every little bit helps—that gives us $175,000 from WIC toward the $2 million we need," Cohan said, beginning a new column on the flip chart (Table 1, Column D). "Now, in regard to the inspection programs, we had the nursing home fire last month that killed three residents, and the papers and the local chapters of the American Association of Retired Persons have demanded that the program be enhanced. I would not recommend we cut that right now. But we could reduce the red tape and be a little less exacting in hospital inspections, and we could also reduce mandated travel, lodging, and outside consultant fees for inspection teams—all of which would only save us about $70,000. Some more furniture and equipment purchase delays could bring that up another $20,000, I figure. All of this means $90,000 cut from the inspection programs."

As the two continued to talk, other points were made concerning what they planned to recommend to the health commissioner.

Enforcement of food safety regulations is required when local health departments decide to close or otherwise sanction restaurants, grocery stores, and food producers—such as a dairy selling tainted cottage cheese. The inspection program was already quietly cut by the previous administration; the remaining pieces of furniture and equipment would only result in a $10,000 savings this late in the fiscal year.

While anti-tobacco and other health promotion programs were probably the most effective programs the department had for reducing death rates in the state, they were seldom mandated by law, as were the inspection programs. Including equipment and furniture, the department could save $300,000 by reducing programs that had significant advertising costs, such as the picnic safety billboard and TV campaign planned for the coming Spring, and the free "Stop Smoking" classes run in each county in cooperation with the local agricultural extension agents. The Stop Smoking program was heavily supported by health advocates, but was opposed by the tobacco farmers, who were disproportionately represented in the governor's political party.

In the commissioner's office two political appointees could be shifted to the new health reform commission the legislature was establishing—assuming approval to do so was granted by the governor's legislative liaison office. Also, the department could cancel the new geographical information system equipment—computers, servers, plotters, and the like. In total, these created another $250,000 in cuts.

The two bureaucrats had made some big reductions, but needed more. Continuing, they concluded that the migrant health clinic marketing program could be terminated, with a $75,000 savings. The communicable disease program and the primary care program had already been sliced to the bone by the previous administration, but some additional monies could be deleted—about $30,000 from both programs for a total of $60,000. As for oral health, it had an educational program for training rural dental hygienists that was to start later that year to examine the teeth of the state's poorest 5th graders. By terminating a program like that—for a savings of $40,000—existing programs with established expectations in the minds of citizens could be saved, and public complaints would be kept to a minimum.

Pontifico and Cohan still had another $1 million to cut from four budget categories that altogether only had a total of $1,812,500 remaining in the current fiscal year (the total of the four question mark cells in Column D of Table 1). They looked at each other and realized they were facing a major policy dilemma.

Discussion Questions

3. What do you think about the cuts so far? Which ones would you change and why?

4. Will the proposed reductions result in increased health problems?

5. What are some reasons why capital expenditures such as those for the new health department building on Vine Street are usually not included in budget cuts such as these?

Pontifico frowned even more deeply and said with a sigh, "We have some tough questions before us. The problems for each of these remaining programs are mostly political—they are not the types of programs usually found at these high funding levels in a state health department, so I figure they are where the real cuts will need to come. Here's a list with my analysis."

1. *Family Planning.* This program is a male reproductive health program that the lieutenant governor has been championing. It is also part of a new wave in state family planning programs, which usually overwhelmingly address women's needs, especially for the diagnosis and treatment of sexually transmitted infection, access to contraceptives such as Depo-Provera shots, IUDs, and condoms, and even arranging for sterilization using federal funds. Each local health department in this state, and there are 60 of them ranging in size from 4 to 400 staff members, has a federally funded Title X clinic and receives Title X funds. The federal bureaucracy has been putting pressure on us to add more state money, and this new male reproductive health program is our first meager effort. To be truthful, it is not working very well—only a slight increase in male enrollment in Title X services has resulted.

2. *Local Health Department Liaison.* About half of this money could be easily saved, as far as I am concerned: The local health department can alter its own fees under most state laws it implements, such as for new septic field approvals, housing condemnations, and inspections of local restaurants and temporary food services, like funnel cake booths at local festivals and fairs. The problem is that the local health departments are also having tax revenue problems because property values have declined, especially in urban areas, and the local health departments in this state live on a portion of the annual county property tax income more than on fees. We can reduce some of the services we provide for them, such as centralized, no-cost laboratory services for analyzing, for instance, the heads of suspected rabid animals—bats, dogs, raccoons, and even cows. They would have to contract with private laboratories for those services. This might create a need to increase local taxes, but that will allow us to cut state taxes in the governor's budget retrenchment plan. The downside is this: The local health departments are fairly well organized, and some are well connected with the state senators and representatives that come from their areas. A local health department has highly trained staff for some rural areas who often help local politicians with their position papers on health matters. Remember, the strongest legislative force is often found in these rural areas from which politicians get re-elected frequently. This gives them seniority and important committee chairmanships in the state capital, while urban areas are more likely, at least in this state, to "throw the bums out" each November. The governor's cuts eventually have to be approved by the state legislature; it may be especially difficult to get them through the state house of representatives' appropriation committee that is headed by a rural local health department supporter.

3. *Arthritis Prevention Program.*   This program is completely expendable, as far as the health department mission is concerned. It was, however, created under a previous administration and has the support of what in the state legislature is sometimes called the "Band of Four." These are the two most senior senators from both parties and they have ear-marked this money for the health department after taking it from the Department of Aging's budget. The previous head of that department had the nerve to cut the program 5 years previously, so the senators had the program moved to our department and reduced the Department of Aging's overall budget by 10% as "punishment" for trying to cut their favorite program. All four senators have arthritis, are heavily supported by the state university's national arthritis center physician group, and use the state programs as augmentations to the money given to the state university medical center to test arthritis prevention initiatives on the state's population. The state has been recognized by national arthritis organizations as the friendliest state for getting high-quality arthritis care and prevention services. One of the Band of Four was also recognized by those same organizations just two months ago with a national award for her efforts "to reduce the suffering and disability caused by arthritis around the world."

4. *The First Lady's State Autism Project.*   The remaining program has not yet been started, but was mentioned with great fanfare in a governor's office press release during the last legislative budget cycle. The First Lady's program, like the arthritis program, is not a natural fit with the mission of the public health department, but it is a pet project of the governor's wife, Mabel Yersinian, who recently became the legal guardian for an 8-year-old cousin who has profound autism.

Discussion Question

6. Which of these remaining four programs do you cut to total another $1 million? Why?

THE MIGRANT HEALTH CLINIC GETS THE BAD NEWS

Henrietta Blevins called the Springfield Migrant Center's senior staff meeting to order. She has been the administrator of this state government– run clinic for 10 years and is candid with her staff. They face important decisions.

"The health department in the capital has sent us a directive to cut our marketing program to zero, and we need to figure out the details and let them know how we will implement these cuts."

Her financial manager made the first comment: "They know that our Medicaid expenditures will be reduced if we are not out there telling the migrants about this clinic and the many health services it provides. These migrants already miss out on a lot of services, even though our state supposedly has a migrant-friendly policy position."

"Yes," said the chief of nursing, "saying the state is migrant-friendly is fine, but if the services we have for them are kept in the shadows, the clinic becomes a sham. We need to be able to get the word out to this often-isolated group of people. As a nurse I cannot in good conscience go along with this obvious and unfeeling cut in medical services."

Blevins pushed the discussion further: "Yes, the state can save money by not offering services that eventually expend state tax monies in the form of state Medicaid matches of federal funds. The state does not have to be as worried about these Medicaid reductions because the state is the provider and cannot politically protest the reductions in the way a private clinic might. As you are all aware, under the federal Hatch Act, government employees usually can't go to the state legislators and argue for programs—they have a conflict of interest and cannot lobby on a particular bill like a budget proposal."

Blevins continued even more energetically: "Okay, but just because the state has cancelled our marketing program does not mean that our humanitarian services have to become a hidden asset to the needy. I suggest that we do the following: (1) step up efforts to get public service announcements on local radio (there are, of course, no local TV stations) and in the newspapers, especially those underground papers that reach many of the foreign-language migrants that come in during the tobacco and tomato harvests; (2) reach out to the faith-based organizations serving the migrants (perhaps I can get a local not-for-profit group to print some more of the pamphlets about our services that we had printed last year in Spanish); and (3) provide more evening hours to increase the convenience of our services while also encouraging more word-of-mouth dissemination of those new hours among the migrants. I have the power to flex the staff hours and to increase my own hours without pay, as an unclassified, at-will employee, and I plan to do it so we can keep our numbers high."

Discussion Question

7. What else can be done to market the programs after the cut? As state employees, do the migrant clinic healthcare professionals, such as physicians and nurses, have a greater ethical (moral) obligation to follow the directives of elected officials—their bosses—than to follow the values of their professions, or the needs of their clients? If they listen to their professions and not to their superiors, are they guilty of insubordination?

3

Flu Vaccine

Mary K. Feeney
University of Illinois at Chicago

GENERAL OVERVIEW

The 2004–2005 U.S. Influenza Vaccine Shortage

Influenza, or the flu, causes roughly 36,000 deaths and 200,000 hospitalizations annually in the United States and costs the American economy between $11 billion and $18 billion each year [#18, pg. 1]. The primary method for preventing influenza is the flu vaccine, which is generally available in a variety of settings, including clinics, hospitals, schools, workplaces, and other convenient locations. The vaccine is typically distributed in October and November in anticipation of the winter flu season, which usually begins in late November and peaks in February. For the 2004–2005 flu season, the Centers for Disease Control and Prevention (CDC) recommended that as many as 185 million Americans receive a flu shot. Among those 185 million, almost half (90 million) are considered high-risk [#14, pg. 2; #19]. The high-risk population includes adults 65 and older, infants 6 to 23 months old, pregnant women, health care workers, those who care for children under 6 months old, and people with compromised immune systems or chronic illnesses, such as asthma, lung cancer, and cystic fibrosis [#14; #19].

In recent years Americans have faced flu vaccine shortages on multiple occasions. For example, at the beginning of the 2000–2001 flu season, demand for the vaccine outstripped supply when problems developing a new viral strain and safety and quality control issues temporarily delayed vaccine delivery by 6–8 weeks [#10; #18]. The reduced supply resulted in an uneven distribution of available vaccines and sharp price increases as the cost of flu shots more than doubled from the previous season [#18, pg. 2]. In 2001–2002, three manufacturers produced 87 million doses, of which almost one-third were not available when demand for the vaccine peaked. The following year supply exceeded demand when only 87% of the 95 million doses produced were purchased. In 2003–2004, demand exceeded supply when 4 million doses were discarded and 87 million doses were inappropriate for that year's flu strain [#8; #18; #19].

The Institute of Medicine (IOM) notes that these recent shortages have "highlighted the fragility of vaccine supply," which is further complicated by declining financial incentives to develop and produce vaccines [#22, pg. 1]. The high-risk market, long-term exorbitant production costs, and low profit margins have reduced the number of vaccine manufacturers in the United States from more than 25 companies 30 years ago to only 5 in 2003 [#22, pg. 1].

The production of the flu vaccine is a risky and long-term venture for numerous reasons.

1.   Opening new facilities can take 5 or more years due to high Federal Drug Administration (FDA) quality standards.

2.   Producing the flu vaccine takes 6 to 8 months, and the formula cannot be altered once production has begun.

3.   Manufacturers must reformulate the vaccine annually to address new influenza strains, preventing manufacturers from reusing excess supplies from the previous season.

4.   There is extensive risk associated with predicting supply and demand for the flu vaccine because there is no mechanism for predicting the market.

5.   Demand and supply in the flu vaccine market tend to be fickle, shifting from year to year or month to month based on the severity of the flu season, public health efforts to promote vaccination, and the timing of vaccine availability.

6.   The profit margin for producing the flu vaccine is low because vaccines are sold at a low price relative to the high time, risk, and cost of producing safe and efficient vaccines.

7.   Producing vaccines is particularly unprofitable in comparison to developing pharmaceutical drugs that patients purchase on a daily basis.

Precipitating Factors in the 2004–2005 Flu Crisis

By 2004, two companies, Aventis and Chiron, produced all of the flu vaccine for the United States and hoped to provide 100 million doses for the

2004–2005 flu season. In August 2004, Chiron, a California-based company, announced to the FDA and the Medicines and Healthcare Products Regulatory Agency (MHRA) in Britain that the 48 million doses produced at Chiron's plant in Liverpool, England, had been contaminated. Concerns about quality and safety at the Liverpool plant emerged as early as 2003 following an FDA inspection. At that time, however, the FDA allowed Chiron to voluntarily fix the problems and, based on reassurances from Chiron, the U.S. government believed the bacterial contamination issue would be resolved. The FDA proceeded to communicate with Chiron via letters, e-mails, and phone calls, while the MHRA took a more proactive approach, including inspections of the plant [#9].

In October 2004, to the surprise of the U.S. government, the MHRA suspended Chiron's license and closed the Liverpool plant. Dr. Schaffner of the National Vaccine Advisory Committee stated that, "we have been reassured on a regular basis" that the contamination at Chiron was not going to be a major problem [#29, pg. 3]. Tommy Thompson, Secretary of Health and Human Services, reported that "we had no idea" this suspension would occur [#28, pg. 1]. By mid-October, the FDA confirmed that none of the Chiron vaccine could be salvaged.

Media frenzy and public outrage followed the announcement that Americans would not receive almost half of the expected 100 million doses of the flu vaccine. Across the nation long lines formed outside health clinics, while others rushed to Canada for the flu shot. As with the 2000–2001 vaccine shortage, when demand surpassed supply, reports of price gouging immediately appeared. For example, a pharmacist was reportedly offered 10 doses that usually cost $67 for $700 [#2]. Meanwhile, Shore Memorial Hospital in New Jersey was offered 8,000 doses, which had been illegally smuggled into the United States, at the price of $60 each [#3]. Besides price gouging, in a more extreme case, 620 vaccine doses were stolen from a Colorado pediatrician's office [#5].

In addition to the rising cost of flu shots, distributing available vaccines quickly became a problem. The distribution issues came as no surprise to federal officials or healthcare workers who have long known about the fragility of the U.S. vaccine market. Following the 2000–2001 vaccine shortage the GAO published a report outlining the issues related to vaccine shortages and recommending policies to prevent future problems. The report's primary concern was that there is "no system to ensure that high-risk people have priority when the supply of vaccine is short" [#18, pg. 3].

Because the production, sale, and distribution of the flu vaccine are private enterprises, the available 2004 vaccine supply was unevenly distributed throughout the nation. Those health facilities that ordered the vaccine from Chiron were left with no doses, while others, supplied by Aventis, had their entire order filled immediately. Distribution is based on type of healthcare provider, not on the level of risk among patients. Public officials know very little about how flu vaccine supplies are shipped and to whom, making it difficult to impossible for the government to intervene in the distribution of the available vaccine produced by Aventis.

The CDC responded to distribution concerns by recommending that healthcare providers ration the vaccine to high-risk patients. However, because the CDC lacks the authority to intervene in the distribution process or enforce guidelines, the recommendation left states, healthcare centers, county health departments, and doctors to determine how to distribute the vaccine. Many flu shot providers asked healthy adults to voluntarily pass up the vaccine, leaving available supplies for high-risk individuals. In Maryland, the state immunization center operated as a vaccine broker to ensure that public health agencies received 100% of their orders. Meanwhile, in Virginia, the state divided available vaccines proportionately to census data [#25]. In rare cases, such as in the District of Columbia, flu shots were strictly reserved for high-risk patients [#24]. However, in general, city and state officials did not deny the vaccine to healthy people who wanted it.

In response to price gouging and distribution issues, the CDC created a panel to investigate the ethics of distributing the flu vaccine. In addition, a federal task force, the Flu Action Task Force, was convened to manage the federal vaccine supply, coordinate efforts, and prevent price gouging [#21]. By mid-October, federal agencies began distributing their store of flu doses to high-risk areas and within 1 week a total of 3.2 million doses had been sent to high-priority groups. That same week many hospitals began sharing flu vaccine supplies. The federal government also diverted an additional 300,000 doses from federal employees and the military to the high-risk civilian population.

Once it was confirmed that the entire Chiron supply was unsalvageable, the federal government began to look overseas for additional doses. Secretary Thompson announced that Aventis would have 2.6 million more doses of the flu vaccine by January 2005. The United States also began negotiating with an ID Biomedical plant in Canada and GlaxoSmithKline in Germany to purchase additional doses. Unfortunately, those purchases were delayed as they awaited FDA approval. By early December, President Bush confirmed that the United States would purchase 1.2 million doses from Germany [#12].[1] The FDA required patients to sign a consent form for the more costly doses from Germany because they were not licensed in the United States.

Many state officials also began looking for alternative methods to obtain the vaccine for their high-risk populations. Illinois Governor Rod Blagojevich (D) located 750,000 doses overseas and requested permission from the FDA to purchase them. In New York City, Mayor Michael Bloomberg (R) requested 500,000 doses of the flu vaccine from federal health agencies for high-risk residents. When that request was denied,

Bloomberg decided to spend $2 million to buy vaccines from manufacturers in Germany and Canada; however, that purchase would also require FDA approval [#11].

Unfortunately, previous experience indicates that people will not rush to purchase these delayed supplies. For example, during the 2000–2001 flu season, the late shipments went unused or sold at very low prices. Rod Watson, president of Prevention MD, an immunization and medical screening company in Seattle, Washington, cancelled numerous flu shot clinics in October, and by December 2004 had excess shots he could barely give away, let alone sell [#4]. The same lack of demand occurred in states such as California, Colorado, and Texas, despite the fact that December vaccinations would still protect many people during the peak flu month of February.

CONCLUSION

Appendices A and B provide summary information about influenza facts and figures and a flu time line for 2004–2005. It is evident that influenza raises a number of healthcare public policy issues, including the following:

- High-risk populations need vaccines.

- The market for flu vaccines is unstable and unpredictable.

- The FDA relies on companies to provide vaccines, but may not be sufficiently monitoring those companies.

- The federal government is aware of the problems associated with the flu vaccine market but has no long-term plan for addressing these problems.

- When a vaccine shortage does occur, there has been a lack of federal coordination to act.

- The United States needs a more competitive flu vaccine production market.

The following role play options can facilitate the discussion of these and other issues:

Option 1: The Flu Vaccine Administration Task Force

Option 2: How Will Georgia Protect Itself Next Year?

Option 3: Writing a Policy Brief

The instructor will assign students to any or all of the options and assign roles within each.

Option 1: The Flu Vaccine Administration Task Force

In the wake of the 2004–2005 flu vaccine shortage, we are convening a federal task force to develop a strategic plan for addressing the issues presented in this case. It is your task to discuss and propose policies to ensure that the 2004–2005 flu vaccine shortage does not happen again. Although this may seem like an easy task, you will soon learn that divergent values and political beliefs will make negotiating this plan challenging.

Each group will identify and outline the problem(s) (if any) that the task force will address, as well as the potential solutions that they support. Some of the goals you should keep in mind include, but should not be limited to, the following:

1. Protect the health of people living in the United States.

2. Ensure fairness in the availability and distribution of the vaccine.

3. Ensure that high-risk populations are protected.

4. Protect the market values you support.

5. Protect the social values you support.

6. Promote competitiveness in markets.

7. Investigate alternatives for flu vaccine production.

Characters

Michael Bloomberg   You are the mayor of New York City. You want to purchase vaccines from Germany to ensure that high-risk individuals receive the vaccine.

Dr. Alex Smith   You are a public health expert working with the Centers for Disease Control. Your primary interest is developing rules and procedures for managing flu vaccine production and distribution.

Sam Jones   You are a representative of the Association of Retirement Homes. You are concerned about getting cheap (or free) vaccines to the older adults of the nation. You are also concerned about the distribution issues involved in getting the vaccines to all those in need.

Kelly North   You are a strict libertarian who firmly believes that the government needs to butt out and allow the market to determine vaccine production and distribution.

Tony Brown   You are the leader of the American Coalition for Universal Healthcare. You want the government to ensure that vaccines will be available annually to all citizens, not just to those who are at high risk.

Option 2: How Will Georgia Protect Itself Next Year?

Since the 2004–2005 flu vaccine shortage, the federal government has decided that it will not take over the vaccine market, manage vaccine distribution, guarantee the purchase of flu vaccines, or pursue other alternatives to protect vaccine producers.

The governor of Georgia, Sunny Perdue, has decided that the state must develop an emergency plan for future flu vaccine shortages. Your task is to meet with other officials and representatives from around the state to develop a plan for purchasing, managing, and distributing flu vaccines in the future. You cannot make recommendations for what the federal government should or could do. You are working under the assumption that the state alone must address this issue without the assistance of the federal government.

Your task includes the following:

1. Outline the challenges facing the state.

2. Outline the interests of each character.

3. Present the committee discussion to the class:

    a. Introduce each character and their interests.

    b. Engage in a discussion about the plan.

4. Develop an emergency management plan that:

    a. Prevents a flu vaccine shortage.

    b. Anticipates what the state will do in the face of a flu vaccine shortage.

5. Participate in a Q&A session with state citizens.

Characters

- Local public health representative
- President of the Public Housing Outreach Organization
- Representative from the Georgia Senior Citizens Association
- State Senate Representative (R)
- State Senate Representative (D)
- President of the state university
- Owner and operator of Pharma Corp., the largest producer of vaccines in the United States
- Other (invent your own).

Class Assignment

The rest of the class members are the citizens of Georgia, who will be called upon to participate in a Q&A session at the end of the presentation. As citizens, you will be given the opportunity to present the committee with questions and suggestions. At the end of the Q&A session, all citizens and committee members will be asked to vote whether they approve of the plan.

Option 3: Writing a Policy Brief

Following the 2004–2005 flu vaccine shortage and subsequent debate about the need for a long-term plan to address vaccine research, production, and distribution, the U.S. Congress has requested that the National Academies of Science (NAS) assemble the Committee for Innovative Vaccine Research, Production, and Distribution to research the issue and make recommendations for a future flu vaccine plan. The committee is developing a report to address the following four areas of interest:

1. Understand market and nonmarket forces that contributed to the previous shortage.

2. Develop a plan to achieve the future frontiers of vaccine research today.

3. Ensure the health of all Americans.

4. Develop a long-term plan for fair distribution of the vaccine.

You have been invited by the Committee for Innovative Vaccine Research, Production, and Distribution to a panel presentation on the issue of flu vaccines in America. Your task is to:

1. Visit the Web site of the NAS and familiarize yourself with the organization history, mission, units, and committees. You should browse a few of their reports to get a better understanding of the outcomes of NAS work.

2. Choose a character from the list that follows, or develop your own relevant persona.

3. Research the topic and develop your position on the issue. You may speak to one of the committee goals or all four; it is your choice.

4. Write a three-page policy brief or position paper presenting your research (the group should send the briefs to their classmates at least 4 days before class).

5. Make a brief presentation to the NAS committee during the class exercise.

6. Field questions from the NAS committee (i.e., your classmates).

Characters

Association of Public Health Officials (APHO)

Association of Retired Folks (ARF)

Libertarian Organization (LO)

People for a Free Market (PFM)

Organization for Free Vaccinations (OFV)

Scientists for Advanced Technology (SAT)

A university professor

Class Assignment

The rest of the class members are the NAS committee. They should all visit the NAS Web site and familiarize themselves with the organization history, mission, units, committees, and reports. They will then act as members of the committee, listen to the presentations from the panel guests, and ask follow-up questions of the panelists on the topic.

APPENDIX A

Influenza Facts and Figures

- Influenza causes roughly 36,000 deaths and 200,000 hospitalizations annually in the United States.

- Nearly 90 million Americans are at high risk for getting the flu.

- Estimated annual costs of the flu to the U.S. economy are $11–$18 billion.

- As of 2004–2005, two companies, Aventis and Chiron, produce all flu vaccines for the United States and deliver the vaccine in October and November.

- In 2003–2004, the United States had 80 million doses of flu vaccine. (Unfortunately, they were not appropriate for that year's flu strain.)

- In 2000–2001, delivery of the flu vaccine was delayed until December because of a vaccine production problem.

- Health officials have warned about the fragile vaccine situation in the United States for decades [#13].

- "The flu vaccine marketplace has been withering for years." [#32]

APPENDIX B

Flu Vaccine Time Line (2004)

Aug. 26, 2004	Bush Administration announces first national plan for how United States can prepare for and respond to an influenza pandemic. Tommy Thompson, Secretary of Health and Human Services, states, "A pandemic virus will likely be unaffected by currently available flu vaccines."
Aug. 27, 2004	Chiron announces contamination of 48 million doses of flu vaccine (nearly half the U.S. supply). Chiron is based in California but manufactures the vaccine in Liverpool, England. About 90% of the vaccines produced at Chiron go to the United States. U.S. government and Chiron both contend that the flu vaccine problem would be resolved by Oct. or Nov., when Americans receive flu vaccinations.
Oct. 5, 2004	United Kingdom suspends Chiron's license. The Chiron license suspension comes as a surprise to the U.S. government. "We had no idea," said Secretary Thompson. Dr. Schaffner of the National Vaccine Advisory Committee states that "we have been reassured on a regular basis" that the contamination at Chiron was not going to be a major problem.
Oct. 7, 2004	CDC recommends rationing flu vaccine to high-risk patients only.
Oct. 8, 2004	CDC says that someone will investigate reports of flu vaccine price gouging, but does not specify what agency. Associated Press reports charges against a Kansas distributor who tried to sell flu vaccine with 1,000% markup.
Oct. 12, 2004	House Government Reform Committee opens investigation of FDA response to August reports of contamination problems at Chiron. CDC and FDA may have known about Chiron's license suspension and shortage as early as Sept. 13th.
Oct. 13, 2004	620 flu vaccine doses stolen in Colorado.
	Feds begin to distribute flu vaccine and divert doses to high-risk areas.
Oct. 15, 2004	District of Columbia denies flu shots to nonhigh-risk people.
Oct. 17, 2004	FDA confirms no flu vaccines from Chiron can be salvaged.
Oct. 18, 2004	Secretary Thompson announces Aventis will have 2.6 million more doses of flu vaccine in Jan. 2005.
	United States begins negotiating with Canada to get 1.5 million more flu vaccine doses.

Oct. 19, 2004	Hospitals start sharing flu vaccine supplies. Federal task force, Flu Action Task Force, will manage vaccine supply, coordinate effort, and prevent price gouging.
Oct. 20, 2004	Canadian doctors begin asking for Canadian ID before giving flu vaccine. Canadians argue Bush Administration is hypocritical for asking for flu doses but not allowing Canadian pharmaceutical drugs into the United States.
Oct. 22, 2004	Secretary Thompson says, "we are prepared," and claims Bush Administration increased spending on flu vaccine from $39 million in 2001 to a *proposed* $283 million for 2002. Thompson argues that the United States has a "healthy" supply of flu vaccine and 61 million doses will be available to the 90 million high-risk Americans. (You do the math.)
Oct. 22, 2004	3.2 million flu vaccine doses sent to be administered to high-risk groups.
	Many Americans go to Canada for flu vaccination.
	United States looks to Europe for flu vaccines.
Oct. 28, 2004	CDC creates panel on ethics of flu vaccine distribution.
	Feds divert 300,000 flu vaccine doses from federal employees and military to high-risk civilian populations.
	United States identifies 5 million flu vaccine doses at Canadian and German plants, but awaits FDA approval, which should come in Dec.
Oct. 30, 2004	Vancouver offers special flu vaccination clinic for Americans at $40 per dose.
Nov. 1, 2004	WHO plans a Nov. 11 summit of flu makers and nations.

Flu Vaccine Time Line (2005)

Aug. 12, 2005	ID Biomedical Corporation's influenza virus vaccine (Fluviral) receives the FDA approval for a fast track designation. Fast track designation, a result of the FDA Modernization Act of 1997, facilitates and expedites the review of new drugs to treat serious or life-threatening diseases and address unmet medical needs.
Oct. 6, 2005	Senators Clinton (D-NY) and Roberts (R-KS) introduce legislation to ensure an adequate flu vaccine supply. "Despite three shortages of seasonal flu vaccine since 2000, we still don't have the flu vaccine production and distribution infrastructure we need to ensure a stable supply and demand for seasonal flu vaccine, raising serious concerns about our ability to respond to a flu pandemic or an outbreak of avian flu," states Senator Clinton.
Oct. 11, 2005	Indiana State Medical Association administers its private stock of flu vaccine to high-risk children. The Indiana State Department of Health uses funds from the federal program Vaccines for Children to stockpile doses for uninsured and underinsured children.

REFERENCES

1. Altman, Lawrence K. 2004a. A Big Maker of Flu Shots Finds Some Contaminated. *New York Times*, August 27, A14.
2. Altman, Lawrence K. 2004b. U.S. Inquiry in Price Rises for Flu Shots. *New York Times*, October 8, A23.
3. Associated Press. 2004a. Flu Shot Supply Grows, but Demand Withers. December 13.
4. Associated Press. 2004b. Flu Vaccine Smugglers Thwarted. November 24.
5. Belluck, Pam. 2004. A Headache and a Fever: Long Lines for Flu Shots. *New York Times*, October 14, A1.
6. Bozeman, Barry. 2002. Public-Value Failure: When Efficient Markets May Not Do. *Public Administration Review 62* (2): 134–151.
7. Brown, David. 2004a. Canada's Vaccine Plan May Be Model for U.S. *Washington Post*, October 25, A03.
8. Brown, David. 2004b. How U.S. Got Down to Two Makers of Flu Vaccine. *Washington Post*, October 17, A01.
9. Brown, David. 2004c. U.S. Knew Last Year of Flu Vaccine Plant's Woes. *Washington Post*, November 18, A01.
10. Cohen, Jon. 2002. U.S. Vaccine Supply Falls Seriously Short. *Science*, March 15, 1998–2001.
11. Connolly, Ceci. 2004a. N.Y. Mayor Has Plans to Import Flu Shots. *Washington Post*, November 10, A03.
12. Connolly, Ceci. 2004b. U.S. to Buy German Flu Vaccine. *Washington Post*, December 8, A02.
13. Cowley, Geoffrey. The Flu Shot Fiasco. *Newsweek*. MSNBC. Retrieved on November 18, 2004, from http://www.msnbc.msn.com/id/6315714/site/newsweek/
14. Department of Health and Human Services. 2004. Interim Influenza Vaccination Recommendation—2004–05 Influenza Season. Atlanta, GA: Centers for Disease Control.
15. Edwards, John. 2004. Senator Edwards Asks GAO to Probe Flu Vaccine Shortage 2003 [cited November 22, 2004]. Available from http://edwards.senate.gov/press/2003/1210-pr.html
16. Enserink, Martin. 2004. Crisis Underscores Fragility of Vaccine Production System. *Science, 306* (5695): 385.
17. Government Accountability Office. 2001a. Flu Vaccine: Steps Are Needed to Better Prepare for Possible Future Shortages. Statement of Janet Heinrich, Director, Health Care-Public Health Issues. In Special Committee on Aging. Washington, DC: United States Government Accountability Office.
18. Government Accountability Office. 2001b. Flu Vaccine: Supply Problems Heighten Need to Ensure Access for High-Risk People. Washington, DC: United States Government Accountability Office.
19. Government Accountability Office. 2004. Infectious Disease Preparedness: Federal Challenges in Responding to Influenza Outbreaks. Washington, DC: United States Government Accountability Office.
20. Harris, Gardiner. 2004a. Advice on Vaccine Shortage Is Lacking, Local Officials Say. *New York Times*, October 22, A12.
21. Harris, Gardiner. 2004b. U.S. Creates Ethics Panel on Priority for Flu Shots. *New York Times*, October 28, A18.

22. Institute of Medicine. 2003. Financing Vaccines in the 21st Century: Assuring Access and Availability. Washington, DC: Institute of Medicine, The National Academies.

23. Kettl, Don. 2004. More than the Flu. *Governing* (on-line), December. Accessed May 25, 2005, from http://www.governing.com/archive/2004/dec/potomac.txt

24. Levine, Susan. 2004a. A Painstaking Parceling: Communities Agonize Over Flu Vaccine Distribution. *Washington Post*, November 21, 01.

25. Levine, Susan. 2004b. D.C. Plans Flu Shot Crackdown: Only High Risk People Get Doses under Emergency Order. *Washington Post*, October 15, 2004, 02.

26. Ozols, Jennifer Barrett. 2004. We Are Clearly Not Prepared. *Newsweek*, October 25, Society Page.

27. Pollack, Andrew. 2004a. More Questions for Producer of Flu Vaccine. *New York Times*, December 11, C3.

28. Pollack, Andrew. 2004b. U.S. Will Miss Half Its Supply of Flu Vaccine. *New York Times*, October 6, A1.

29. Pollack, Andrew. 2004c. Vaccines Are Good Business for Drug Makers. *New York Times*, October 29, C1.

30. Ruethling, Gretchen. 2004. In Minnesota, Flu Vaccines Go Waiting. *New York Times*, November 12, A16.

31. Simon, Herbert A., Victor A. Thompson, and Donald W. Smithburg. 1950. *Public Administration*. New Brunswick, NJ: Transaction Publishers.

32. Thompson, Tommy G. 2004. Flu Vaccines and Antivirals. Remarks by Secretary of Health and Human Services. United States Department of Health and Human Services. October, 19. Hubert H. Humphrey Building, Washington, DC. Retrieved from http://www.hhs.gov/news/speech/2004/191004.html on October 29, 2005.

33. Vedantam, Shankar. 2004. U.S. to Direct Flu Shot Shipments. *Washington Post*, October 13, 01.

34. Waxman, Henry A. 2004. Flu Vaccine Crisis: The Role of Liability Concerns. Washington, DC: U.S. House of Representatives, Committee on Government Reform.

ENDNOTE

1. Ceci Connolly. 2004. "U.S. to Buy German Flu Vaccine," *Washington Post*, December 8, A02, reports 1.2 million. Pollack, Andrew. 2004. "More Questions for Producer of Flu Vaccine." *New York Times*, December 11, C3, reports up to 4 million.

4

Medicare and Drug-Eluting Stents[1]

David M. Currie
Mark Arundine

Richard Ivey School of Business
The University of Western Ontario

IVEY

On April 24, 2003, the United States Food and Drug Administration (FDA) approved the Cypher stent for use in surgical procedures in the United States.[2] Approval was based on the results of U.S. and European research showing that the Cypher stent significantly reduced the incidence of restenosis, the narrowing of a coronary artery following angioplasty. The Cypher stent is the first of a group of drug-eluting stents, which have a coating of a chemical that inhibits formation of scar tissue following surgery. According to medical experts, drug-coated stents represent a major breakthrough in the treatment of heart disease, the major cause of death in the United States.

Medicare, the health insurance plan funded by the United States government and the major purchaser of stents, had taken the unprecedented step of stating in advance of the FDA's approval that it would increase the amount it would reimburse hospitals for an angioplasty procedure involving coated stents. Unfortunately, the amount that Medicare would reimburse was less than the cost of a procedure using the Cypher stent. Because hospitals could not recover the cost of inserting the Cypher stent, they would lose money each time a procedure was performed.

Studies indicated that in the short term, the value of a procedure using the Cypher stent rather than a traditional, uncoated stent did not justify the additional cost, which seemed to justify Medicare's position. Over the longer term, the stent might have a positive impact for two reasons: first, the Cypher stent would avoid one of the major problems associated with angioplasty surgery—repeat procedures to overcome the body's natural tendency to heal itself following surgery; second, the stent almost certainly would postpone the need for heart bypass surgery. Although these results were advantages to patients, they represented the loss of a major source of revenue for hospitals.

The stent's medicinal and economic values to patients, hospitals and insurers such as Medicare, in both the long and short terms, present an opportunity to explore some of the ethical and financial dilemmas occurring in health care in all developed countries, and particularly in the United States. Furthermore, the stent could have a positive impact on one segment but a negative impact on others, so the stent's overall value to society was not clear.

HEART DISEASE

Heart disease is the number one cause of death in the United States.[3] The heart is the muscle in the human body responsible for distributing blood, which provides oxygen that cells use to generate energy. The heart itself needs oxygen, so two small tubes—the coronary arteries—wrap around the heart to provide blood (see Exhibit 1). Over time, plaque—fat, cholesterol or other substances—may accumulate inside an artery, causing the passage to narrow—a process called stenosis (see Exhibit 2). As the passage narrows, the quantity of blood flowing to the heart decreases, reducing the amount of oxygen the heart receives. If the heart is unable to receive oxygen sufficient to meet its needs, the result is a chest pain, termed angina. If the passage becomes completely blocked, no blood flows to that portion of the heart (ischemia), and the cells die—a heart attack or myocardial infarction.

In 1968, medical researchers developed a method for replenishing the heart's blood supply when a coronary artery became blocked.[4] The procedure

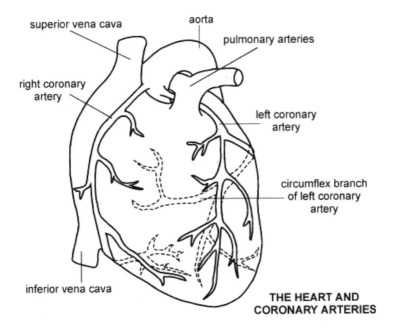

Exhibit 1. Schematic of the heart showing coronary arteries.
Source: www.patient.co.uk/showdoc/21692419/.

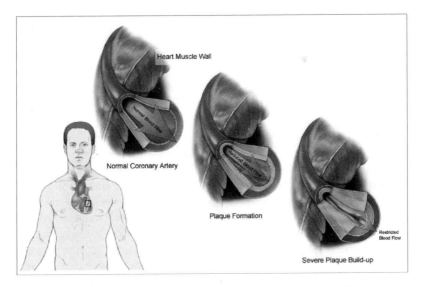

Exhibit 2. Image of a coronary artery plaque (stenosis). Illustration by Bob Morreale, permission granted by the American Health Assistance Foundation. *Source:* www.ahaf.org/hrtstrok/about/CoronaryHeartDisease_2003.htm.

involves removing an artery or vein from another location in the body and grafting it around the blocked coronary artery. The procedure, known as a heart bypass (or coronary artery bypass graft), is considered major surgery because it requires opening the patient's chest to gain access to the heart. A bypass involves a lengthy stay in hospital, which increases the cost of the procedure. Although there were more than 540,000 bypass procedures in the United States in 2000, the frequency of bypass surgery has been declining since 1996, due to development of less-invasive, lower-cost alternatives.[5]

ANGIOPLASTY AND STENTS

One alternative for overcoming stenosis was developed by medical researchers in 1977. Balloon angioplasty is a procedure in which a small tube containing a balloon is inserted into the artery at the point of stenosis.[6] Inflating the balloon compresses the plaque against the wall of the artery, widening the passage and allowing improved blood flow. Following the procedure, the balloon and tube are removed. In the 25 years since its development, angioplasty has become such a common procedure for treating early stages of heart disease that in 2003, approximately 650,000 balloon angioplasty procedures were performed in the United States, a number that had grown 320 per cent since 1987.[7] Balloon angioplasty is considered less invasive than bypass surgery, requires fewer days in hospital and in some circumstances may be performed on an outpatient basis. Consequently, it is less expensive.

Unfortunately, the angioplasty procedure creates a different problem. The human body has a natural tendency to heal itself after a traumatic event, such as surgery. In 40 to 50 per cent of patients undergoing balloon angioplasty, the artery becomes blocked again within three to six months following surgery, in a process called restenosis.[8] A major reason for restenosis is the buildup of scar tissue at the location of the trauma caused by the angioplasty. In 1993, researchers developed a technique to overcome restenosis by inserting a metal scaffold to prop open the artery.[9] The scaffold, known as a stent, is a wire mesh tube similar to the spring in a ballpoint pen. The stent is compressed when inserted, but expands when it is released inside the artery, holding the artery open (see Exhibit 3). Stents proved so popular with physicians and patients wishing to avoid restenosis that stent installation grew 147 per cent from 1996 (when first records were kept) until 2000.[10] The American Heart Association estimates that 70 to 90 per cent of angioplasty procedures involve insertion of a cardiac stent.[11] Basic stents subsequently have become known as bare metal or uncoated stents because they do not have a chemical coating. Although the uncoated stent reduces restenosis, it does not eliminate it.

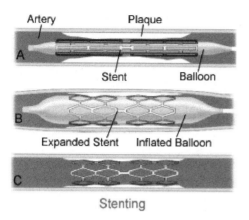

A. A catheter is guided through the groin toward the heart, then to the area of plaque buildup in a coronary artery. The catheter is followed by an uninflated balloon inside a collapsed stent.

B. The balloon is inflated, expanding the stent and widening the artery.

C. The balloon is deflated and the balloon and catheter are withdrawn. The stent remains open in place, allowing blood to flow through the artery.

Exhibit 3. Schematic illustrating the stent procedure. Permission granted: Image © Texas Heart Institute, www.texasheart.org. *Source:* www.tmc.edu/thi/cad.html.

Restenosis still occurs in 20 to 30 per cent of patients within three to six months following uncoated stent surgery, again due largely to the buildup of scar tissue.[12]

In the 1990s, medical researchers developed stents coated with chemicals that were discovered to prevent the buildup of scar tissue. The first drug-eluting stent—the Cypher stent—was approved for use in Europe in 2002.[13] (The Cypher stent's chemical agent, sirolimus, is a fermentation product of a bacterium isolated from a soil sample collected from Easter Island.) In the United States, new medical technologies must be approved by the FDA, which approved the Cypher stent in April 2003, following publication of results of tests of the stent's safety and effectiveness. A second drug-eluting stent, the Taxus Express, was approved in 2004, and other drug-eluting stents are undergoing clinical trials as of 2005.[14] (Paclitaxel, the active chemical in the Taxus stent, is derived from a scarce yew tree that grows in the Pacific Northwest United States.)

Drug-eluting stents reduce the risk of restenosis by slowly releasing high concentrations of the chemical agent directly at the point of the trauma. The high concentration of the drug helps overcome the body's natural tendency to form scar tissue. Because the concentration is localized, it does not have the serious side effects that might result if the high concentration was distributed throughout the body by taking a pill or receiving an injection. As with uncoated stents, drug-eluting stents reduce the incidence of restenosis, but they do not eliminate it. Restenosis occurs in approximately eight per cent of patients following angioplasty using drug-eluting stents.[15]

Although drug-eluting stents currently are viewed as the most effective tool for inhibiting restenosis, there is no evidence that they influence rates of either mortality (death) or myocardial infarctions (heart attacks).[16] Tendency toward death or heart attack depends on the patient's underlying health factors, such as diet and lifestyle. Stents may postpone the need for alternative surgeries, but they do not address the underlying causes of heart disease.

Even before introduction of the Cypher stent in the United States, public and professional reaction to the drug-eluting technology was immediate and enthusiastic. Patients, attracted by the prospect of avoiding repeat procedures, demanded to have drug-eluting stents rather than only balloon angioplasty or uncoated stents. Some patients with heart disease postponed surgery in anticipation of FDA approval of the drug-eluting stents, which caused unfortunate effects, as some patients suffered heart attacks because of the delay.[17] Many physicians shared the public's enthusiasm. One cardiologist said it "would be unethical to use anything other than a drug-coated stent."[18] An article reviewing the procedure said that drug-eluting stents represent an "amazing technologic and pharmacologic advance" in treating coronary heart disease.[19]

UNITED STATES HEALTH-CARE SYSTEM

The United States places a high value on the quality of health care. As a result, the United States spends a larger percentage of its gross domestic product (GDP) on health care than do other industrialized countries (see Exhibit 4). In U.S. dollar equivalents, the United States spends more than $4,000 per person annually on health care, an amount that is more than 80 per cent higher than that of Germany, the country in second place.

However, the high level of spending has not resulted in increased life expectancy for U.S. citizens (see Exhibit 5). Life expectancy at birth in the

Country	Health Expenditure (% of GDP)	Per Capita Health Expenditures Purchasing Power Parity (PPP) (US$)
United States	13.10	$4,539
Germany	10.60	2,671
Canada	8.90	2,503
France	9.30	2,456
Japan	7.60	2,971
United Kingdom	7.30	1,833

Exhibit 4. Health spending indicators—selected countries, 2000. *Source:* Organization for Economic Cooperation and Development, *OECD Health Data 2003*, OECD, Paris, 2000.

Country	At birth (all sexes)	At age 65 (females)	(males)
Japan	81.2	22.7	17.8
Canada	79.3	20.6	17.1
France	79.0	21.3	16.9
Germany	78.0	19.6	16.0
United Kingdom	77.9	18.9	15.7
United States	76.8	19.3	16.2

Exhibit 5. Life expectancies at birth and age 65—selected countries, 2000 (years). *Source:* Organization for Economic Cooperation and Development, *OECD Health Data 2003*, OECD, Paris, 2000.

United States trails that of the same cohort of countries. The United States does not fare much better according to another indicator of longevity, life expectancy of age 65. Furthermore, the United States ranks 24th among all countries according to an indicator developed by the World Health Organization that measures life expectancy in full health.[20]

The emphasis on quality drives technological innovation and results in higher prices for medical care over time. In 2001, spending on health care increased 8.7 per cent at a time when U.S. inflation was only 1.6 per cent.[21] The increase in health-care spending results from several causes, including population demographics. Because older people typically consume more medical care, the aging U.S. population leads to more spending on medical care. At the same time, the use of outpatient services, diagnostic tests, prescriptions and new technology is increasing. Coupled with price increases, the total amount spent on medical care has increased continually in recent years.

The American Heart Association estimates the cost of heart disease and strokes at $394 billion in 2005.[22] The estimate includes direct costs, such as physician and hospital services, and indirect costs, such as mortality and lost productivity. (Similar estimates for 2004, for all forms of cancer, amounted to $190 billion.) More cardiac stent procedures are conducted in the United States than in other countries: in 2002, approximately 454,000 procedures were conducted in the United States, of an estimated 900,000 worldwide.[23] The worldwide market for stents of all types was estimated at $3.3 billion in 2003.[24]

Medical care in the United States is provided and financed through a variety of channels. The United States historically has preferred privately rather than publicly provided and financed health care, but most people in the United States do not purchase health care directly. Instead, most people purchase health insurance through privately owned insurance providers. People older than 65 years of age are eligible for the government-provided insurance plan, Medicare. Although many insurance providers exist within the United States, it is estimated that 41 million people do not have health insurance.[25] Uninsured individuals bear the financial burden for medical care from their own resources or are subsidized by hospitals or charity organizations.

MEDICARE

Medicare was created in 1965, to provide health insurance for people over the age of 65. Medicare covered approximately 39 million people in the United States in 2002.[26] Initially, Medicare partially reimbursed physicians, hospitals and other health-care providers for their costs of providing care. However, reimbursing for costs did not provide an incentive for health-care providers to control costs. As medical-care costs escalated, many people called for Medicare to change its payment system. In 1983, Medicare began to establish rates that it would pay for services. Each year, the Centers for Medicare and Medicaid Services survey hospitals nationally to determine costs of procedures, products and services. Medicare then determines the amount it will reimburse for a procedure and pays a portion of that amount to the provider of the service. The amount reimbursed may be more than, but frequently is less than, the actual cost of providing the services. On average, Medicare reimburses hospitals 98 cents for each dollar worth of Medicare services they provide.[27] One study indicates that 67 per cent of hospitals lose money on the Medicare services they provide.[28] Medicare reimburses physicians separately from hospitals.

This arrangement does not mean that all Medicare services lose money, however. As part of the rate-setting process, a committee of physicians and health-care professionals determines the relative amounts Medicare will reimburse for the variety of procedures Medicare covers. For example, the committee might determine that Medicare will pay $7,200 for a balloon angioplasty procedure, but will pay $28,000 for a heart bypass procedure. (These numbers are approximate. Medicare's actual reimbursement rates vary according to many factors, including the location of the hospital in which the procedure is performed.) The balloon angioplasty procedure may be profitable for a hospital at those rates, but the bypass procedure may be even more profitable. Medicare typically pays well for cardiac procedures.[29]

In effect, the committee determines how Medicare's budgetary pie will be allocated. Because Medicare's total budget is determined annually by Congress, the only way to raise the reimbursement rate for a balloon angioplasty procedure would be to lower the reimbursement for a bypass or some other procedure. Because Medicare's budget is determined during Congress's spending deliberations, there are occasions when members of Congress influence the procedures and services that Medicare will cover.[30]

Some critics argue that Medicare's rate-setting process leads to a bias in favor of specialists over basic health care.[31] Other critics point out that Medicare's reimbursement plan bears little relation to the actual cost of a procedure.[32] For example, Medicare's reimbursement of $7,200 for a stent procedure assumes that each patient receives 1.5 stents during each procedure. The 1.5 stent assumption is based on the fact that some patients receive one stent during a procedure, while others receive more than one stent. (In some patients, the area of stenosis may be so long that more than one stent is required to prop open the artery.) Thus, the hospital makes money if a patient needs only one stent, but may lose money if a patient needs two or more stents.

THE STENT'S BUDGETARY IMPACT

Drug-eluting stents present a perplexing problem for private insurers and for Medicare. Studies showed that when the Cypher stent was compared against uncoated stents, the cost of the procedure increased approximately $2,800.[33] The increased cost was primarily attributable to the higher cost of the stent, but also to the fact that patients needed longer treatment of anti-clotting drugs during recovery. Thus, using drug-eluting stents in place of uncoated stents would certainly drive medical care costs up, at least in the short run. Both private and public insurers would have to cover the cost increase by raising rates or decreasing payments for other services.

Because patients covered by Medicare are older and thus the most frequent consumers of coronary procedures, approximately 50 per cent of all stent procedures in the United States are covered by Medicare. Medicare's decision about the new stents would have an important impact on its budget of approximately $100 billion for inpatient hospital care in 2003.[34] In anticipation of the stent's higher cost, Medicare stated that it would increase the reimbursement amount by $1,800 if and when the FDA approved drug-eluting stents: each stent procedure using drug-eluting stents would cost more than the amount that Medicare reimburses, even with the $1,800 increase. Because the amount Medicare chose to reimburse did not cover the total cost of the procedure, stent procedures using coated rather than uncoated stents would decrease profits for hospitals.

The short-run cost increase was partially offset in the long run by the stent's benefits. Because drug-eluting stents reduced the level of restenosis, patients would not have to undergo as many repeat procedures. Studies showed that one year from the operation, when most of the benefits would occur, the Cypher stent saved approximately $2,500, which almost offset the higher initial cost.[35] Drug-eluting stents, however, were money losers under current assumptions about prices and the number of repeat procedures and bypass surgeries. If each of the 650,000 balloon angioplasty procedures performed annually lost a net $300 (the difference between the $2,800 higher cost and the $2,500 savings), the total loss would exceed $190 million.

In addition, because drug-eluting stents reduce the risk of restenosis, oxygen flow to the heart can be maintained for longer periods, postponing the need for bypass surgery. Therefore, patients would not have to undergo as many bypass procedures as in the absence of drug-eluting stents, which would save Medicare millions of dollars in future expenditures even though current expenditures might increase.

The long-run impact on Medicare's budget also depended on the reaction of physicians and patients to drug-coated stents. The success of drug-coated stents in reducing restenosis encourages physicians to take preventive measures by stenting partially obstructed segments of arteries that they previously would not have deemed worthwhile. Because Medicare pays more for procedures involving drug-coated stents, the increased usage leads to more revenue for physicians and hospitals and higher payments by Medicare.

The situation facing hospitals was just as perplexing as the one facing insurers. Procedures involving drug-eluting stents would cost the hospital money in both the short and long runs. In the short run, hospitals would not receive reimbursement equal to the cost of the procedure under Medicare's existing guidelines. Therefore, hospitals would lose money on each procedure involving drug-eluting stents. In the long run, hospitals would face a decline in revenue and profits if fewer bypass procedures were performed. One source predicted that bypass surgeries could decline 20 per cent.[36] Under Medicare's existing guidelines, bypass procedures were a source of significant revenues and profits to hospitals. In fact, some hospitals specialized in such coronary procedures because of their profitability, leaving less-profitable procedures to other hospitals. A *New York Times* article noted that at one hospital, cardiac procedures have the highest contribution margin, accounting for 13 per cent of patient volume but 28 per cent of profits.[37] In January 2005, at the 41st annual meeting of the Society of Thoracic Surgeons, it was reported that a major theme focused on the "growing concern" caused by the decline in surgery volumes.[38]

ENDNOTES

1. This case has been written on the basis of published sources only. Consequently, the interpretation and perspectives presented in this case are not necessarily those of the U.S. Food and Drug Administration or any of its employees.

2. "FDA Approves Drug-eluting Stent for Clogged Heart Arteries," media release, Food and Drug Administration, Rockville, MD, April 24, 2003.

3. "Heart Attack," American Heart Association, 2005, www.americanheart.org/presenter.jhtml?identifier=1200005, accessed April 4, 2005.

4. H. Arjomand et al., "Percutaneous Coronary Intervention: Historical Perspectives, Current Status, and Future Directions," *American Heart Journal*, November 2003, pp. 787–796.

5. A. B. Bernstein et al., *Health Care in America: Trends in Utilization*, National Centre for Health Statistics, Hyattsville, MD, 2003, www.cdc.gov/nchs/data/misc/healthcare.pdf, accessed April 4, 2005.

6. P.P. Dobesh et al., "Drug-eluting Stents: A Mechanical and Pharmacologic Approach to Coronary Artery Disease," *Pharmacotherapy*, November 2004, pp. 1554–1577.

7. American Heart Association, *Heart Disease and Stroke Statistics: 2005 Update*, American Heart Association, Dallas, TX, 2005, www.americanheart.org/downloadable/heart/1105390918119HDSStats2005Update.pdf, accessed March 31, 2005.

8. P.P. Dobesh et al., "Drug-eluting Stents: A Mechanical and Pharmacologic Approach to Coronary Artery Disease," *Pharmacotherapy*, November 2004, pp. 1554–1577.

9. R. Kerber, "The Making of a Blockbuster: How Boston Scientific Gambled on Its New Taxus Stent," *The Boston Globe*, April 26, 2004, p. C1.

10. A.B. Bernstein et al., *Health Care in America: Trends in Utilization*, National Centre for Health Statistics, Hyattsville, MD, 2003, www.cdc.gov/nchs/data/misc/healthcare.pdf, accessed April 4, 2005.

11. American Heart Association, *Heart Disease and Stroke Statistics: 2005 Update*, American Heart Association, Dallas, TX, 2005, www.Americanheart.org/downloadable/heart/1105390918119HDSStats2005Update.pdf, accessed March 31, 2005.

12. P.P. Dobesh et al., "Drug-eluting Stents: A Mechanical and Pharmacologic Approach to Coronary Artery Disease," *Pharmacotherapy*, November 2004, pp. 1554–1577.

13. One-Year SIRIUS Trial Analysis Confirms Cost-Effectiveness of CYPHER Sirolimus-eluting Coronary Stent, news release, Johnson & Johnson, New Brunswick, NJ, March 31, 2003, www.investor.jnj.com/releaseDetail.cfm?ReleaseID-105263&year=2003, accessed March 9, 2005.

14. P.P. Dobesh et al., "Drug-eluting Stents: A Mechanical and Pharmacologic Approach to Coronary Artery Disease," *Pharmacotherapy*, November 2004, pp. 1554–1577.

15. "FDA Approves Drug-eluting Stent for Clogged Heart Arteries," media release, Food and Drug Administration, Rockville, MD, April 24, 2003.

16. J. Pache et al., "Drug-eluting Stents Compared with Thin-strut Bare Stents for the Reduction of Restenosis: A Prospective Randomized Trial," *European Heart Journal*, July 2005, pp. 1262–1268.

17. "Unraveling the Cypher: An Angioplasty.org Editorial on the FDA Warnings About Johnson and Johnson's Drug Eluting Stent," ptca.org/articles/cipher_fda_f.html, accessed April 4, 2005.

18. R.N. Fogoros, "Problems with the Drug-Coated Stent?: A Letter to Doctors Warns of Early Clotting, and How to Avoid It," July 20, 2003, heartdisease.about.com/cs/coronarydisease/a/DrgCoatStnt2.htm, accessed March 9, 2004.

19. P.P. Dobesh et al., "Drug-eluting Stents: A Mechanical and Pharmacologic Approach to Coronary Artery Disease," *Pharmacotherapy*, November 2004, pp. 1554–1577.

20. "WHO Issues New Health Life Expectancy Rankings: Japan Number One in New 'Healthy Life' System," press release, World Health Organization, Geneva, Switzerland, June 4, 2000, www.who.int/inf-pr-2000/en/pr2000-life.html, accessed August 15, 2005.

21. R. Pear, "Spending on Health Care Increased Sharply in 2001," *New York Times*, January 8, 2003, p. A12.

22. American Heart Association, Heart Disease and Stroke Statistics: 2005 Update, American Heart Association, Dallas, TX, 2005, www.Americanheart. org/downloadable/heart/1105390918119HDSStats2005Update.pdf, accessed March 31, 2005.

23. A.B. Bernstein et al., *Health Care in America: Trends in Utilization*, National Centre for Health Statistics, Hyattsville, MD, 2003, www.cdc.gov/nchs/data/misc/healthcare.pdf, accessed April 4, 2005.

24. R. Kerber, "The Making of a Blockbuster: How Boston Scientific Gambled on Its New Taxus Stent," *The Boston Globe*, April 26, 2004, p. C1.

25. R. Pear, "Spending on Health Care Increased Sharply in 2001," *New York Times*, January 8, 2003, p. A12.

26. M. Scalise, "Medicare History," www.curehealthcare.com/MedicareHistory.htm, accessed March 19, 2005.

27. R. Abelson, "Hospitals Say They're Penalized by Medicare for Improving Care," *New York Times*, December 5, 2003, p. 1.

28. R. Pear and W. Bogdanich, "Some Successful Models Ignored as Congress Works on Drug Bill," *New York Times*, September 4, 2003, p. 1.

29. R. Abelson, "Generous Medicare Payments Spur Specialty Hospital Boom," *New York Times*, October 26, 2003, p. 1.

30. R. Pear and W. Bogdanich, "Some Successful Models Ignored as Congress Works on Drug Bill," *New York Times*, September 4, 2003, p. 1.

31. G. Kolata, "Patients in Florida Lining Up for All That Medicare Covers," *New York Times*, September 13, 2003, p. 1.

32. R. Abelson, "Hospitals Say They're Penalized by Medicare for Improving Care," *New York Times*, December 5, 2003, p. 1.

33. D.J. Cohen et al., "Cost-Effectiveness of Sirolimus-Eluting Stents for Treatment of Complex Coronary Stenoses," *Circulation*, August 3, 2004, pp. 508–514.

34. R. Abelson, "Generous Medicare Payments Spur Specialty Hospital Boom," *New York Times*, October 26, 2003, p. 1.

35. D.J. Cohen et al., "Cost-Effectiveness of Sirolimus-Eluting Stents for Treatment of Complex Coronary Stenoses," *Circulation*, August 3, 2004, pp. 508–514.

36. H. L. Davis, "New Heart Remedy Puts Hospitals in a Cost Bind," *Buffalo News*, August 4, 2003, p. B1.

37. R. Abelson, "Generous Medicare Payments Spur Specialty Hospital Boom," *New York Times*, October 26, 2003, p. 1.

38. M. M. Conroy, "STS: Introduction of Drug Eluting Stents Triggers Decline in Coronary Artery Bypass Graft Procedures," www.pslgroup.com/dg/2499b6.htm, accessed April 23, 2005.

5

Merck's Crixivan

Kimberly A. Rucker
Health Care Consultant, Washington, D.C.

Kurt Darr
The George Washington University,
Washington, D.C.

ORGANIZATIONAL BACKGROUND

Merck & Co., Inc., is a research-driven pharmaceutical products and services company headquartered in Whitehouse Station, New Jersey. Merck's activities can be broken down into the following four major product groups that are aimed toward improving human and animal health:

Research—Discovery and development of human and animal health products are conducted at eight major research centers in the United States, Europe, and Japan.

Manufacturing—Chemical processing, drug formulation, and packaging operations are carried out in 31 plants in the United States, Europe, Central and South America, the Far East, and the Pacific Rim.

Product marketing—Products are sold in the United States, Europe, Central and South America, the Middle East, the Far East, and the Pacific Rim.

Services marketing—The Merck-Medco Managed Care Division manages pharmacy benefits for more than 65 million Americans, encouraging the appropriate use of medicines and providing disease-management programs.

Merck's mission statement[1] reads as follows:

The mission of Merck is to provide society with superior products and services—innovations and solutions that improve the quality of life and satisfy customer needs—to provide employees with meaningful work and advancement opportunities and investors with a superior rate of return.

In addition, Merck states that it embraces the following values:

- Preservation and improvement of human life

- Commitment to the highest standards of ethics and integrity

- Dedication to the highest level of scientific excellence and commitment of their research to improving human and animal health and the quality of life

- Expectation of profits, but only from work that satisfies customer needs and benefits humanity

- Recognition that the ability to excel—to most competitively meet society's and customers' needs—depends on the integrity, knowledge, imagination, skill, diversity, and teamwork of employees, and we value these qualities most highly

George W. Merck, the company's founder, is quoted as saying, "We try never to forget that medicine is for the people. It is not for the profits. The profits follow, and if we have remembered that, they have never failed to appear."[2] In 2000, Merck booked $6.822 billion in net income.[3]

THE SITUATION

The History

Merck had spent several years and several hundred million dollars to develop an acquired immunodeficiency syndrome (AIDS) drug called Crixivan, a promising treatment for HIV infection in adults when antiretroviral therapy is warranted. "It's the largest research and manufacturing project we've ever undertaken," said Raymond Gilmartin, Merck's chairman and chief executive.[4] AIDS was first diagnosed in 1981 in the United States among homosexual men. HIV, the virus that causes AIDS, was later identified in 1983. AIDS is late-stage HIV infection. The overwhelming majority of HIV-infected individuals eventually develop AIDS. Individuals with AIDS have severely weakened immune systems that can no longer defend against opportunistic infections and cancers. Deterioration of the immune system is the reason for most deaths associated with AIDS.

Merck began its search for an antiretroviral therapy in 1986, but several years elapsed before it discovered indinavir sulfate, the active ingredient in Crixivan. During those years, Merck experienced several setbacks, none of which was as devastating as the death of Irving Segal, Merck's leading scientific investigator on the project, who died in the bombing of Pan Am flight 103 in 1988. Yet the project continued and indinavir sulfate was discovered in 1992. By 1995, Crixivan's clinical trials had progressed to Phase III. Completing Phase III clinical trials is the last step required by the Food and Drug Administration (FDA) prior to requesting approval for a drug's public distribution. In January of 1996, Merck's Emilio Emini presented some of the initial data from Phase III studies on protocol 035 at the Third Conference on Retroviruses and Opportunistic Infections. Protocol 035 showed that Crixivan alone caused HIV levels to drop to undetectable levels in four out of nine (44%) patients after 6 months of treatment. When Crixivan was combined with AZT and 3TC (two previously discovered, less effective anti-HIV drugs), the percentage of patients with undetectable blood HIV levels was even more dramatic. Patients receiving the triple-combination therapy displayed undetectable virus levels in 86% of the cases (six out of seven patients), nearly doubling the effectiveness of the drug. These results marked the first instance where an AIDS drug was shown to decrease the level of HIV to such an extent that it was undetectable. Never before had such promising AIDS treatment data been presented. The drug marked a breakthrough in AIDS treatment.

Crixivan's success was an enormous relief to Merck's management. Two months prior to obtaining the approval to begin Phase III trials, and before knowing with certainty that the drug would be successful, Merck's management team had taken an immense risk by beginning expansion efforts on two facilities that would be entirely dedicated to the production of Crixivan. Management was therefore elated when the drug passed successfully through Phase III clinical trials. The company could now obtain approval to begin distribution of Crixivan under the FDA's accelerated approval process. The approval came just 42 days after Merck submitted the FDA application and was the fastest approval in FDA history. After obtaining approval, Merck was eager to begin Crixivan sales, and the company was sure that the public would respond positively to the introduction of the drug that could extend so many lives.

The Competition

AZT and 3TC were the antiviral predecessors to Crixivan and the group of anti-HIV drugs that emerged in the mid-1990s. AZT in combination with 3TC was an effective drug therapy for its time. However, the class of drugs known as protease inhibitors, of which Crixivan is one, is much more potent. By the time Merck obtained FDA approval, Crixivan was one of three protease inhibitors approved by the FDA and available to the public. Merck's competitors, Abbott Laboratories and Roche Holding, LTD, produced the other two drugs, Invirase and Norvir, respectively. All three drugs interrupt the HIV virus's life cycle. Crixivan had an advantage over the other two drugs in that Crixivan was considered more potent than Invirase and had less severe side effects than Norvir.

Because the FDA's approval to distribute Crixivan was 6 months earlier than its executives expected, Merck was still months away from having production plants ready to produce the drug at levels that would satisfy demand. Yet, the competitive pressure was mounting since both Invirase and Norvir were already on the market. Crixivan's clear advantages in potency and decreased side effects would not be enough to gain a substantial foothold in the market if the competing drugs had a significant lead time in their distribution to the public. Merck felt it essential to introduce Crixivan as soon as possible and was committed to introducing the drug closely following Invirase and Norvir. Merck's limited production capability, however, would prove difficult to overcome.

The AIDS Epidemic: The Number of Patients to Potentially Benefit from Crixivan

Based on information from the Joint United Nations Program on HIV/AIDS, the number of new HIV infections worldwide in 1996 was 3.1 million and the number of people living with HIV/AIDS was 22.6 million.[5] It was estimated that from the start of the epidemic until 1996, 1.0 to 1.5 million cumulative HIV infections had occurred in North America. At the time, HIV infection was one of the major causes of death for individuals between the ages of 25 and 44. Among men in this age group, it was the leading cause of death in the U.S. In 1994, HIV infection was the third leading cause of death among 25- to 44-year-old women in the U.S., with an additional estimated 12,000 children living with the virus. The characteristics of those infected with HIV were also changing. AIDS cases related to heterosexual contact represented an increasing proportion of newly diagnosed cases in North America. The Centers for Disease Control and Prevention estimated that there were more than 1 million Americans who were HIV-positive, and could thus benefit from taking the medication.[6]

With such a large number of persons requiring drug treatment for AIDS, there would be a high demand for Crixivan once it was learned that the drug could substantially extend life without the high dosage and adverse side effects associated with the other two drugs on the market. High demand for the drug would pose a difficult problem for Merck on many levels. The difficulties were due to the limited production capacity and the medically disastrous consequences that could result if Crixivan patients could not continue their treatments due to limited supply.

Production Capacity

Crixivan is a difficult drug to mass-produce because of its complicated molecular structure. Whereas most Merck pharmaceuticals are made in about four steps over 2 weeks, Crixivan requires a 6-week process that entails 15 steps. Seventy-seven pounds of 30 raw materials are needed to produce just 2.2 pounds of the drug, which is only enough to supply one patient for 1 year.[7] The huge quantities of Crixivan that would be required to meet patient demand made matters worse. Patients are required to take six 400-milligram pills a day, in combination with other AIDS drugs, to achieve the desired reduction of HIV in the blood. Due to the above factors, the supply of Crixivan would be temporarily very limited. Initially, Merck could only produce enough Crixivan to treat 25,000 to 30,000 patients. Yet thousands more would be likely to demand the drug because of its efficaciousness.

Due to the lack of available capacity, Merck could have outsourced the manufacturing of the drug to other companies. However, Merck had earlier decided to use its own plants in order to control quality. On previous occasions, for less complicated drugs, Merck had outsourced drug production and was displeased with the quality. The company feared the outcome if it used an outsourced supplier for its most complex production activities to date.

FDA's Conditions

Due to the drug's limited availability, the FDA made its approval of Crixivan contingent on Merck's ability to monitor how Crixivan was supplied or made available to AIDS patients. This requirement was added as a result of the serious consequences if patients discontinued taking the drug or took fewer than the 2.4 grams a day as prescribed. "If therapy is discontinued, the virus will likely re-emerge, perhaps in a form resistant to the drug. . . . Then the drug will be useless to the patient. . . . Worse, that raises the risk that a drug-resistant strain could cross over into the general population," said a researcher at the Aaron Diamond AIDS Research Center in New York.[8]

Selection of the Distributor: Stadtlanders Pharmacy

To quell the concerns surrounding the serious consequences that could result from interrupted drug treatment, Merck assured the FDA it would take precautions to monitor supply and ensure that an adequate volume of the drug was available to treat patients who started the Crixivan regimen. To guarantee an adequate supply for those who started Crixivan, the majority of prescriptions were to be channeled through a single distributor, a major mail-order seller named Stadtlanders. In the spring of 1996, Merck spokesperson Jan Weiner explained that the limited distribution was a temporary measure: "We intend to use Stadtlanders as a primary distribution outlet until we have adequate supplies. . . . We believe we will have adequate supplies in the fall."[9] Once full production was achieved, Crixivan would be available through retail pharmacies, wholesalers, and other sources.

Stadtlanders Pharmacy (formerly Stadtlanders Drug Distribution) provides mail-order pharmaceuticals for customers with special needs, including those with HIV and AIDS or with organ transplants or those undergoing fertility treatments who need assistance in complying with drug regimens. Stadtlanders' services include customer monitoring and counseling and working with insurance plans and assistance programs to help customers with paperwork and billing.[10] Based on Stadtlanders, highly specialized services in providing drugs to high-risk patients and the tailored services that the pharmacy could provide AIDS patients, it was decided that Merck's limited production volume would be monitored primarily through Stadtlanders. Also a limited amount of Crixivan would be sold to the Department of Veterans Affairs hospitals and some managed-care organizations that Merck determined would track and control the number of patients on the drug.

Merck executives reportedly agonized over the decision of how to distribute Crixivan. One of the alternatives considered was holding back the drug until the plants could reach full production. However, in light of the pressure from AIDS activists to provide the drug to HIV-positive patients as soon as possible in addition to the competitive pressures from Abbott and Roche Holding, that option was not pursued.

Nor could Merck pursue a broader distribution system. A broader distribution might have led to a disruption in patients' drug schedules. In coming to the decision to use a single distributor, Merck officials sought a distribution system that would allow the company to control the number of patients who started the drug and guarantee refills for them. Merck representative Michael Watts explained the reasoning behind the selected distribution strategy: "We selected to go through a single distributor on a temporary basis because the drug is so difficult to make. With a limited supply to work with, Merck needed to make sure that people who began the therapy had a sufficient supply." Watts added, "Going through one distributor is not just a matter of tracking who's on it . . . but [in addition], we can track the amount of drug we have."[11] Merck made the decision to use a single distributor in an effort to monitor the number of patients on the drug in the most efficient, effective, and controlled manner.

In effect, however, Stadtlanders Pharmacy would be given a temporary virtual monopoly since it was the only pharmacy permitted to distribute the drug. Those interested in obtaining Crixivan were required to register with Stadtlanders, or had to belong to one of the few VA hospitals or managed-care organizations that had obtained distribution rights. Stadtlanders, being the primary distributor of the drug, was responsible for controlling the number of new patients when there was not enough Crixivan to maintain current patients.

Pricing of Crixivan

When Crixivan was introduced, pharmaceutical prices were already a hotly debated issue. The Working Group on Pharmaceuticals and National Health Care Reform, an independent committee of academics, advocates, and policy makers, had pushed for government controls on pharmaceutical pricing. The group acknowledged that research and development costs could not be ignored, but that the pharmaceutical industry as a whole was too profit-oriented when lives were at stake. The pharmaceutical industry is one of the nation's largest profit makers. According to *Fortune 500* listings, it was the most profitable industry every year from 1988 to 1994.[12] It had been ranked as first or second most profitable in 30 of the last 38 years. Merck alone enjoyed a net income of more than $3 billion in 1995, up 11% from the previous year.[13] The rate of return on equity in the same year was 14%.[14] According to a 1994 United Kingdom Department of Health study, drug prices through much of Europe averaged 4%–78% lower than in the United States.[15]

Analysts believed that Crixivan could generate half a billion dollars or more in annual sales in a few years, but Merck initially priced the drug far lower than the industry expected. Crixivan was 24% less than Invirase and 33% below Norvir. A Merck spokesman said the price was set to be "competitive, to facilitate access, and to assure usage of the product."[16] Jules Levin, who directs the National AIDS Treatment Advocacy Project in New York, praised Merck for its pricing of the drug saying, "Merck has done a very humane thing with the price it's charging."[17]

Stadtlanders, however, was imposing a 37% mark-up on the price of the drug to consumers. Stadtlanders paid Merck $365 for a patient's 1-month supply of Crixivan that had a list price of $501.88. Stadtlanders stated that its actual profit was closer to 14% because most customers received discounts under various health plans. Stadtlanders claimed that the profit from Crixivan would be further decreased because it had to hire 400 additional employees to monitor distribution of Crixivan. However, AIDS activists were angered by the fact that non–health plan patients were required to pay the full retail price. Merck's lawyers determined that negotiating a price with Stadtlanders or pressuring it to lower its price would be vertical price fixing, because the producer and the distributor involved in the sale of the product negotiated its price. This is a *per se* violation of Section 1 of the Sherman Antitrust law, which deems every "contract, combination in the form of trust or otherwise, or conspiracy, in restraint of trade or commerce . . . illegal."[18]

Uncompensated Care Provisions

Merck's philosophy is that its overall business mission is to enhance health. Merck has stated that it believes that an essential component of its corporate responsibility is to provide support to charitable organizations that benefit society.[19] In keeping with its corporate philosophy, Merck developed a patient assistance program called SUPPORT™ that specifically assisted patients who needed Crixivan and provided free Crixivan to those who were unable to pay for it if certain conditions pertaining to third-party payers were met as described below. Merck realized the difficulty that many patients had in identifying and securing drug coverage, and therefore wanted to help find resources to pay for Crixivan. Using a toll-free number, physicians and their patients could obtain assistance on many levels. The SUPPORT™ program assisted insured patients in obtaining maximum reimbursement for Crixivan and assisted uninsured patients in locating and applying for alternate coverage sources. Program counselors were assigned to individual cases and provided the following services:

- Answered questions regarding insurers' policies, regardless of whether one had private insurance, was part of an HMO, or had insurance through public programs, such as Medicaid or AIDS Drug Assistance Programs (ADAPs)

- Assisted patients in identifying and applying for alternate insurance coverage for Crixivan

- Assisted physicians, their patients, and patients' families with the application process for patient assistance

- Arranged for eligible patients to have Crixivan sent to the prescribing physician's office

- Assisted physicians with billing, claim form completion, and coding for Crixivan

- Worked with physicians or patients to resolve specific issues related to payment, reimbursement, or claims denials for Crixivan

For patients with no alternate insurance, the program could provide Crixivan at no cost when medically indicated and certain conditions were met such as having an income of less than $20,000 per year. In addition, Merck planned to offer Crixivan free of charge to those who had participated in most of its Phase II and one of its Phase III studies.

There were, however, limitations to the SUPPORT™ program. Merck had implemented a policy that stipulated that if a state ADAP or private insurance company chose not to cover Crixivan, Merck would block all patients in that state's ADAP or insurance program from entering its patient assistance program, regardless of financial need. Merck believed that otherwise payers would refuse to pay for Crixivan because Merck would pick up the costs for people who could not pay out-of-pocket.

The Public Outcry

Merck believed that it had acted in good faith to make decisions that would benefit Crixivan users and, accordingly, had developed a fair and comprehensive distribution plan. During the early years of Crixivan's development, Merck had built what it thought was a strong, positive relationship with AIDS activists. A community advisory board was created to keep the AIDS community informed on the drug's development process and, after receiving increasing pressure from the AIDS activist community, Merck created a compassionate use program that was implemented to allow access to Crixivan to patients who were dying. In addition, Merck had cooperated with AIDS activists when they accused Merck of conducting the Crixivan development process too slowly. Merck responded by allowing an independent drug-manufacturing consultant to evaluate Merck's production efforts. The consultant later reported to AIDS activists that Merck was doing all it could to make the drug ready for public consumption. Despite Merck's efforts, the company has received a great deal of bad press.

Distribution and Pricing

Once Merck's plan to distribute Crixivan primarily through Stadtlanders was known, AIDS activists called for public protests against Merck and Stadtlanders. A spokesman for a prominent AIDS activist group said that it has made the restricted distribution of Crixivan one of its "target issues" in its meetings with legislators and with the Federal Trade Commission. The group is seeking to have a provision added to the FDA reform bill that ensures that all FDA-approved drugs will be available to all licensed pharmacies in the United States.[20] The group is calling for a review of the Crixivan distribution system and an investigation as to why the FDA approved it and how the Crixivan approval was obtained so quickly.

The National Alliance for the Restoration of Democracy (NARD) called the decision to distribute the drug through a single distribution agent "anticompetitive," "ill-conceived," "ludicrous," and "cynical and preposterous." NARD's president has asked Merck to dismantle the program and to immediately open the distribution of Crixivan to all community pharmacies that wish to dispense it.[21] NARD's president feels that if Merck wanted to encourage accountability, it could have set out clinical guidelines as was done for other drugs that require limited distribution. Yet, Merck feels that there is a critical difference between the two situations; in earlier cases of limited drug supply, having continuous drug treatment was not as crucial.

Furthermore, AIDS activists and pharmacists accused Stadtlanders of using its virtual monopoly to price-gouge AIDS patients. Kate Krauss, the spokesperson for the AIDS activist group ACT UP Golden Gate, commented, "We want to send a message to Merck, Hoffman La Roche and Abbott that price gouging is unacceptable. . . . Boycotting Stadtlanders, which survives because of the goodwill of the AIDS community, would be easy for us to do."[22] The group accused Stadtlanders of imposing a 37% mark-up on the drug when the average profit on drugs sold in pharmacies is 15%. Moreover, local pharmacies feel that Stadtlanders has an unfair advantage in that it has a mailing list of HIV-infected patients that it can use for direct marketing. As noted, Stadtlanders acknowledged that Crixivan is marked up 37%, but added that most patients would not pay full price because they had discounts under various health plans.

To a lesser extent, Merck is also receiving criticism for its decision to prevent entry into its indigent-patient program if a person's insurance plan or state ADAP program won't pay for Crixivan. Opponents feel that it is unfair to block entry into the program on this basis regardless of a person's financial need. Many believe that this policy prevents the already vulnerable HIV-positive population from obtaining a drug that could extend their lives. Patients are caught between Merck and health care payer organizations that are disputing who should pay for drug treatment.

The accusation that the limited distribution system is in violation of antitrust law seems unfair to both Merck and Stadtlanders. Some AIDS activists agree. Martin Delaney, founding director of the AIDS activist group Project Inform, defended Merck by saying that "People should understand that the reason they [Merck] did it this way was a patient-oriented one: to guarantee that no patient would be cut off. Everyone agrees there had to be some tracking method. I don't know if this was the only way to do it or not."[23] Merck has received similar support from other AIDS activists who say that the company is trying to be responsible. Negative press has been more prevalent, however.

Pharmacist/Patient Relationship

Merck is being accused of insensitivity to how heavily AIDS patients rely on their local pharmacists to counsel them about taking their medicines properly and to provide allowances for price breaks when patients have financial problems. The editor and publisher of the *Journal of the International Association of Physicians in AIDS Care* stated that AIDS patients "rely on their pharmacists as much as they rely on their doctors. Merck wasn't sensitive to this at all."[24] Critics do not believe that a single, mail-order pharmacy across the country can provide the same amount of support that neighborhood pharmacies provide. Yet, in Merck's opinion, that view is untrue.

As to the accusation that Merck has not been sensitive to the needs of AIDS patients for a relationship with their local pharmacists, none of the critics seems to mention that Stadtlanders is unique in providing specialized support services to its customers. Stadtlanders specifically provides mail-order pharmaceuticals for customers with special needs, including those with HIV and AIDS. Although a mail-order pharmacy, Stadtlanders provides support that caters to the needs of HIV/AIDS patients by providing medical counseling as well as assistance with financial issues. Stadtlanders' mission is to be a partner in the successful management of high-risk disease.

In addition, AIDS activists feel that not enough information is being provided to the public about Crixivan and its dosage requirements. This accusation is particularly distressing to Merck because its publications department has written the literature about the drug, but the documents must be approved by the FDA and have been delayed by the approval process. The literature gives specific instructions on usage of the drug and how it can be accessed.

Retail Pharmacy Industry

Retail pharmacists are fearful that pharmaceutical companies that grant exclusive distribution rights to single pharmacies could be the beginning of a trend that threatens them. Pharmacists are particularly wary of drug chains that obtain exclusive rights to AIDS drugs because the profit that can be obtained on HIV-inhibiting drugs is substantially greater than that of most other common drugs sold by pharmacies. In response to the limited distribution of Crixivan, pharmacy trade groups have initiated a letter-writing campaign to federal regulators and have begun lobbying Congress to prohibit pharmaceutical companies from being able to restrict drug distribution. Lobbyists argue that exclusive distributorship agreements are unlawful if they decrease competition and do not include other pro-competitive justifications.

NEXT STEPS

Merck's mission and vision statements seem to prohibit the actions of which the company is accused. Its philosophy includes the following:

- Merck's mission is to provide innovations and solutions that improve the quality of life and satisfy customer needs.

- Merck is committed to the highest standards of ethics and integrity. "In discharging our responsibilities, we do not take professional or ethical shortcuts. Our interactions with all segments of society must reflect the high standards we profess."

- Merck has an expectation to make profits, but only from work that satisfies customer needs and benefits humanity.

Merck cannot believe that such a public outcry has erupted over a temporary measure that will last only until Merck's plants are able to produce sufficient supplies of Crixivan. Merck has called an emergency meeting of the board to discuss how it should handle the situation.

ASSIGNMENT

You are the CEO and have been asked to brief the board on the situation by summarizing the facts, giving your opinion as to how the public relations debacle should be handled, and providing suggestions as to what should be the company's next steps. In addition, although the public relations dilemma is the most immediate problem, consideration must be paid to other issues such as:

- Addressing the board's concern over public policy changes that may result from this controversy and that may influence the manner in which drugs are introduced to the public

- Deciding whether changes should be made to the decision-making process when introducing drug products to the public in the future to avoid the problems that resulted from this situation

- Identifying other countervailing groups that may find fault with the way in which Merck conducts business in an attempt to proactively address the potential concerns that those groups may raise

REFERENCES

AIDS Activists/Merck-4-: HMOs could negotiate lower cost. (1996, April 11). Message posted to *Dow Jones News Service*.

AIDS Activists/Merck-2-: Stadtlanders main distributor. (1996, April 11). Message posted to *Dow Jones News Service*.

A Program of Reimbursement Support and Patient Assistance Services. Retrieved from http://www.crixivan.com/indinavir_sulfate/crixivan/consumer/patient_resources/support.jsp

Barnett, A.A. (1996). Protease inhibitors fly through FDA. *The Lancet, 347*, 678.

Breu, J. (1996). AIDS drug distribution eases—By a crack. *Drug Topics, 140*(9), 30.

Breu, J. (1996). R.Ph.s steamed over AIDS drug's limited distribution. *Drug Topics, 140*(8), 32.

Gottschalk, K. (1996). Protease inhibitors—The cost of AIDS drugs. *Consumer News, 1*(5). Retrieved September 1, 2001 from http://cidronline.com/cnews_/healthcare/9605.html

James, J.S. (1996, April 5). *Indinavir (Crixivan®) access and distribution.* Posted to http://www.immunet.org/immunet/atn.nsf/page/a–244–03

MacPherson, K., & Silverman, E.R. (1996, February 27). Business makers chase profits in quest for AIDS drug. *The Plain Dealer,* p. 4C.

Tanouye, E. (1997, November 5). Medicine: Success of AIDS drug has Merck fighting to keep up the pace. Posted to http://www.pulitzer.org/year/1997/national-reporting/works/6.html

Tanouye, E., & Waldholz, M. Pharmaceuticals: Merck's marketing of an AIDS drug draws fire. (1996, May 7). *The Wall Street Journal,* p. B1.

Womack, A. AIDS activists may boycott pharmacy over sale of Merck product. (1996, April 11). Posted to *Dow Jones News Service.*

ENDNOTES

1. Merck's corporate web site. 01 September 2001 http://www.merck.com/about/mission.html

2. Merck's corporate web site. 01 September 2001 http://www.merck.com/about/cr/

3. Merck's corporate web site. 01 September 2001 http://www.anrpt2000.com/financialhighlights.htm

4. MacPherson, K., & Silverman, E.R. "Business makers chase profits in quest for AIDS drug." *The Plain Dealer.* 27 February 1996, 4C.

5. HIV/AIDS Global Epidemic Fact sheet. Online Posting. Retrieved 1 September 2001: http://www.unaids.org/publications/documents/epidemiology/estimates/situat96kme.html

6. Womack, Anita. "AIDS activists may boycott pharmacy over sale of Merck product." *Dow Jones News Service.* 11 April 1996.

7. Tanouye, Elyse. "Medicine: Success of AIDS drug has Merck fighting to keep up the pace." Online posting. 5 November 1997. The Pulitzer Board. 1 September 2001 http://www.pulitzer.org/year/1997/nationalreporting/works/6.html

8. Tanouye, Elyse and Michael Waldholz. "Pharmaceuticals: Merck's marketing of an AIDS drug draws fire." *The Wall Street Journal.* 07 May 1996, B1.

9. "AIDS Activists/Merck-2-: Stadtlanders main distributor." *Dow Jones News Service.* 11 April 1996.

10. Stadtlanders Pharmacy Profile. 21 September 2001. The Industry Standard. http://www.thestandard.com/companies/dossier/0,1922,264504,00.html

11. Gottschalk, Kurt. "Protease inhibitors—The cost of AIDS drugs." *Consumer News.* 1.5 (1996). Retrieved 1 September 2001 http://cidronline.com/cnews_/healthcare/9605.html

12. Ibid.

13. Ibid.

14. Merck's corporate web site—1997 Financial Highlights: http://merck.com/overview/97ar/p3.htm
15. Gottschalk, 1.
16. Waldholz, Michael. "Merck's newly approved AIDS drug is priced 30% below rival medicine." *The Wall Street Journal.* 15 March 1996, B5.
17. *Ibid*
18. Greenberg, Warren. *The Health Care Marketplace* (New York: Springer-Verlag, 1998), 103.
19. Merck's corporate web site. 01 September 2001 http://www.merck.com/overview/philanthropy/13.htm
20. Breu, Joe. "AIDS drug distribution eases—By a crack." *Drug Topics.* 140.9 (1996): 30.
21. Breu, Joe. "R.Ph.s Steamed Over AIDS Drug's Limited Distribution." *Drug Topics.* 140.8 (1996): 32.
22. "AIDS Activists/Merck -2-: Stadtlanders Main Distributor." 1996.
23. "AIDS Activists/Merck -4-: HMOs Could Negotiate Lower Cost." *Dow Jones News Service.* 11 April 1996.
24. Tanouye, et al., B1.

PART II

Strategic Management

6

Riviera Medical Center

Riviera Wellness Services

Michael J. King
Doctors Medical Center of Modesto, Modesto, California

Robert C. Myrtle
University of Southern California, Los Angeles, California

Alex Harrington joined Riviera Medical Center (RMC) as CEO 18 months ago. RMC is a 350-bed acute care hospital located in Northern California. It is part of a nonprofit chain of hospitals that has had financial challenges over the past several years that have redirected some of RMC's earnings to support capital investment at other locations. As a result, RMC has not had adequate funds available to reinvest in facilities and equipment.

In addition, approximately 5 years ago RMC entered into a contract with the county to provide services to medically indigent adult patients who are the responsibility of the county. The county contract and inadequate reinvestment have damaged RMC's image in the region.

Harrington is aggressively looking for ways to improve the hospital's image in the community without making significant capital investment. He believes the opportunity to partner with employers to help control the cost increases associated with employee health benefits is a way to align

---

This case is based on actual events. The organization, its location, and the names of people have been disguised.

91

more closely with employers and improve the hospital's image with that constituency. He knows that when employers select the health plans for their companies, cost is a central component in their decision making.

During recent months, Harrington has led efforts to develop a workplace wellness program, which he calls Riviera Wellness Services (RWS). He is considering whether it is time to present the concept to the RMC board of directors and seek their approval of the new program. His consideration includes one more review of the business plan developed for RWS and another opportunity to think about how RMC came to develop the plan for RWS. He settles into his office on a Saturday morning and begins his review, starting with some of the history of RMC.

RMC HISTORY

Through the 1980s and much of the 1990s, RMC grew to become the hospital of choice and technological leader in its region. It developed itself as a cardiac specialty center, and was the dominant women and children's hospital in the region. The facilities were the best in the area, the equipment was state of the art, the nursing staff was highly trained, and the medical staff was on the cutting edge. The hospital was also financially very successful.

There was only one primary competitor in RMC's region—Northern Valley Medical Center (NVMC). That competitor had started a strategy focused on developing a foundation model medical group practice as a way to develop a referral base. NVMC reinvested its hospital earnings into the development of its medical group practice rather than facilities. In contrast, RMC focused on the independent physicians who were entrepreneurial and were attracted to the high-quality technology leadership offered by RMC.

When RMC negotiated the contract with Riviera County to purchase and close the old County Hospital, the action prevented the county from selling the hospital to another party and increased RMC's census, which used some of its excess capacity. The addition of the uninsured or underinsured population, however, created a risk of changing the hospital's demographics. Administration had determined that the benefits of adding the additional volume outweighed the risk associated with patient demographics; however, the changes that took place over the next several years proved that management grossly underestimated the impact of the changing patient demographics. The contract with Riviera County remains in place through 2012.

One of the most immediate impacts of the county contract was the growth in emergency department activity. The emergency department was built in the early 1990s for a capacity of around 40,000 visits annually. By 1998, the department added about 15,000 visits and was seeing a total of about 55,000 visits annually. Most of the growth was in uninsured patients or patients covered by the Medicaid program. The emergency department was quickly overloaded and many insured patients felt uncomfortable around the newly added clientele.

The medical staff was extremely upset with the change and many doctors looked to shifting some or all of their practices to NVMC. That hospital had established a strong foundation medical group, and was in fact attracting private physicians who had been loyal to RMC, resulting in a shift of insured business to NVMC. This shift permitted NVMC to begin a construction campaign to modernize its facilities and expand capacity.

In addition, during the decade of the 1990s, Western Health System aggressively marketed in the Riviera service area and expanded its membership to cover approximately 20% of the population. Western is a fully integrated health system that insures its members and provides physician services and hospital services to its population of enrollees. In 2005, Western commenced construction of a new 200-bed hospital, which opened in late 2008.

Following the county contract, the demographics in the community got worse as far as RMC was concerned, with the uninsured population exceeding 25% by 2007. RMC required significant increases in managed care rates to offset the increased cost of care for uninsured or underinsured patients. NVMC more aggressively increased rates to finance several hundred million dollars in new facilities, making employers in the region unhappy with the rate of increase in healthcare costs. Much of their dissatisfaction was directed toward the hospitals. The more sophisticated employers, however, saw that the costs associated with NVMC were higher than with RMC.

RMC lost profitability and the system it was a part of had other priorities for the funds it was generating. Capital reinvestment ran at approximately 50% of depreciation during the most recent decade. Competing hospitals made significant investments during the same period.

RMC has followed a strategy focused on quality of care and has achieved notably higher quality scores on publicly reported data than competitors in the region. Harrington thought that this was an important advantage for RMC. This accomplishment was recognized by others, as the hospital achieved numerous quality awards, including from the American Heart Association, health plans, and other organizations. Harrington was especially pleased that RMC had received trauma certification as a level II trauma center from the American College of Surgeons. He felt strongly that from a quality standpoint RMC occupied a leadership position. He also told himself that although quality is important to health plans and employer groups, it is often not well understood or fully appreciated by the general consumer. Harrington concluded that although RMC does not have the newest hospital, it does have a reputation with employers as being a good alternative for quality and cost.

His thoughts turned to a point of considerable concern. Over the past decade RMC has gone from the premier institution in the region to third in image with patients. Still, in Harrington's view RMC has the opportunity to be identified as the hospital of choice by working with employers.

He reminded himself that RMC has plans for building replacement hospital beds to create modern facilities that can compete with the other two hospitals in the immediate area, but turned his thoughts to another potentially important strategic step—the plan he is reviewing to introduce a worksite wellness program to help employers lower their healthcare costs while improving the overall health and well-being of their workforces.

PLANS FOR RMC'S WORKSITE WELLNESS PROGRAM

Harrington thought about the importance of his vision for the hospital to be a partner with the community, and especially to develop relationships with local employers in the hospital's service area. As a part of this effort, RMC has worked with the California Health Collaborative (CHC), an organization representing mostly union health and welfare funds that are primarily self-funded for health insurance. CHC's goal is to improve health and lower costs for its members and their employees. With approximately 3 million Californians represented by CHC, Harrington had, in his view, wisely sought involvement with the organization.

An important accomplishment from working closely with CHC was the development of a model direct contract between the hospital and those employer and payer groups represented by CHC. The contract covers inpatient and outpatient services provided by the hospital, and there is an annual pay-for-quality component of the contract. RMC has significantly higher quality scores than other hospitals in the area, which CHC members benefit from. CHC and their members have recognized that improved quality translates into fewer complications and ultimately lower costs.

Harrington believes RWS will build on and extend the past accomplishments made possible by working with CHC. In his view, RWS will allow increased direct interaction with employers and employees at their place of business, which is a powerful opportunity for RMC to establish itself as a partner in health for the community.

He concluded that the combination of high-quality healthcare services and a position as a partner for wellness for the community should translate into an improved image in the community and ultimately result in increased market share. Harrington believes these efforts are part of an overall value proposition that RMC brings to the community.

Harrington mentally reviewed how far his plans for RWS had come, acknowledging that some aspects of the plans are still under way. Initial plans call for RWS to send a team of healthcare professionals to an employer's worksite to conduct comprehensive screenings of employees. A personal wellness profile will be prepared for each employee who chooses to participate in the screening process. An aggregate wellness profile will be prepared for the employer to summarize the state of wellness for those employees who participate in the screenings.

The RWS team will help employees and employers to establish individual and aggregate wellness improvement plans. Employees deemed at high risk of developing a chronic disease will be referred to their physician or to a participating RMC physician. To protect employee privacy rights, individual information will not be available to employers.

RMC's administration shares Harrington's view that the hospital needs to develop and implement strategies to help the hospital be seen as an attractive partner for the employers in Riviera County. They are convinced that RWS will provide one such strategic advantage in the hospital's service area, especially because it will be the first program of its kind in the region.

As he reviewed the status of RWS, Harrington's thoughts turned to some of the larger influences in the healthcare industry that have brought RMC to the point of presenting plans for RWS to the governing board.

THE INDUSTRY

RMC's administration has identified the renewed awareness of healthy living and wellness as an opportunity to work with employers throughout California and to develop programs designed to improve the health of their workforces and reduce their insurance cost through health improvements. There is a significant increased awareness of how healthy behaviors can improve the quality of life through increased energy and reduced health complications.

Harrington remembered that he was especially influenced by release of an important study by the Partnership for Prevention, a nonprofit, nonpartisan organization that develops evidence-based solutions to major national health challenges. The study, Leading by Example, evaluates numerous CEOs' views on the business case for worksite health promotion. The study pointed out that the primary driver of soaring health costs is inadequate investment in health through primary prevention, health risk reduction, and disease management. It further noted, "Some forward-thinking organizations are integrating employee health as a business strategy that enables them to manage costs effectively, while investing in the potential of their human capital." Harrington concluded that this information is highly supportive of plans for RWS.

THE SERVICE

In reviewing the business plan for RWS, Harrington recalled that the essence of the service is to provide health assessments for employees with a focus on risks for chronic disease, and to establish programs to help employees minimize the risks associated with such chronic diseases. The initial phase of the program is planned to be a series of medical screenings conducted at various stations manned by experts in the respective medical or clinical areas involved. Prior to conducting such screenings, the employees will be required to provide blood for laboratory tests that will be reviewed the following day as a part of the screening process. Separate stations will be set up for: (1) Cardiac Care; (2) Oncology; (3) Orthopedics/Bone Density; (4) Exercise and Conditioning; (5) Nutrition and Diet; (6) Sleep and Respiratory; (7) Diabetes; and (8) Women's Health.

Based on the results of the screenings, a tailored healthy lifestyle program will be established for each employee. Chronic conditions such as diabetes and obesity will be addressed through education in group settings, such as weight management and diabetes classes or support groups. For employees who need more in-depth attention, RMC will use its certified diabetes clinic and Cardiac Center of Excellence. These specific resources can be used where appropriate to help prevent further deterioration of the chronic conditions identified in people who are screened. Other areas of concern will be addressed on an individual basis or by referral to a primary care physician.

RWS's screening results will be accumulated and a health rating determined for each employee at the beginning and the end of the year. The data will be aggregated for the participants in an employer's workforce and an aggregate average score established for its workforce. The employers will be able to present their aggregate data to managed care companies when negotiating annual health insurance rates; measured improvements should lower health insurance costs.

Recognizing that individual health is a highly confidential topic and subject to the privacy provisions of the Health Insurance Portability and Accountability Act (HIPAA), Harrington was satisfied that RMC's plans for individual health information to be maintained anonymously with access available only to those developing and implementing the individually tailored wellness programs as well as the physician overseeing the program were consistent with HIPAA. He had made certain that the intent of the program is to help employees of participating companies improve their health through lifestyle changes, and not to create a health record that is available to their employers.

RMC administrators are convinced that their worksite wellness program will be unique with tailored health improvement plans for each employee and oversight by a uniquely qualified team of professionals headed by a primary care physician. They also plan for specially trained local primary care physicians to be available for consultation for employees who require special attention. In addition, the measures used to rate employee health are supported by evidence that they are primary indicators of individual health and wellness.

KEY ASPECTS OF RIVIERA WELLNESS SERVICES

Harrington reviewed several of the key aspects of RWS that he and other RMC administrators had developed during their planning, including the following:

Organizational Mission Coordinate efforts with employers to improve the wellness of their workforce. This will be accomplished through easily accessible health screenings and development of tailored health improvement plans for individual employees.

Vision Statement Our vision is to establish the standard for employers and employees to make health improvement and wellness a continuous priority.

Objectives Objectives of the worksite wellness program are: (1) to limit the increase in health insurance cost to 5% or less by Year 3 for self-funded employers that participate in the program; and (2) to reduce absenteeism due to illness by 3% during Year 2 for employers that participate in the program.

Culture The desired organizational culture for RWS includes: (1) RWS's employees will have an enthusiasm for wellness; (2) employees will present an image of a professional and well-coordinated healthcare team; (3) employers will have a service orientation and will go out of their way to make the service convenient and user-friendly; and (4) employees will be active participants in community events and organizations focused on health and wellness.

Entry and Growth Strategy   A team of specialists representing each of the eight focus areas will be available to begin screenings at client sites by January Year 1. The teams will be comprised of registered nurses and will be aided by a phlebotomist who will assist with blood drawing for laboratory work. As demand for the service grows, the number of teams available for the screenings will be increased. The initial targeted population is the self-funded PPO employer groups. To the extent that major health reform plans include incentives and possibly funding for wellness improvement among the lower-income populations in California, demand for services should substantially increase, perhaps far in excess of RMC's initial expectations.

Once the program is launched in Riviera County, it can quickly be expanded to surrounding counties. Riviera County has more than 450,000 residents. There are more than 1 million people in the RMC extended service area, which is within 30 miles of the hospital. Growth of the service will be more controlled by the desire to have manageable growth than by maximizing potential growth. In order to be successful in the long term, the service must be delivered with quality. RMC's administration believes that controlled growth of the service is the most certain way to ensure excellence.

Being first to market in the local service area is strategically important. RMC's administrators plan to market to key employers immediately, and strive to bring wellness to the workplace in a more focused way than has previously been experienced in the community.

Once this initiative has been rolled out, it can be duplicated by RMC's competition within a period of about 6 months. By developing the foothold as the hospital bringing wellness to employers and employees, RMC's administrators believe that the hospital will be in a position to have a competitive advantage for delivering the service over the next several years. First to market can erect barriers to entry and may deter other hospitals from offering similar services.

MARKET RESEARCH AND ANALYSIS

Customers

Harrington recalled that initial target clients will be members of the CHC. He remains convinced that because they are determined to reduce health costs and improve quality without degrading benefits, RWS is a close fit with CHC's objectives.

Harrington also recalled that additional potential customers include employers or employer groups with self-funded health insurance plans. These groups typically see the direct correlation between the improved health of their members and lower health costs. Another group of potential customers is the HMO populations within employer groups. Well-documented health status of a workforce will be a selling point to HMOs.

Competition and Competitive Edge

Nationally, Comprehensive Health Services and Ceridian Corporation are the two largest players in the area of workforce health assessment and health management programs. Comprehensive Health Services is based in Vienna, Virginia, and Ceridian Corporation is based in Minnesota. Neither organization has an office in California. There are wellness plans developed by many larger employers. However, in Harrington's thinking, there is significant opportunity to provide these services to employers with fewer than 1,000 employees.

There appears to be minimum competition in communities throughout California with populations below 500,000 and for companies between 100 and 1,000 employees. This will give RWS a competitive edge in those initial target markets.

Estimated Market Share and Sales

In Harrington's view, market share will start on a small scale and grow as the service gains a positive reputation, as evaluation teams are developed, and as marketing and sales efforts take hold. RMC's administrators believe that the initial target, CHC, can generate approximately $300,000, $500,000, and $700,000 in revenue for Years 1 through 3, respectively. (See Tables 1–4.)

Table 1. Riviera Wellness Services, Financial Projections

	Year				
	One	Two	Three	Four	Five
Employee Screenings	1,500	2,500	3,500	4,500	7,500
Revenue	$ 300,000	500,000	700,000	900,000	1,500,000
Direct Screening Costs	108,928	176,640	247,296	317,952	529,920
Admin Salaries	189,000	194,666	201,483	208,535	215,834
Supplies & Forms	34,500	47,864	87,500	112,500	187,500
Sales & Marketing	40,000	30,000	25,000	25,000	25,000
Other Admin	24,000	24,000	24,000	24,000	24,000
Total Costs	396,428	473,170	585,279	687,987	982,254
EBITDA	$ −96,428	26,830	114,721	212,013	517,746
percent	−32.14%	5.36%	16.39%	23.56%	34.52%

Table 2. Riviera Wellness Services, Financial Projections (with cash flow)

Year One

						Month							
	One	Two	Three	Four	Five	Six	Seven	Eight	Nine	Ten	Eleven	Twelve	Year
Employee Screenings	80	80	120	120	120	120	120	120	124	164	164	168	1,500
Revenue	$ 16,000	16,000	24,000	24,000	24,000	24,000	24,000	24,000	24,800	32,800	32,800	33,600	300,000
Direct Screening Costs 8 RN Per Diems (40 to 44 screenings/day)	5,888	5,888	8,832	8,832	8,832	8,832	8,832	8,832	8,832	11,776	11,776	11,776	108,928
Admin Salaries	15,750	15,750	15,750	15,750	15,750	15,750	15,750	15,750	15,750	15,750	15,750	15,750	189,000
Supplies & Forms	1,840	1,840	2,760	2,760	2,760	2,760	2,760	2,760	2,852	3,772	3,772	3,864	34,500
Sales & Marketing	4,000	4,000	4,000	4,000	3,000	3,000	3,000	3,000	3,000	3,000	3,000	3,000	40,000
Other Admin	2,000	2,000	2,000	2,000	2,000	2,000	2,000	2,000	2,000	2,000	2,000	2,000	24,000
Total Costs	29,478	29,478	33,342	33,342	32,342	32,342	32,342	32,342	32,434	36,298	36,298	36,390	396,428
EBITDA	-13,478	-13,478	-9,342	-9,342	-8,342	-8,342	-8,342	-8,342	-7,634	-3,498	-3,498	-2,790	-96,428
Increase in A/R	-16,000												-16,000
Increase in A/P													
Free Cash Flow	-29,478	-13,478	-9,342	-9,342	-8,342	-8,342	-8,342	-8,342	-7,634	-3,498	-3,498	-2,790	-112,428
Capital Expenditures	-40,000												-40,000
Interest													
Debt Service													
Net Operating Cash Flow	-69,478	-13,478	-9,342	-9,342	-8,342	-8,342	-8,342	-8,342	-7,634	-3,498	-3,498	-2,790	-152,428
Cash from hospital	100,000		50,000					25,000					175,000
Cash from borrowing													
Cash Balance	$ 30,522	17,044	57,702	48,360	40,018	31,676	23,334	39,992	32,358	28,860	25,362	22,572	22,572

Table 3. Riviera Wellness Services, Financial Projections (with cash flow)

Year Two

							Month						
	One	Two	Three	Four	Five	Six	Seven	Eight	Nine	Ten	Eleven	Twelve	Year
Employee Screenings	168	168	210	210	210	210	210	210	210	210	242	242	2,500
Revenue	$ 33,600	33,600	42,000	42,000	42,000	42,000	42,000	42,000	42,000	42,000	48,400	48,400	500,000
Direct Screening Costs	11,776	11,776	14,720	14,720	14,720	14,720	14,720	14,720	14,720	14,720	17,664	17,664	176,640
Admin Salaries	16,223	16,223	16,222	16,222	16,222	16,222	16,222	16,222	16,222	16,222	16,222	16,222	194,666
Supplies & Forms	3,864	4,000	4,000	4,000	4,000	4,000	4,000	4,000	4,000	4,000	4,000	4,000	47,864
Sales & Marketing	2,500	2,500	2,500	2,500	2,500	2,500	2,500	2,500	2,500	2,500	2,500	2,500	30,000
Other Admin	2,000	2,000	2,000	2,000	2,000	2,000	2,000	2,000	2,000	2,000	2,000	2,000	24,000
Total Costs	36,363	36,499	39,442	39,442	39,442	39,442	39,442	39,442	39,442	39,442	42,386	42,386	473,170
EBITDA	−2,763	−2,899	2,558	2,558	2,558	2,558	2,558	2,558	2,558	2,558	6,014	6,014	26,830
Increase in A/R													
Increase in A/P			−10,000										−10,000
Free Cash Flow	−2,763	−2,899	−7,443	2,558	2,558	2,558	2,558	2,558	2,558	2,558	6,014	6,014	16,830
Capital Expenditures													
Interest													
Debt Service													
Net Operating Cash Flow	−2,763	−2,899	−7,443	2,558	2,558	2,558	2,558	2,558	2,558	2,558	6,014	6,014	16,830
Cash from hospital													
Cash from borrowing													
Cash Balance	$ 19,809	16,910	9,467	12,025	14,583	17,141	19,699	22,257	24,815	27,373	33,387	39,401	39,401

Table 4.   Riviera Wellness Services, Daily Revenue and Variable Cost Detail

	# of employees per day	Rate per employee	Per day amount	# of days annually	Annual totals
Revenue	40	200	8,000	38	$304,000

Cost	Hours	Rate per hour	Per day amount		
Oncology Screen	8	46	$368		
Cardiac Testing	8	46	$368		
Diabetes Screening	8	46	$368		
Nutrition Evaluation	8	46	$368		
Weight Management	8	46	$368		
Ortho Screen	8	46	$368		
Sleep & Respiratory	8	46	$368		
Women's Health	8	46	$368		
total cost			$2,944	38	$111,872
Contribution Margin			$5,056		$192,128
Percentage			63.20%		63.20%

ECONOMICS AND BUSINESS

Harrington quickly reviewed some of the key business variables in the plans for RWS, including the following:

Gross and Operating Margins   Employee health assessment and wellness program development are the primary initial markets to be pursued by RWS. Contribution margin percent is expected to be more than 60% from the primary activities. Years 2 through 5 of operations are expected to generate progressively improving earnings before interest, taxes, depreciation, and amortization (EBITDA) margins ranging from 5% to 34%.

Profit Potential and Durability   RMC administrators project achieving EBITDA of $500,000 in Year 5, while serving only 1% of the target market. This model will have highly sustainable profits so long as RWS can demonstrate that the healthcare cost savings its clients are achieving are a result of healthier lifestyles and reduction of chronic diseases.

Fixed and Variable Costs   Variable costs primarily consist of the service delivery teams that provide the screening services to groups of employees. Each service delivery team consists of eight professionals. It is anticipated that this team screens 48 employees during an 8-hour day. The service teams cost $2,900 per day to conduct the screenings. Other variable costs relate to health risk–appraisal packages, which cost $12 per screening, and lab testing, which costs $11 per screening. Fixed costs relate primarily to administrative services and marketing costs.

Months to Breakeven   RMC's administrators project achieving breakeven status by month 16. The service teams will develop slowly and gain productivity as sales efforts start to take hold.

MARKETING PLAN

Harrington's thoughts next turned to marketing RWS and to some of the critical components of the marketing plan being developed for the service.

Overall Marketing Strategy

RWS's service is directly tailored to help employees change their lifestyles and achieve health cost savings and incentives for themselves and their employers. The sales and marketing focus will be directed to employers with self-funded health insurance plans. These employers will see immediate and direct savings and should be eager to hear how RWS can help improve the health of their workforce.

Initial target employers will have between 100 and 1,000 employees and will be identified through coordination with CHC or through local Chambers of Commerce. The program manager will identify key markets and prospective customers.

Pricing

In Harrington's view, there is little competition that is directly comparable to RWS. The initial pricing is based on a full-day screening of 40 employees per day per team, and a margin of approximately 50% based on direct cost of services. A price of $200 per employee for the screening service achieves the margin objective, allows for support of the administrative functions, and provides for marketing costs. The cost considers the need to involve expensive medical professionals in the screening process. The pricing is expected to be at a level that RMC can ultimately demonstrate a return on investment of at least 500% through the combination of reduced healthcare costs and reduced absenteeism. It is possible the return to employers could be much higher than the initial estimate.

Advertising and Promotion

RMC's administrators plan for advertising and promotion to be designed to support the sales team's efforts. A professionally designed brochure will describe the service to be provided, the employee health scorecard, and the aggregate employee health report. This will also demonstrate anticipated savings in health costs attributable to the improved health of the workforce. As an example, Safeway Stores (SWY), a large grocery store chain with $45 billion in revenue and 197,000 employees, has implemented a wellness program to reward healthy choices and activities. The program was estimated to decrease total healthcare costs by 30% over a two-year period. Results will also be tracked from RWS's clients and will be used in ongoing sales brochures.

IMPLEMENTATION

In his review of how implementation of RWS was to unfold, Harrington thought about several aspects of implementation that he and his administrative colleagues had focused on, beginning with the tools they planned to use in implementing RWS.

Reporting Tools

RMC will purchase the software and services of Wellsource, Inc., to provide reporting to clients. Wellsource is a wellness company that offers software and Internet services that generate individual wellness profiles and aggregate wellness reports. Their Personal Wellness Profile Software will allow the RWS team to present health risks, target risk groups, track progress, and evaluate cost–benefit performance. The software is a proactive tool to manage the wellness of individuals and groups. It considers lifestyle, health factors, and measurements of health risk, including personal and family medical history, nutrition, stress, and biometrics. Assessment scores and recommendations are based on optimal health factors rather than risk of death.

The Wellsource tools also include a weight and health profile, a coronary risk profile, a diabetes risk profile, and a HealthStyle Index, which is a comprehensive lifestyle and health assessment.

Service Delivery

RWS will start with a single-service delivery team, which will include a few individuals formally trained in using the Wellsource tools. Once the sales team engages a customer for the screening and health-scoring services, a date or dates will be set for the screening services, and scheduling will be based on customer preference first and availability second. The individual wellness profile is a detailed report of health and wellness and will be made available to each employee who has a screening. Aggregate reports are prepared and presented to clients to identify health risks in their organization. Trend reports can also be prepared over time after follow up visits to demonstrate progress within the organization.

Intervention plans can be designed to establish one-to-one coaching for those who desire such structured interaction. Also, classroom instruction and self-study can be made available to those who prefer such intervention methods. Interventions can be tailored to the needs and desires of the individual and can also be coordinated with the employer in an effort to help address the needs of the workforce.

Screenings and interventions will be conducted at the employer's worksite whenever possible. If the employer does not have adequate facilities, screenings and interventions can be performed at the hospital. If space is a limiting factor to selling the service, RMC will invest in a mobile unit for future use.

There will also be tools available to help motivate individuals and employees, such as e-mail notices and reminders. There are also wellness challenges that can be issued to help keep target groups focused on their goals.

Tools can also be made available to track health activity. A personal health diary is available for participants to log health, exercise, and nutrition practices. These tools make it easy to track individual and organization progress. Rewards and recognition programs can be introduced to motivate individuals and organizations as they accomplish their goals.

The Wellsource software allows clients to track changes and improvements. Employers should also track trends and savings in productivity, work-loss time, and healthcare expenses.

All of these efforts should help employers to modify their corporate culture to promote a healthy work environment and healthy lifestyles.

Development Plan

A key component of the health assessment is the process for health screening and development of the health report card. The reporting will be a combination of the data from the Wellsource software and some proprietary reporting. RWS administration will work with patent and trademark counsel to ensure that proprietary processes and documents are adequately protected. The process for such assessment and patent and trademark filings must be completed before RWS becomes operational.

The health assessment team qualifications have been identified and RMC's administrators are in the early phases of locating qualified candidates for such positions. It is anticipated that the first screenings will not take place until the first quarter of Year 1.

A marketing brochure is a key component of the sales team's effort. The brochure is being developed with the assistance of a professional public relations and marketing firm. This brochure will be available at the beginning of Year 1.

Organization

RWS will be a division of RMC. The clinical staff will be recruited out of the RMC workforce, which currently stands at about 2,000 individuals. A program manager will be hired to oversee all aspects of operations of the program. This individual will likely have a background and training in wellness. Candidates include exercise physiologists with training in nutrition. This individual will also be supported by a program coordinator, a sales manager, and an administrative assistant.

Harrington is comfortable that RWS will have joint reporting to Debbie Pike, RMC's Director of Public Relations and Marketing, and John Morse, Chief Operating Officer. This joint reporting was decided on because of the emphasis on having RWS benefit the community, which is part of Harrington's larger strategy for the hospital.

HARRINGTON'S CONCLUSIONS AND THOUGHTS ABOUT PRESENTING RWS PLANS TO THE BOARD OF DIRECTORS

Following his review of the business plan for RWS and his more general thinking about the environment facing RMC, Alex Harrington concluded that it is indeed time to share plans for RWS with the board of directors and to ask for their approval of the plan. His rationale includes a conviction, based on the significant planning that has gone into development of RWS, that this is a service opportunity that will be in strong demand in the current environment. He believes that the fact that there is little immediate competition helps make this an attractive business prospect for RMC. RWS complements the RMC hospital strategy and provides value to the community, employers, and their employees. The opportunity to provide a roadmap to improved health to numerous individuals will be widely valued. Along with RMC's leading quality of care, which is publicly reported by numerous sources, the RWS initiative will help RMC achieve its objective of being the hospital of choice for employers in Riviera County.

Although Harrington feels the proposed program is ready to present to the board of directors, he wonders how the board will react. Specifically he wonders if they will see the wellness service as merely viable or as a significant strategic advance for the hospital. He also wonders if the business community will be pleased by RWS's availability.

7

Medical Center of Southern Indiana

Community Commitment and Organization Revival

Jonathon S. Rakich

Alan S. Wong
Indiana University Southeast, New Albany, Indiana

At the signing of the Declaration of Independence, it is reported that Benjamin Franklin told John Hancock, "We must indeed all hang together, or, most assuredly we shall hang separately." The words of our Founding Fathers were indeed noble. They were, however, more than mere words; they reflected a deep and abiding commitment to creating something unprecedented. It was their collective spirit, their devotion to a common good, that made a revolutionary notion viable.

In an interview with the case writers, Kevin Miller, the current President and CEO of the Medical Center of Southern Indiana (MCSI) (www.mcsin.org), reflected on the results of the hospital's performance for the

Note to the reader: Historical portions of this case are largely based on local newspaper accounts and internal hospital documents. These sources are cited throughout. To enhance readability, there is liberal use of accounts' wording absent quotation notation. Observations and statements attributed to persons identified in the case carry quotation notation.

year ending 1998. He stated, "We feel very much the same about our hospital that the nation's Founding Fathers did. Of course, our revolutionary notion—to build, and preserve a hospital dedicated to enhancing the quality of life of the community—pales before that of creating a new nation. However, our local founding fathers, that is, our tight-knit community, has fought over the years to plan, build, and sustain our hospital, and, more critically, has fought to keep it open when all odds pointed to its closure just a few years ago. Through the commitment of business leaders, local government, physicians, hospital employees, and citizens, our hospital forged a new beginning when the community purchased it in 1991, weathered the 'critical care' years through 1997, and accomplished the turnaround with a 1998 operating profit of $480,545, our largest ever."[1]

Miller further observed, "It was that irrepressible will that carried our hospital and community through the toughest of times. This unconquerable spirit forms the foundation of the partnership—between the hospital and its constituents, between its physicians and management—that has brought our hospital back from the brink of extinction to a position of unparalleled growth and unmatched station in a growing, forward-looking community."[2]

When asked, "What's new?" at the MCSI, the answer is "plenty." As reported in the June 25, 1993, issue of the *Evening News*, "There's a new owner, new management, a renewed commitment to the community, new services, a new look and, of course a new name! The facility was formerly known as North Clark Community Hospital."[3] Miller observed, "It is evident that the strategy of investing over $3.0 million between 1992 and 1998 in new equipment, new services, and expanded operations finally paid off. The MCSI was built, suffered setbacks, recovered, and made an impressive comeback, and now has a promising future."

In 1998, MCSI had a bed complement of 96 beds, 270 full-time equivalent (FTE) employees, and $22.6 million in net patient revenues, with an operating profit of $480,545. It had achieved its highest ever number of patient days (15,915), outpatient surgeries (883), and primary care clinic visits (11,314). Its occupancy rate was 45.4%.[4]

HISTORY

The Dream

The building of a hospital in the city of Charlestown, Indiana, was the dream of many community members, especially Eli Goodman, a local physician, and John K. Bowen, the city's mayor then. From its inception in 1973, the hospital was known as North Clark Community Hospital

(NCCH). Its name was changed in late 1991 to the Medical Center of Southern Indiana when the facility was purchased by the City of Charlestown. Initial plans for a 120-bed, acute-care hospital plus a 118-bed extended care facility were announced by Mayor Bowen in July of 1973.[5] Events that precipitated this ambitious project were the desire by community members and local physicians to have their own hospital; the donation of a 21-acre site by a local citizen, Mrs. Sylvester Greissel; and a decision by Clark Memorial Hospital, the county's only other acute-care hospital, not to oppose the building of the facility. On September 17, 1973, the board of Clark Memorial Hospital, a 232-bed, county-owned, acute-care hospital, indicated that it would not seek to expand satellite services to the northern portion of the county, nor would it lodge an objection with the area's comprehensive planning agency—the Southeast Indiana Comprehensive Planning Council—to the building of a new facility in the northern part of the county, in which the city of Charlestown is located.[6]

In September 1973, the non-profit Charlestown North Clark Community Corporation (CNCCC) was formed to operate the planned hospital. William L. Voskuhl, M.D., was elected chair and Mayor John K. Bowen as vice chair of the board of trustees. Initial consideration was given to having the hospital built by the Denver Corporation, with financing by a City of Charlestown revenue bond issue. Ownership would revert to the city after the retirement of the bonds in 20–25 years. In the interim, the hospital would be leased by the non-profit CNCCC.[7]

The next 9 months of planning resulted in substantive changes, including scaling back the size of the facility. The CNCCC was reincorporated as the North Clark Community Hospital Board (NCCHB) and in July of 1974, a contract was signed with The Planned Systems Technology Company (PlanTech) of Indiana to build the hospital.[8] The agreement with PlanTech included a 2.5% development fee and a 1-year management contract. In January, the NCCHB entered into an agreement with the John Nuveen Company of Chicago to sell $8.1 million in tax-free revenue bonds for the building of a 96-bed, acute-care hospital. Finally, the dream of so many community members had become a reality. Ground breaking occurred in July of 1975. North Clark Community Hospital opened its doors in September 1976. Among the 200 individuals attending the ceremony were Dr. William L. Voskuhl, Mayor John K. Bowen, and Col. Harlan Sanders, the founder of Kentucky Fried Chicken.[9]

The Struggle

As reported in the November 29, 1977, issue of the *Indiana Times*, North Clark Community Hospital ran into troubled times. It had lost money since its opening 14 months before. On an average day, only 40–50 of its 96 beds were filled—62 filled beds were required to meet expenses—and only 5 of the county's 50 physicians used the hospital exclusively. Furthermore, the other large hospital located in the southern part of the county, Clark Memorial Hospital, announced a planned expansion of an additional 26 beds to its existing complement of 232 beds.

The combination of losses, low census, and potential increased competition did not bode well for NCCH. The board considered several alternatives, including selling the facility or retaining a professional hospital management company to manage the hospital.[10] The board chose the latter by signing a 3-year contract with the Hospital Corporation of America (HCA) to manage NCCH. At the time, HCA owned or managed 95 hospitals that operated in 25 states. Thomas F. Frist, President of HCA, stated, "This [North Clark Community Hospital] is an excellent hospital with an outstanding medical staff, a fine group of employees and a superior reputation for high quality care. We do not anticipate any major changes in the hospital operating philosophy . . . except to incorporate the systems and procedures which we have developed and used effectively throughout our own [HCA] hospital network."[11]

The Sale

North Clark Community Hospital's struggle for survival continued during the next 6 years until its sale to HCA for $15 million in March 1985. Benefits of being part of HCA were access to purchasing systems, physician recruitment, capital, and other resources of HCA. At the time, HCA owned 4 hospitals in Southern Indiana and it owned or managed more than 400 hospitals nationwide.[12] At the time of purchase, HCA was pursuing a strategy of horizontal and vertical integration.

The Spin-Off

Restructuring by HCA in mid-1987 through an Employee Stock Ownership Plan (ESOP) resulted in the creation of HealthTrust. This company, owned principally by employees with minority interest by HCA, was formed by the spin-off of 100 HCA hospitals, including North Clark Community Hospital.[13] Based in Nashville, HealthTrust hospitals had aggregate revenues of $1.5 billion. With continued poor financial performance, however, HealthTrust indicated in May of 1991 that North Clark Community Hospital would be divested, that is, either sold or closed. The reasons for this action were declining census caused by encroachment of larger Louisville, Kentucky, hospitals into NCCH's service area, outmigration of patients traveling to larger city facilities, the impact of managed care contracting by Indiana businesses with Kentucky insurers, the economic climate, and Medicare cutbacks.[14] The stark reality was that in fiscal year 1991 (ending August 31), the 96-bed North Clark Community Hospital had an average occupancy of 15.6 patients per day and a net loss of $1,743,000.[15]

Beginning the Turnaround

As in the past, the community rallied around its hospital. With citizen and hospital employee support, the City of Charlestown purchased NCCH from HealthTrust for $2 million on December 31, 1991. The hospital was renamed the Medical Center of Southern Indiana, was leased to a newly formed non-profit company, Charlestown Hospital Inc., and was managed by American MedTrust of Atlanta.[16] A new chapter in the hospital's history had begun.

MEDICAL CENTER OF SOUTHERN INDIANA

The Setting

Clark County, Indiana, is predominately rural. It covers 369 square miles of the southern portion of the state with its southernmost border on the Ohio River, separating it from Kentucky. The city of Louisville is the closest large metropolitan area, with a population of approximately 300,000.[17] Clark County is one of seven counties in the Louisville Standard Metropolitan Statistical Area with a population of 1 million, and, consequently, its proximity to Louisville results in patient outmigration to the large number of medical facilities in the city. In 1998, Clark County's population was 93,805, having increased approximately 9% since 1990.[18] The employed labor force was 50,000 with a low unemployment rate of just 2.7%.[19] Nearly 75% of Clark County's residents live in rural areas. The county's largest cities are Jeffersonville with a population of 27,000; Clarksville with a population just over 20,000; along with Sellersburg and Charlestown with populations of 6,000 each.[20] In 1997, county household income was $36,726, ranking 49th among Indiana's 92 counties.[21] Two institutions of higher education are located in the area. Ivy Tech's Sellersburg campus, which is part of Indiana's 23 regional campus, vocational and associate-degree educational system, enrolled 2,000 students in 1997. Indiana University Southeast, part of the eight-campus Indiana University system, enrolled approximately 6,000 students. Even with these institutions of higher education, only 11% of the county's population has earned a bachelor's degree or higher.[22] Thus, the county is predominately rural, has a Medicare population percentage equal to that in the state as a whole, has a low household income, and has relatively few numbers of individuals who have earned higher education degrees.

In 1998, medical facilities in Clark County included Clark Memorial Hospital, located in Clarksville in the southern portion of the county. It is a full-service, acute-care facility with 285 beds including 52 skilled nursing beds, a 47-bed inpatient psychiatric unit, and an active medical staff of 132 physicians.[23] The second full-service hospital located in the northern part of the county is the Medical Center of Southern Indiana with 96 beds, including 18 skilled nursing beds, and an active medical staff of 75 physicians. Employment at MCSI was 270 full-time equivalents making it the largest employer in the city of Charlestown. Other facilities include Jefferson Hospital—a 100-bed psychiatric and substance abuse facility—and Lifespring Mental Health Services, an outpatient mental health facility located in Jeffersonville.[24] Even though MCSI's primary competitor is Clark Memorial Hospital, substantial numbers of residents seek treatment in Louisville, which is 15 miles from Charlestown.

The 1992–1998 Years

A 1992 article in the *Community Showcase Evening News* (6/23/92) headlined the Medical Center of Southern Indiana as the "Pride of Charlestown." Rebounding from the 1991 fiscal year loss of $1,743,000 and purchase of the hospital by the City of Charlestown from HealthTrust to prevent its closure, Donna Mullins, Director of Human Resources and the hospital's first employee, stated, "We felt small; we were a tax write-off for HealthTrust, and that attitude extended to staff, doctors and patients. It was devastating. Despite the divestiture by HealthTrust, the community that had fought to build the hospital fought even harder to keep it open. The community spirit was overwhelming."[25] The purchase of the hospital by the city, its leasing to a non-profit organization, and the retaining of a for-profit firm, American MedTrust, to manage the hospital was, as indicated by Mullins, "an act of courage on the part of Mayor Bob Braswell and the city. The mayor—a long time supporter of the hospital and a hospital board member—had no hesitation in making the partnership with American MedTrust work."[26]

American MedTrust

American MedTrust (AMT), which took over the management of the Medical Center of Southern Indiana in 1992, is an Atlanta-based for-profit management corporation that specializes in revitalizing community hospitals. It is composed of experienced executives who have a track record of successfully turning around troubled hospitals. The firm's operating philosophy is to ". . . enhance customer satisfaction by integrating the hospital management team, the community, and the medical staff. AMT's core concept is to establish a strong value-based relationship with key constituencies (i.e., physicians, patients and their families, employees, and the community) that are both personal and effective." The revitalization initiatives AMT pursues are as follows:[27]

- Providing a rapid assessment plan based on operating priorities, including initiating new financial and operating systems to control costs immediately

- Increasing revenues by increasing the number of managed care contracts

- Investing in new equipment and renovations to support growth in programs and services

- Developing simple, accurate cost and statistical systems to track patient outcomes and the success of new programs

- Assisting affiliated physicians and group practices manage their practices more effectively

- Forming affiliations with large, integrated delivery systems to expand market reach, provide better access to care, and solidify links with hospital medical staff

Kevin J. Miller, a principal with AMT, became President and CEO of the Medical Center of Southern Indiana in 1994. Prior to accepting that position, he held senior corporate development positions for two major health care systems and had occasionally served as an interim director of hospitals in transition. He holds a master's degree in health services administration and is a Fellow in the American College of Healthcare Executives.[28]

In an interview with the case researchers, Miller indicated that "1992 was a do or die year for the Medical Center of Southern Indiana. The time immediately after the buyout was critical. By laying important groundwork right away, AMT was able to turn an operating profit of $197,499 on net patient revenues of $7,822,046 the first year without any layoffs." He stated further, "Under ownership of HealthTrust, the previous administration backed off on marketing. There were no public relations, no meetings with groups in the community, and no meetings with businesses. Furthermore, with the anticipated closing of the hospital, managed care contracts were not renewed. In this business, managed care contracts are critical for survival."

Health Care Expenditures and Managed Care

Aggregate health care expenditures in the United States were $1,146 billion in 1998, representing 13.0% of Gross Domestic Product (GDP) and $4,093 on a per capita basis. Of aggregate health care expenditures, 54.4%

were private and 45.6% were publicly paid by federal, state, and local governments. Medicare, the health insurance program for the elderly and certain individuals with disabilities, accounted for $213.6 billion. Medicaid, a joint federal–state program for indigent individuals, had expenditures of $186.9 billion.

Broken down by sector, the 1998 aggregate health care expenditures for hospital care were $377.1 billion; physician and clinical services were $254.2 billion; nursing home care was $88.0 billion; and home health care was $33.5 billion. Projections for 2003 are aggregate health care expenditures of $1.591 billion, representing 15.2% of GDP and $5,456 per capita.[29]

In 1997, there were 6,097 hospitals of all types in the United States. Of that number, 5,057 were classified as community general hospitals, which are nonfederal and short term, with an average length of stay of less than 30 days. Twenty-two percent of the community general hospitals had a bed size between 50 and 99 beds. Seventeen percent were sized 25–49 beds and 5.5% had fewer than 25 beds. Correspondingly, there were only 807 (16%) that had more than 300 beds.[30]

During the period from 1980 to 1997, there were a large number of hospital closures. In aggregate, the 1980 base of 5,830 community general hospitals decreased by 13% by 1997 with the largest number of closures occurring in the 50 to 99 bed size. This category, the one in which the Medical Center of Southern Indiana falls, decreased by 24%. The implication is that the health care environment was not sympathetic to smaller hospitals, especially those with less than 100 beds. The health care delivery landscape turned more onerous for these institutions. In the mid-1980s, the federal government instituted a fixed-price reimbursement program for paying provider organizations that treated Medicare beneficiaries. The implementation of the prospective pricing system based on diagnosis-related groups replaced the cost-based reimbursement system previously used by the federal government. The implication was that hospitals had to decrease costs. Furthermore, the 1990s witnessed the rise of managed care. The fact that the MCSI survived during this turbulent period is a testament to its strengths and the commitment of the community to the hospital.

Managed care is an insurer's arrangement with physicians, hospitals, and other health care providers to provide a defined set of health care services to plan members for a fixed annual amount or prospectively agreed fees and charges. Managed care plans can take on many forms ranging from health maintenance organizations (HMOs), in which providers receive a fixed capitated amount and enrolled beneficiaries must use plan specified providers, to preferred provider organizations (PPOs), in which beneficiaries' copayments and deductibles are generally less if the plan's approved providers are used; they are higher if providers outside the network are used by patients. In an HMO or PPO managed care plan, a hospital, for example, will negotiate a set fee for its services with the plan. The net effect of managed care plans was to direct its subscribers (i.e., those covered individuals) to hospitals and physicians that had prenegotiated fees, which are quite frequently substantially lower than traditional charges. As Miller previously indicated, a hospital without managed care contracts with insurers is at a distinct disadvantage since potential patients would be directed (as in the case of an HMO) or have a large financial incentive (as in the case of a PPO) to seek services at a participating hospital.[31]

Most of the nation's 269 million people had employer-provided or government-provided health insurance in 1998. Sixteen percent, or 42 million, had no insurance. Of those insured, Medicare covered 30.9 million people and Medicaid covered 24.5 million.[32] Of the estimated 214 million people insured through private insurance programs, mostly through employment, an astounding number were members of managed care programs. HMO enrollment, for example, was 105.3 million people in 1998, having increased from 12.5 million in 1983. PPO enrollment was 98.3 million people, having increased from 28.5 million in 1987.[33]

Rebuilding the MCSI Managed Care Business

"My primary priority when assuming the position of CEO in January 1994 was to increase the number of managed care contracts," said Miller when being interviewed by the case writers. Since HealthTrust planned to close the hospital, it canceled existing contracts. In 1994, the hospital had only two. In 1998 it had 25. Miller indicated that it has taken a great deal of effort to restore relationships with managed care companies. "I pulled out all the stops," he said, "by being sensitive to insurers, earning their respect, and proving to them why it was to their benefit to contract with MCSI. Initially, a lot of plans wouldn't even return my phone calls. Because of our past track record under HealthTrust, many of them wouldn't give me the time of day." Enlisting the support of the local state senator, a bill titled *Any Willing Provider* was passed by the Indiana legislature in 1995 that required managed care companies to negotiate with providers such as MCSI. With the assistance of that legislation and persuasion from the state insurance commissioner, Miller worked with the legislature to require insurers to present the conditions under which they contract with hospitals, and to give written notice explaining why they declined to sign up with hospitals. This initiative not only helped MCSI but also dozens of other hospitals around the state. "As a policy," Miller indicated, "MCSI will continue to do what is appropriate to keep the trust of managed care insurers." Today, relations with insurers are much improved and the hospital's affiliation with the Norton Health System, a major regional hospital system located in Louisville, is an added boost to MCSI's managed care business. "The alliance provides the acceptance of more insurers, treatment in new areas (including chemotherapy and teleradiology), access to more physicians and, most importantly," Miller said, "it has driven up the hospital's status with the community, physicians, and managed care plans."[34]

The Mission

The published mission of the Medical Center of Southern Indiana follows:

> We at the Medical Center dedicate our lives, our hearts, and resources to enhancing the quality of life in southern Indiana. The Medical Center's physicians and employees commit to providing excellent medical care, community education and advanced diagnostic and emergency services to the communities of southern Indiana. We will bring together medical technology and compassion to treat each of our patients competently and with dignity.[35]

As outlined in its 1998 strategic plan document, the objectives of the MCSI are to (1) improve the quality of services provided, (2) improve market share in its service area; and (3) improve the hospital's image. Specific initiatives to accomplish these objectives follow:[36]

1. *Increase physician recruitment, retention, and collaboration:* Among the action plans are developing a primary care physician office site and specialty clinic in nearby Scottsburg; expanding and aggressively marketing a physician referral and health information program; aggressively marketing primary care physicians, family practice centers, and specialty clinics through direct mail and print ads; and exploring options for development of two new primary care clinics in the western part of the service area.

2. *Continue managed care contracting:* The action plans include developing North Clark Physicians, Inc. (NCP), by adding new physicians, marketing the medical staff organization services, and matching the hospital's managed care list with the NCP managed care list; pursuing a managed care contract with Humana, a major health insurance company, to facilitate servicing Medicare patients who are members of Humana's Medicare Select program; obtaining managed care contracts for specialty services (i.e., skilled nursing, home health, and behavioral health services); increasing occupational medicine contracts; improving financial and clinical information systems; and investigating and developing a community-based insurance product and/or direct contracting with employers.

3. *Improve existing services and pursue new product/service development and marketing:* Planning activities include increasing utilization of the

emergency department through aggressive marketing; increasing out-patient visits and ancillary services volumes; growing the occupational medicine program by providing on-site services and marketing of hand surgery availability; developing a wound care center; implementing a quality improvement team to examine and improve dietary services, environmental services, antibiotic usage review, and clinical informa-tion reports; developing a senior care program and investigating a geriatric assessment center; and continuing to expand the hospital's "quality of caring" program and enhance patient/customer relations.

Other potential service area expansion programs to undergo prelimi-nary feasibility studies are an assisted living center, adult day care, child care (for-profit), migraine headache center, counseling, and a retail phar-macy. In addition, the 1998 strategic plan dealing with improving and expanding services calls for investigating: the possibility of affiliating key products with branded services (i.e., oncology with Sloan-Kettering Can-cer Center); the development of disease specific outreach programs such as cancer and diabetes; the development of women's and men's services (i.e., gynecology, an alternative birthing center, a urological center); and devel-oping affiliation with the community hospice program and local long-term care facilities. Finally, a major initiative to be considered is a feasibility study of AMT acquiring Charter-Jefferson Hospital and referral of adult psychiatric and geropsychiatric patients to MCSI.

The Organization and Medical Staff

In 1998, the Medical Center of Southern Indiana had 329 employees rep-resenting 270 full-time equivalents. Due to community "ownership," both literally and figuratively, turnover among its employees was a low 11%. The hospital's structure is characterized by a lean organization. This is in keeping with AMT's operating policy of controlling costs. Exhibit 1 pre-sents the MCSI organization chart and identifies the hospital's various functions.

The medical staff is composed of 140 individuals, 75 of whom are active. One AMT initiative upon assuming management of the hospital was to rebuild physician–administration relationships. Under HealthTrust, these relationships had deteriorated. As a result, a partnership—independent prac-tice association (IPA)—was formed with 10 primary care physicians. The main objective was to enable these physicians to keep their own practices, yet compete through the IPA for managed care contracts. Furthermore, the IPA offers practice management services to these physicians.[37]

Miller observed, "Over the years we have helped our medical staff expand access to patients. There are three primary care and two specialty clinics located throughout the county and owned by MCSI. Our biggest

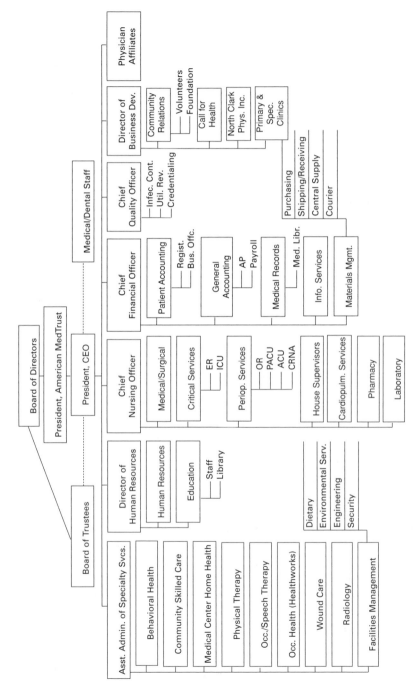

Exhibit 1. The Medical Center of Southern Indiana organization chart.

118

improvement, however, has been involving physicians in issues central to quality and their day-to-day practices. Our attitude is one of cooperation and involvement in major organizational decisions that affect the medical staff." He went on to say, "Just as managed care contracts are critical to the survival of any hospital, so too is medical staff relations. Nothing happens in a hospital until a patient is admitted and a physician orders treatment. Doctors are absolutely critical to our hospital's success. Consequently, we are continuously seeking to have more physicians join our medical staff." To make the point, he referred to the data in Exhibit 2. It shows the hospital's 1998 revenue generated by physicians.

Service Enhancement and Investment

As a full-service hospital, MCSI offers inpatient medical/surgical care, outpatient diagnostic testing and care, 24-hour emergency services, radiology, skilled nursing care, psychiatric care, home health care, laboratory services, occupational medicine, pain management therapy, social services/discharge planning, and specialty clinics. Exhibit 3 presents the full range of services.[38] It is not surprising that the service lines were expanded under the management of American MedTrust. In fact, it is consistent with its operating philosophy to invest in new programs and services and is essential to the hospital fulfilling its mission. CEO Miller indicated that "beyond expanding traditional inpatient and outpatient medical/surgical services, it was critical to respond to the needs of our Medicare patient base through the creation of 3 cost-based programs: a home health agency (1993), a skilled nursing facility (1993) with 24 beds, and a geriatric psychiatry inpatient/outpatient hospitalization program in 1994. These programs have made a significant impact on patient care, meeting community needs, and our bottom line."[39]

Home Health Agency

MCSI's accredited home health agency filled a chronic community need for care outside the hospital. In 1998, more than 15,000 visits were made to patients in a five-county region. Even though visits dropped from 21,000 in 1997 due to government funding cutbacks, the agency enhances continuity of care by providing basic care, psychiatric care, respite care, physical therapy, and homemaker services. In the past 4 years, its gross revenue has grown from about $422,000 to $1.75 million in 1998. Home health and homemaker respite visits totaled 28,700 in 1998.

Skilled Nursing Facility

MCSI's skilled nursing facility also serves a critical need in the larger community, receiving referrals in the region and throughout the metropolitan

Physician	Discharges	Patient Days	O/P Registration	Revenue (in dollars)
1	243	2,313	1,355	$4,667,850
2	199	3,570	207	4,634,015
3	376	2,312	1,786	4,464,752
4	45	260	3,310	3,477,125
5	128	1,028	1,205	2,236,740
6	131	1,770	6	2,084,305
7	220	942	109	1,974,429
8	142	910	594	1,806,472
9	96	596	1,500	1,615,923
10	75	340	2,877	1,369,355
11	33	159	2,645	1,123,274
12	74	527	121	964,095
13	–	–	470	868,175
14	64	441	184	776,929
15	38	153	3,861	760,447
16	4	54	65	443,268
17	18	40	189	342,562
18	17	40	80	336,688
19	5	24	608	324,944
20	21	96	306	303,228
21	5	26	125	298,867
22	–	–	174	242,421
23	10	30	613	235,524
24	3	11	114	210,477
25	19	56	381	189,882
26	1	2	165	148,272
27	–	–	52	134,660
28	4	2	259	133,885
29	–	–	120	132,508
30	1	1	333	128,175
31	4	14	77	120,848
32	1	1	47	108,640
33	3	24	31	101,881
All others	36	172	5,785	2,918,740
Total	2,016	15,914	29,754	$39,679,356

Exhibit 2. MCSI 1998 physician utilization and gross hospital revenue generated by physician.

Behavioral Health Services (inpatient geropsychiatric unit, outpatient counseling)

Call for Health (physician referral service)

Cardiopulmonary

Community Education

Community Skilled Care (skilled nursing and subacute care unit)

Diabetic Education

Echocardiography/TEE

Electrocardiography (EKG, stress test)

Electroencephalography (EEG)

24-hour Emergency Services

Endoscopy

Home Health Care (nursing, physical therapy, respite/homemaker, mental health, pediatric nursing)

Inpatient/Outpatient Surgical Services (cardiology-pacemaker, ENT, gastroenterology, general surgery, GYN, neuro-surgery, orthopedic, plastic/reconstructive, pediatric, thoracic, vascular)

Intensive Care Unit

Laboratory Services

Leatherman Spine Center

Medical-Surgical Unit (pediatric, adult, geriatric)

Nutritional/Dietary Counseling

Occupational Medicine

Occupational Therapy

Orthopedic Options (joint replacement program, sports medicine)

Outpatient Chemotherapy

Outpatient Diagnosis and Treatment Services

Pain Management

Physical Therapy

Podiatry

Pulmonary Function Lab

Radiology (bone densitometry, CT scanning, magnetic resonance imaging, mammography, nuclear medicine, ultrasound)

Respiratory Therapy

Social Services/Discharge Planning

Speakers' Bureau

Specialty Clinic (Charlestown)

Speech Therapy

Urology

Volunteer Services

Wound Care

Exhibit 3. Services offered by MCSI.

area. The 18-bed unit is fully Medicare certified, having received two deficiency-free survey ratings since its opening in March 1994. The program provides extensive care for stroke and postsurgical patients, and has proven an excellent complement to both hospital and community nursing home programs. Its gross revenues increased from $1.07 million in 1994 to $4.7 million, with 262 admissions in 1998 and an average length of stay of 16.8 days.

Geropsychiatric Services

In 1994, an inpatient geropsychiatry partial hospitalization program was implemented. The 17-bed facility is equipped to treat adults over the age of 54 who require 24-hour monitoring. The partial hospitalization program provides intensive, adult day-care services and helps reduce inpatient hospitalization. Gross revenue for behavioral health programs totaled $4.56 million in 1998, based on 337 admissions and an average length of stay of 19.1 days.

Outpatient Mall

In response to the need to provide the most cost-efficient, accessible care possible to the community, an outpatient mall was created in the hospital. Nearly $300,000 was spent to remodel and equip 4,000 square feet of storage space and to open the mall in the fall of 1995. The multi-departmental facility provides the one-stop outpatient shop that patients need, and enhances radiology, physical therapy, cardiopulmonary, and laboratory services. One room in the center doubles as a daytime room for partial psychiatric therapy and as a nighttime public education facility.

Capital Expenditures and Improvements

It takes money to make money. When Mr. Miller became CEO in 1994, he found that very little had been spent to make improvements in the hospital. During the period of 1995–1998, management spent about $2.25 million on equipment and renovations to support newly implemented programs and services. Included in those purchases was $450,000 to lease an advanced computerized tomography system (CT scanner) to support the radiology department's ability to care for patients on site, without having to refer them to hospitals 20 minutes or more away. A new mammography system, a new SPECT nuclear medicine camera, a new remote primary and specialty care clinic, and numerous other ventures were funded.

Key Indicators and Finances

1998 was the first year in many in which MCSI had an operating profit. It was $480,545, based on net patient revenues of $22.4 million and gross patient revenues of $39.6 million. The difference between gross and net patient revenue is known in the trade as contractual allowances and discounts (the difference between charges for services and the amount received). Peter Feimer, Assistant Administrator of Specialty Services, likened it to the difference between list price and negotiated price. Essentially a phenomenon of managed care contracting, it is not uncommon for hospitals to have such a large disparity between charges and contracted prices. Consequently, for analysis purposes, net patient revenue is a better indicator of a hospital's fiscal status.

Exhibit 4 presents selected operating statistics for the MCSI for the years from 1994 to 1998. Inspection reveals increasing trends in net patient revenue, FTE employees, patient admissions, patient days, outpatient surgeries, and occupancy rate.

Financial information for the seven-year period of 1992–1998 is presented in the following exhibits. Exhibit 5 contains the MCSI's balance sheet. Exhibit 6 presents each balance sheet item as a percentage of the total assets. Exhibit 7 contains the income statement and Exhibit 8 presents the income statement items as a percentage of net revenue. Exhibit

STATISTIC	1994	1995	1996	1997	1998
Net patient revenue (in millions)	$13.0	$14.3	$15.8	$18.9	$22.4
Total patient revenue (in millions)	$19.5	$23.7	$27.7	$34.3	$39.6
Accounts receivable (days)	64	66	80	66	66
Total employee hours	380,668	444,497	478,400	548,958	581,906
Total number (full, part, and PRN)	264	294	380	351	329
Full-time equivalent employees	183	214	230	258	270
Total patient admissions	1,471	1,871	1,936	2,086	2,016
Total patient days	11,335	14,194	15,402	15,680	15,915
Outpatient surgeries	529	600	573	709	883
Primary care clinic visits	2,085	3,197	6,831	8,694	11,314
Home health visits	8,067	12,928	16,967	21,104	15,197
Medical staff	–	104	121	129	119
Occupancy rate (based on 96 beds)	32.4	40.5	44	44.7	45.4
Occupancy rate (based on 77 beds)	40.3	50.5	54.8	55.8	56.6
Outpatient visits	8,883	11,793	10,447	10,501	10,851
Wages and benefits (in millions)	$6.3	$7.3	$8.5	$9.9	$11.2

Exhibit 4. MCSI operating statistics, 1994–1998.

Balance Sheet—MCSI

	1992	1993	1994	1995	1996	1997	1998
Assets:							
Cash & Cash Equivalents	$ 357,266	$ 312,769	$1,032,531	$ 631,844	$ 905,077	$ 639,558	$ 447,297
Receivables	1,748,403	1,966,056	2,276,182	2,034,829	3,410,861	3,379,851	2,479,264
Inventories	289,995	291,333	349,260	378,020	342,441	333,041	395,347
Other Current Assets	27,688	39,062	48,439	54,864	53,757	43,633	60,697
Total Current Assets	$2,423,352	$2,609,220	$3,706,412	$3,099,557	$4,712,136	$4,396,083	$3,382,605
Prop., Plant & Equip (net)	$ 252,185	$ 572,818	$1,059,143	$1,791,723	$2,300,939	$2,444,674	$2,791,278
Net Acquisition & Start Up Costs (net)	268,268	394,236	385,472	291,768	198,552	127,681	56,950
Other Assets	100	2,000	0	0	0	0	0
Total Assets	$2,943,905	$3,578,274	$5,151,027	$5,183,048	$7,211,627	$6,968,438	$6,230,833
Liabilities and Fund Balance:							
Current Maturities of LT Debt	$ 103,983	$ 158,814	$ 196,748	$1,222,637	$1,192,278	$ 702,032	$ 665,314
Account Payable	305,134	893,943	969,486	812,054	986,736	694,982	1,289,160
Accrued Salaries & Wages	216,136	265,092	363,575	143,203	320,134	167,982	375,647
Accrued compensated absences					163,521	202,398	201,786
Due to Affiliate	329,341	422,515	1,174,463	1,044,947	1,344,625	1,394,119	1,767,346
Estimated 3rd Party Settlements, Net		(69,650)	746,389	1,011,684	1,944,301	2,667,118	433,320
Other Current Liabilities	185,724	198,022	236,755	293,075	478,488	516,336	410,333
Total Current Liab.	$1,140,318	$1,868,736	$3,687,416	$4,527,600	$6,430,083	$6,344,967	$5,142,906
LT Debt, Less Curr. Mat.	$1,165,128	$1,175,052	$1,331,454	$ 565,504	$ 776,541	$ 937,662	$ 976,689
Total Liabilities	$2,305,446	$3,043,788	$5,018,870	$5,093,104	$7,206,624	$7,282,629	$6,119,595
Deferred Revenue	$ 440,960	$ 385,839	$ 330,723	$ 275,604	$ 220,307	$ 165,372	$ 110,256
Fund Balance	197,499	148,647	(198,566)	(185,660)	(215,304)	(479,563)	982
Total Liabilities & Fund Balance	$2,943,905	$3,578,274	$5,151,027	$5,183,048	$7,211,627	$6,968,438	$6,230,833

Exhibit 5. MCSI balance sheet for the years 1992–1998.

Common Size Balance Sheet—MCSI

	1992	1993	1994	1995	1996	1997	1998
Assets:							
Cash & Cash Equivalents	12.1%	8.7%	20.0%	12.2%	12.6%	9.2%	7.2%
Receivables	59.4%	54.9%	44.2%	39.3%	47.3%	48.5%	39.8%
Inventories	9.9%	8.1%	6.8%	7.3%	4.7%	4.8%	6.3%
Other Current Assets	0.9%	1.2%	0.9%	1.0%	0.7%	0.6%	1.0%
Total Current Assets	82.3%	72.9%	71.9%	59.8%	65.3%	63.1%	54.3%
Prop., Plant & Equip (net)	8.6%	16.0%	20.6%	34.6%	31.9%	35.1%	44.8%
Net Acquisition & Start Up Costs (net)	9.1%	11.0%	7.5%	5.6%	2.8%	1.8%	0.9%
Other Assets	0.0%	0.1%	0.0%	0.0%	0.0%	0.0%	0.0%
Total Assets	100.0%	100.0%	100.0%	100.0%	100.0%	100.0%	100.0%
Liabilities and Fund Balance:							
Current Maturities of LT Debt	3.5%	4.4%	3.8%	23.6%	16.5%	10.1%	10.7%
Account Payable	10.4%	25.0%	18.8%	15.7%	13.7%	10.0%	20.7%
Accrued Salaries & Wages	7.3%	7.4%	7.1%	2.8%	4.4%	2.4%	6.0%
Accrued compensated absences	0.0%	0.0%	0.0%	0.0%	2.3%	2.9%	3.2%
Due to Affiliate	11.2%	11.8%	22.8%	20.2%	18.6%	20.0%	28.4%
Estimated 3rd Party Settlements, Net	0.0%	-1.9%	14.5%	19.5%	27.0%	38.3%	7.0%
Other Current Liabilities	6.3%	5.5%	4.6%	5.6%	6.6%	7.4%	6.5%
Total Current Liab.	38.7%	52.2%	71.6%	87.4%	89.1%	91.1%	82.5%
LT Debt, Less Curr. Mat.	39.6%	32.8%	25.8%	10.9%	10.8%	13.4%	15.7%
Total Liabilities	78.3%	85.0%	97.4%	98.3%	99.9%	104.5%	98.2%
Deferred Revenue	15.0%	10.8%	6.5%	5.3%	3.1%	2.4%	1.8%
Fund Balance	6.7%	4.2%	-3.9%	-3.6%	-3.0%	-6.9%	0.0%
Total Liab. & Fund Bal.	100.0%	100.0%	100.0%	100.0%	100.0%	100.0%	100.0%

Exhibit 6. Balance sheet items as a percentage of the total assets for the years 1992–1998.

125

Income Statement—MCSI

	1992	1993	1994	1995	1996	1997	1998
Unrestricted Rev., Gains, & Others:							
Net patient service revenue	$7,822,046	$8,395,734	$13,014,714	$14,377,223	$15,874,463	$18,941,727	$22,458,259
Income on investments	14,446	9,682	2,746	23,818	33,403	42,475	34,735
Rental income	63,202	56,827	28,452	53,028	50,910	60,946	71,965
Gains on sale of assets	55,120	55,121	55,116	55,116	65,511	68,366	55,116
Other revenue	108,795	100,200	112,154	106,451	63,261	107,410	106,604
Unrestricted gifts & bequests	10,000						
Total Unrestricted rev, gains & others	$8,073,609	$8,617,564	$13,213,182	$14,615,636	$16,087,548	$19,220,924	$22,726,679
Expenses:							
Salaries & wages	$3,331,447	$3,954,002	$5,622,103	$6,660,827	$7,644,074	$8,731,566	$9,882,526
Employee benefits	420,665	540,080	718,876	857,072	883,645	1,129,760	1,345,784
Professional fees	920,021	1,061,889	2,071,691	1,721,574	2,397,032	2,720,071	3,121,787
Supplies and other	1,959,520	2,048,803	3,022,647	3,522,281	3,230,159	4,167,609	4,610,041
Maintenance and utilities	302,438	293,644	401,017	244,250	481,402	452,080	241,587
Lease expense	200,000	200,000	200,000	200,000	200,000	250,000	250,000
Depreciation & amortization	71,089	88,275	226,695	328,103	438,628	577,776	663,130
Interest	147,511	151,481	214,670	228,943	255,878	281,878	293,225
Provision of bad debt	523,419	328,242	1,082,696	839,680	586,424	1,174,443	1,838,054
Total expenses	$7,876,110	$8,666,416	$13,560,395	$14,602,730	$16,117,192	$19,485,183	$22,246,134
Excess (Defic.) of Rev. Over Exp.	$197,499	($48,852)	($347,213)	$12,906	($29,644)	($264,259)	$480,545
Unrestricted net assets (deficit), begin.	$0	$197,499	$148,647	($198,566)	($185,660)	($215,304)	($479,563)
Unrestricted net assets (deficit), year end	$197,499	$148,647	($198,566)	($185,660)	($215,304)	($479,563)	$982

Exhibit 7. MCSI income statement for the years 1992–1998.

126

Common Size Income Statement—MCSI

	1992	1993	1994	1995	1996	1997	1998
Unrestricted Rev., Gains, & Others:							
Net patient service revenue	96.9%	97.4%	98.5%	98.4%	98.7%	98.5%	98.8%
Income on investments	0.2%	0.1%	0.1%	0.2%	0.2%	0.2%	0.2%
Rental income	0.8%	0.7%	0.2%	0.4%	0.3%	0.3%	0.3%
Gains on sale of assets	0.7%	0.6%	0.4%	0.4%	0.4%	0.4%	0.2%
Other revenue	1.3%	1.2%	0.8%	0.7%	0.4%	0.6%	0.5%
Unrestricted gifts & bequests	0.1%	0.0%	0.0%	0.0%	0.0%	0.0%	0.0%
Total Unrestricted rev., gains & others	100.0%	100.0%	100.0%	100.0%	100.0%	100.0%	100.0%
Expenses:							
Salaries & wages	41.3%	45.9%	42.5%	45.6%	47.5%	45.4%	43.5%
Employee benefits	5.2%	6.3%	5.4%	5.9%	5.5%	5.9%	5.9%
Professional fees	11.4%	12.3%	15.7%	11.8%	14.9%	14.2%	13.7%
Supplies and other	24.3%	23.8%	22.9%	24.1%	20.1%	21.7%	20.3%
Maintenance and utilities	3.7%	3.4%	3.0%	1.7%	3.0%	2.4%	1.1%
Lease expense	2.5%	2.3%	1.5%	1.4%	1.2%	1.3%	1.1%
Depreciation & amortization	0.9%	1.0%	1.7%	2.2%	2.7%	3.0%	2.9%
Interest	1.8%	1.8%	1.6%	1.6%	1.6%	1.5%	1.3%
Provision of bad debt	6.5%	3.8%	8.3%	5.6%	3.7%	6.0%	8.1%
Total expenses	97.6%	100.6%	102.6%	99.9%	100.2%	101.4%	97.9%
Excess (Defic.) of Rev. Over Exp.	2.4%	-0.6%	-2.6%	0.1%	-0.2%	-1.4%	2.1%

Exhibit 8. MCSI Income statement items as a percentage of net revenue for the years 1992–1998.

Statement of Cash Flow—MCSI

	1992	1993	1994	1995	1996	1997	1998
CF from Operating Activities							
Excess (deficiency) of Rev. Over Expense	$197,499	($48,852)	($347,213)	$12,906	($29,644)	($264,259)	$480,545
Adjust. to Reconcile above to Net Cash:							
Depreciation & Amortization	$71,089	$88,275	$226,695	$328,103	$438,628	$577,776	$663,130
Disposal of fixed assets							
Provision for bad debt	$523,419	$328,242	$1,082,696	$839,680	$586,424	$1,174,443	$1,838,054
Changes in:							
Receivables					($1,962,456)	($1,143,433)	($937,467)
Inventories					$35,579	$9,400	($62,306)
Other current assets					$1,107	$10,124	($17,062)
Accounts Payable					$174,682	($291,754)	$594,178
Estimated 3rd Party settlements					$932,617	$722,817	($2,233,798)
Accrued salaries & wages					$825,543	($25,933)	$474,277
Deferred Revenue					($55,296)	($54,935)	($55,116)
Total Changes	($228,218)	$113,080	$322,620	($819,037)	($48,224)	($773,714)	($2,237,294)
Amortization of Gains	($55,120)	($55,121)	($55,116)	($55,116)			
Net Cash Provided by Operating Activities	$508,669	$425,624	$1,229,682	$306,536	$947,184	$714,246	$744,435
CF from Investing Activities							
Purchase of property & equipment	($243,143)	($211,182)	($283,995)	($532,945)	($298,743)	($478,855)	($939,005)
Acquisition & Start-up Costs	($19,528)	($169,503)	($73,398)	($76)			
Net Cash Provided by Investing Activities	($262,671)	($380,685)	($357,393)	($533,021)	($298,743)	($478,855)	($939,005)
CF from Financing Activities							
Proceeds from issuance of long term debt	$302,170					$914,125	$832,543
Principal payments on long term debt	($340,902)	($89,436)	($152,527)	($174,202)	($375,208)	($1,415,035)	($830,234)
Net Cash Provided by Financing Activities	($38,732)	($89,436)	($152,527)	($174,202)	($375,208)	($500,910)	$2,309
Net Increase (Decrease) in Cash	$207,266	($44,497)	$719,762	($400,687)	$273,233	($265,519)	($192,261)
Cash & Cash Equivalents, beg. Of year	$150,000	$357,266	$312,769	$1,032,531	$631,844	$905,077	$639,558
Cash & Cash Equivalents, end Of year	$357,266	$312,769	$1,032,531	$631,844	$905,077	$639,558	$447,297
Supplemental Disclosures of CF Informat.							
Cash Paid for Interest	$62,742	$120,654	$245,497	$207,083	$257,552	$303,085	$293,225
Suppl. Discl. Of Non-Cash Inv. & Fin. Activit							
Capital lease obligat. incurred for Equip	$36,696	$154,191	$346,863	$434,140	$555,886	$171,785	
Debt obligation incurred for building							

Exhibit 9. MCSI statement of cash flow for the years 1992–1998.

128

9 contains the statement of cash flows. Finally, Exhibit 10 presents selected financial ratios for MCSI and industry averages.[40]

When asked why the hospital had operating losses in four of the last seven years, Miller provided the following reasons:

1. During the past 7 years, the MCSI made substantial expenditures to expand services, not only by type, but also in satellite locations, and to improve technology. Obviously, the startups have taken time to break even. Absent such initiatives, the hospital's financial performance would have been worse. In fact, the hospital would not have survived. The initiatives were included in the MCSI's 1998 strategic plan to provide evidence of just how aggressively MCSI has pursued expansion. A critical mass and mix of services are necessary in order to provide the level of patient care consistent with its mission.

    Referring to the financial exhibits, Miller noted, in 1992, the percentage of net property, plant, and equipment over total assets was just 8.6% (see Exhibits 5 and 6). It jumped to 34.6%, however, in 1995 and the percentage continued to rise until it reached 44.8% in 1998. As a result of the investments over time, the MCSI was able to offer more services and the net patient service revenue increased from $7.8 million in 1992 to $22.5 million in 1998. The 1998 revenue was almost three times the 1992 revenue.

    With the increase in revenue, expenses also increased (see Exhibits 7 and 8). Salaries and wages increased from $3,331,447 in 1992 to $9,882,526 in 1998, almost three times that of 1992. Employee benefits, professional fees, and provision for bad debts also increased by the same magnitude. As expected, depreciation and amortization expenses increased about nine times, from $71,089 in 1992 to $663,130 in 1998. Interest expenses led to several years of negative income.

    Net cash obtained from operating activities primarily funded the increase in investments. Although MCSI experienced negative income in 4 out of 7 years of operations from 1992 to 1998, the annual net cash provided by operating activities has been positive (see Exhibit 9). The free-operating-cash-flow-over-revenue and the free-operating-cash-flow-over-assets ratios indicate a brighter picture than the income statement (statement of operations and changes in net assets). The increasing burden of servicing debt and leases, and investing in equipment and property, however, has largely absorbed the net cash provided by operating activities.

    MCSI has done an efficient job of managing its assets. All asset efficiency ratios show that MCSI has outperformed the industry average in this area. It also holds true for the fixed assets and current assets (see Exhibit 10).

Selected Financial Ratios—MCSI

	1992	1993	1994	1995	1996	1997	1998
Profitability Ratios:							
Total Margin	2.45%	-0.57%	-2.63%	0.09%	-0.18%	-1.37%	2.11%
Industry		*3.80%*	*3.90%*	*4.40%*	*5.00%*	*5.80%*	*3.80%*
ROI	6.71%	-1.37%	-6.74%	0.25%	-0.41%	-3.79%	7.71%
Industry		*3.87%*	*1.92%*	*8.01%*	*1.25%*	*1.64%*	*2.07%*
Free Oper CF Over Revenue				4.70%	2.90%	2.40%	0.70%
Industry							
Free Oper CF Over Assets		5.17%	3.03%	21.10%	2.69%	3.43%	6.52%
Industry				*4.60%*	*3.60%*	*2.60%*	*0.60%*
Liquidity Ratios:							
Current Ratio	2.13	1.40	1.01	0.68	0.73	0.69	0.66
Industry		*2.23*	*2.20*	*2.19*	*2.19*	*2.19*	*2.21*
Days in Patient Accounts Receivable	81.59	85.47	63.84	51.66	78.43	65.13	40.29
Industry		*65.70*	*67.90*	*64.20*	*62.10*	*63.20*	*65.00*
Days Cash On Hand	17.91	13.84	30.76	17.17	21.89	13.16	8.27
Industry		*24.00*	*22.50*	*25.30*	*27.70*	*34.70*	*27.90*
Capital Structure Ratios:							
Fixed Asset Financing Ratio	223.87%	121.51%	92.17%	27.14%	31.07%	36.45%	34.29%
Industry		*42.60%*	*44.10%*	*42.50%*	*40.80%*	*37.70%*	*38.10%*
Cash Flow to Total Debt	11.65%	1.30%	-2.40%	6.70%	5.68%	4.30%	18.69%
Industry		*26.50%*	*26.50%*	*29.80%*	*29.50%*	*33.90%*	*25.20%*
Times Interest Earned	2.34	0.68	-0.62	1.06	0.88	0.06	2.64
Industry		*4.24*	*4.43*	*5.08*	*5.25*	*4.69*	*3.14*
Debt Service Coverage	0.85	0.79	0.26	1.41	1.05	0.35	1.28
Industry		*3.16*	*3.36*	*3.39*	*3.56*	*4.24*	*4.07*
Asset Efficiency Ratios:							
Total Asset Turnover	2.74	2.41	2.57	2.82	2.23	2.76	3.65
Industry				*1.13*	*1.12*	*1.04*	*1.03*
Fixed Asset Turnover	15.49	8.91	9.15	7.01	6.44	7.47	7.98
Industry				*2.44*	*2.52*	*2.29*	*2.33*
Current Asset Turnover	3.33	3.30	3.56	4.72	3.41	4.37	6.72
Industry		*3.52*	*3.47*	*3.51*	*3.52*	*3.40*	*3.36*
Inventory Turnover	27.81	29.58	37.83	38.66	46.98	57.71	57.49
Industry		*44.18*	*43.84*	*44.49*	*45.69*	*46.47*	*46.35*
Other Financial Ratio:							
Capital Expense Growth Rate Ratio		130.61%	97.79%	75.79%	38.10%	20.97%	25.06%
Industry		*6.20%*	*6.50%*	*5.80%*	*6.40%*	*6.90%*	*7.40%*
Gross Property & Equipment	279740.00	64513.00	1275971.00	2243056.00	3097684.00	3747184.00	4686189.00

Exhibit 10. Selected financial ratios for MCSI and industry averages for the years 1992–1998.

130

2. MCSI needed to offer managed care contract allowances (difference between charges such as list price and contractual amounts) in order to reobtain managed care contracts. Because so much of its patient base is covered by these types of plans, it was essential to aggressively pursue managed care contracts in order to survive.

3. Because 65% of MCSI's patient base is Medicare, the federal government's cutbacks on fixed reimbursement have hurt MCSI's revenue stream as well as that of all other hospitals. In the industry, few hospitals were reporting positive net income.

THE FUTURE

On a hot summer day as Miller met with the case writers in his office, he looked out the window and commented, "The Medical Center of Southern Indiana is like the mythical Phoenix—it was near death and arose again. This hospital, the pride of Charlestown, has gone through very difficult times and multiple phases in its organizational life cycle: conception in 1973; birth in 1976 when it opened; adoption by HCA and HealthTrust through acquisitions; abandonment when it was divested by them; and finally, revival, growth, and maturity since being purchased by the City of Charlestown in 1991. As evidenced by our 1998 strategic plan and positive financial results, we aggressively expanded services to meet the needs of our patients, medical staff, employees, and the community of Charlestown. I believe that we have made the investment in our core services that will allow MCSI to thrive in the future." In thinking about the future, Miller wondered:

1. Should MCSI slow down its aggressive expansion strategy of adding new services and consolidate the gains from those presently in place, or continue the aggressive expansion strategy of adding and investing in even more services?

2. Should MCSI reassess present services and retrench those that are not yet breaking even?

3. Should MCSI change its fiscal orientation and focus on cost reduction versus revenue enhancement?

4. Should MCSI pursue a joint venture with physicians in limited partnerships?

ENDNOTES

1. Quotes attributed to Kevin Miller are from interviews with the case writers or from published sources, in which case the sources are cited.

2. "The Comeback," an internal hospital document, p. 1.
3. "Medical Center of Southern Indiana is Pride of Charlestown," Evening News, June 25, 1992.
4. Internal hospital records.
5. "Progress Report: City to Own Hospital," *The Leader*, 17:34, September 20, 1973, pp. 1, 3.
6. "Progress Report: City to Own Hospital," *The Leader*, 17:34, September 20, 1973, pp. 1, 3 and "Experts Take Part in Medical Complex Hearing," The Leader, 17:35, September 27, 1973, pp. 1–2.
7. "Progress Report: City to Own Hospital," *The Leader*, 17:34, September 20, 1973, pp. 1, 3.
8. "Low Bid Accepted for Hospital Plan," *The Leader*, 18:23, July 11, 1974, pp. 1, 3.
9. "Agreement Signed for Bond Sale to Finance New Hospital in C-Town," *The Leader*, July 23, 1975, pp. 1+.
10. "North Clark Hospital May Go on the Block," *Indiana Times*, November 29, 1977, p. 1.
11. "HCA Takes Over: New Management Contract Signed for North Clark Community Hospital," *The Charlestown Courier*, January 19, 1979, p. 1.
12. "Hospital Sale is Closed," The Evening News, March 6, 1985.
13. "North Clark Hospital Becomes Part of New ESOP Company," *The Leader*, 31:11, June 10, 1987, p. 1.
14. "HealthTrust Negotiating to Sell North Clark Hospital," *The Leader*, 35:10, May 22, 1991, p. 1.
15. "North Clark Hospital Has New Owner," *The Leader*, 35:43, January 8, 1992, p. 1.
16. "HealthTrust Negotiating to Sell North Clark Hospital," *The Leader*, 35:10, May 22, 1991, p. 1.
17. "Stats Indiana," Southern Indiana Development Corporation Fact Sheet.
18. www.stats.Indiana.edu/profiles.pr1809.html, p. 1.
19. "1987–2000 Labor Force Estimates Clark and Floyd Counties," Indiana, Southern Indiana Development Council.
20. "1987–2000 Labor Force Estimates Clark and Floyd Counties," Indiana, Southern Indiana Development Council.
21. www.stats.indiana.edu/profiles.pr1809.html, p. 2.
22. www.stats.indiana.edu/profiles.pr1809.html, p. 2.
23. "Health Care Facilities Clark and Floyd Counties, Indiana," Southern Indiana Development Council.
24. "Health Care Facilities Clark and Floyd Counties, Indiana," Southern Indiana Development Council.
25. "The Comeback," an internal hospital document.
26. *Ibid.*
27. American MedTrust Corporate Document, 2000, p. 3 and Web www.medtrust.com.
28. American MedTrust Corporate Document, 2000, p. 3.
29. Health Care Financing Administration, Office of the Actuary, National Health Statistics Group. Tables 1, 2, and 10. www.hcfa.gov/stats/nhc-oatc/.
30. American Hospital Association, *Hospital Statistics*, various years: Chicago, AHA—tables appearing in Longest, B., Rakich, J., and Darr, K., *Managing Health Services Organizations and Systems*, 4th edition, 2000: Baltimore, Health Professions Press, p. 171.

31. Longest, Rakich, and Darr, pp. 189–191.
32. Longest, Rakich, and Darr, p. 91.
33. Managed Care Digest Series, 2000, Aventis, pp. 3, 13; see also Web site www.managedcaredigest.com. *Note:* Segments of the Medicare/Medicaid population were enrolled in HMO and PPO managed care programs.
34. "The Comeback," an internal hospital document.
35. MCSI Web site: www.mcsin.org.
36. MCSI Internal 1998 Strategic Plan, pp. 1–4.
37. "The Comeback," an internal hospital document.
38. MCSI Web site: www.mcsin.org.
39. "The Comeback," an internal hospital document.
40. *Note and source:* Industry averages in the Exhibit 10 are from *2001 Almanac of Hospital Financial & Operating Ratios*, Ingenix Publishing Group/Center for Healthcare Industry Performance Studies (CHIPS). Benchmark ratios used are rural hospitals with fewer than 100 beds.

8

The Case of the
Unhealthy Hospital

Anthony R. Kovner
New York University, New York, New York

Bruce Reid, Blake Memorial Hospital's new CEO, rubbed his eyes and looked again at the budget worksheet. The more he played with the figures, the more pessimistic he became. Blake Memorial's financial health was not good; it suffered from rising costs, static revenue, and declining quality of care. When the board hired Reid 6 months ago, the mandate had been clear: improve the quality of care and set the financial house in order.

Reid had less than a week to finalize his $70 million budget for approval by the hospital's board. As he considered his choices, one issue, the future of six off-site clinics, commanded special attention. Reid's predecessor had set up the clinics 5 years earlier to provide primary health care to residents of Marksville's poorer neighborhoods; they were generally considered a model of community-based care. However, although they provided a valuable service for the city's poor, the clinics also diverted funds away from Blake Memorial's in-house services, many of which were underfunded.

As he worked on the budget, Reid's thoughts drifted back to his first visit to the Lorris housing project in early March, just 2 weeks into his tenure as CEO.

Reprinted by permission of *Harvard Business Review*. An excerpt from "The Case of the Unhealthy Hospital" by A.R. Kovner, 69(5) (September–October, 1991). Copyright © 1991 by the Harvard Business School Publishing Corporation; all rights reserved.

The clinic was not much to look at. A small graffiti-covered sign in the courtyard pointed the way to the basement entrance of an aging six-story apartment building. Reid pulled open the heavy metal door and entered the small waiting room. Two of the seven chairs were occupied. In one, a pregnant teenage girl listened to a Walkman and tapped her foot. In the other, a man in his mid-thirties sat with his eyes closed, resting his head against the wall.

Reid had come alone and unannounced. He wanted to see the clinic without the fanfare of an official visit and to meet Dr. Renee Dawson, who had been the clinic's family practitioner for 6 years.

The meeting had to be brief, Dawson apologized, because the nurse had not yet arrived and she had patients to see. As they marched down to her office, she filled Reid in on the waiting patients: the girl was 14 years old, in for a routine prenatal checkup, and the man, a crack addict recently diagnosed as HIV positive, was in for a follow-up visit and blood tests.

On his hurried tour, Reid noted the dilapidated condition of the cramped facility. The paint was peeling everywhere, and, in one examining room, he had to step around a bucket strategically placed to catch a drip from a leaking overhead pipe. After 15 years as a university hospital administrator, Reid felt unprepared for this kind of medicine.

The conditions were appalling, he told Dawson, and were contrary to the image of the high-quality medical care he wanted Blake Memorial to project. When he asked her how she put up with it, Dawson just stared at him. "What are my options?" she finally asked.

Reid looked again at the clinic figures from last year: collectively they cost $1.1 million to operate, at a loss of $256,000. What Blake needed, Reid told himself, were fewer services that sapped resources and more revenue-generating services or at least services that would make the hospital more competitive. The clinics were most definitely a drain.

Of course, there was a surfeit of "competitive" projects in search of funding. Blake needed to expand its neonatal ward; the chief of surgery wanted another operating theater; the chief of radiology was demanding a magnetic resonance imaging (MRI) unit; the business office wanted to upgrade its computer system; and the emergency department desperately needed another full-time physician—and that was just scratching the surface.

Without some of these investments, Blake's ability to attract paying patients and top-grade doctors would deteriorate. As it was, the hospital's location on the poorer, east side of Marksville was a strike against it. Blake had a high percentage of Medicaid patients, but the payments were never sufficient to cover costs. The result was an ever-rising annual operating loss.

Reid was constantly reminded of the hospital's uncompetitive position by his chief of surgery, Dr. Winston Lee. "If Blake wants more paying patients—and, for that matter, good department chiefs—it at least has to keep up with St. Barnabas," Lee had warned Reid a few days ago.

Lee complained that St. Barnabas, the only other acute care hospital in Marksville, had both superior facilities and better technology. Its financial condition was better than Blake's, in part because it was located on the west side of the city, in a more affluent neighborhood. St. Barnabas had also been more savvy in its business ventures: it owned a 50% share in an MRI unit operated by a private medical practice. The unit was reportedly generating revenue, and St. Barnabas had plans for other such investments, Lee had said.

Although Reid agreed that Blake needed more high-technology services, he was also concerned about duplication of service; the population of the greater Marksville area, including suburban and rural residents, was about 700,000. When he questioned Richard Tuttle, St. Barnabas's CEO, about the possibility of joint ventures, however, he received a very cold response. "Competition is the only way to survive," Tuttle had said.

Tuttle's actions were consistent with his words. Two months ago, St. Barnabas allegedly had offered financial incentives to some of Marksville's physicians in exchange for patient referrals. Although the rumor had never been substantiated, it had left a bad taste in Reid's mouth.

Reid knew he could either borrow or cut costs, but the hospital's ability to borrow was limited as a result of an already high debt burden. His only real alternative, therefore, was to cut costs.

Reid dug out the list of possible cuts from the pile of papers on his desk. At the top of the page was the heading "internal cuts," and halfway down was the heading "external cuts." Each item had a dollar value next to it representing the estimated annual savings (see Table 1).

Reid reasoned that the internal cuts would help Blake become a leaner organization. With 1,400 full-time equivalent (FTE) employees and 350 beds, there was room for some cost cutting. Reid's previous hospital had 400 beds and only 1,300 FTE employees. Reid recognized, however, that cutting personnel could affect Blake's quality of care. As it was, patient perception of Blake's quality had been slipping during the last few years, according to the monthly public relations office survey, and quality was an issue that the board was particularly sensitive to these days. Eliminating the clinics, conversely, would not compromise Blake's internal operations.

Everyone knew the clinics would never generate a profit. In fact, the annual loss was expected to continue to climb. Part of the reason was rising costs, but another factor was the city of Marksville's ballooning budget deficit. The city contributed $100,000 to the program and provided the space in the housing projects free of charge. Reid had heard from two city councilmen, however, that funding would likely be cut in the coming year.

680,000

Table 1.   Reid's list of possible cuts and savings

Internal cuts	Savings
Cut 2% from nursing staff	$340,000
Cut 2% from support and ancillary staff	$290,000
Cut maximum of 3% from business office staff	$50,000
Freeze all wages and salaries at current level	$1.5 million
Eliminate weekly in-house clinics	$100,000
External cuts	**Savings**
Eliminate all off-site clinics	$256,000

Less city money and a higher net loss for the clinic program would only add to the strain on Blake's internal services.

Reid had to weigh this strain against the political consequences of closing the clinics. He was well aware of the possible ramifications from his regular dealings with Clara Bryant, the recently appointed commissioner of Marksville's health services. Bryant repeatedly argued that the clinics were an essential service for Marksville's low-income residents.

"You know how the mayor feels about the clinics," Bryant had said at a recent breakfast meeting. "He was a strong supporter when they first opened. He fought hard in City Hall to get Blake Memorial the funding. Closing the clinics would be a personal blow to him."

Reid understood the significance of Bryant's veiled threat. If he closed the clinics, he would lose an ally in the mayor's office, which could jeopardize Blake's access to city funds in the future or have even worse consequences. Reid had heard through the City Hall rumor mill that Bryant had privately threatened to refer Blake to Marksville's chief counsel for a tax status review if he closed the clinics. He took this seriously; he knew of a handful of hospitals facing similar actions from their local governments.

When Reid tried to explain to Bryant that closing the clinics would improve Blake's financial condition, which, in turn, would lead to better quality of care for all patients, her response had been unsympathetic: "You don't measure the community's health on an income statement."

Bryant was not the only clinic supporter with whom Reid had to reckon. Dr. Susan Russell, Blake's director of clinics, was equally vocal about the responsibility of the hospital to the community. In a recent senior staff meeting, Reid sat stunned while Dr. Winston Lee, Blake's high-tech champion, exchanged barbs with Russell.

Lee had argued that the off-site clinics competed against the weekly in-house clinics that Blake offered under- and uninsured patients. He proposed closing the off-site clinics.

The four in-house clinics—surgery, pediatrics, gynecology, and internal medicine—cost Blake $200,000 a year in physician fees alone, Lee said. And because Medicaid was not adequately covering the costs of these services, the hospital lost about $100,000 a year from the in-house clinics. Furthermore, in-house clinic visits were down 10% so far this year. A choice had to be made, Lee concluded, and the reasonable choice was to eliminate the off-site clinics and bolster services within the hospital's four walls. "Instead of clinics, we should have a shuttle bus from the projects to the hospital," he proposed.

Russell's reaction had been almost violent. "Most of the clinics' patients wouldn't come to the hospital even if there was a bus running every 5 minutes," she snapped back. "I'm talking about pregnant teenage girls who need someone in their community they recognize and trust, not some nameless doctor in a big, unfamiliar hospital."

Russell's ideas about what a hospital should be were radical, Reid thought, but he had to admit they did have a certain logic. She espoused an entirely new way of delivering health care that involved the mobilization of many of Blake's services. "A hospital is not a building, it's a service. And wherever the service is most needed, that is where the hospital should be," she had said.

In Blake's case, that meant funding more neighborhood clinics, not cutting back on them. Russell spoke of creating a network of neighborhood-based preventive health care centers for all of East Marksville's communities, including both the low-income housing projects and the pockets of middle-income neighborhoods. Besides improving health care, the network would act as an inpatient referral system for hospital services.

Lee had rolled his eyes at the suggestion, but Reid had not been so quick to dismiss Russell's ideas. If a clinic network could tap the paying public and generate more inpatient business, it might be worth looking into, he thought. Besides, St. Barnabas was not doing anything like this.

At the end of the staff meeting, Reid asked Russell to give him some data on the performance of the clinics. He requested numbers of inpatient referrals, birth weight data, and the number of patients seen per month by type of visit—routine, substance abuse, prenatal, pediatric, violence-related injury, and HIV.

Russell's report had arrived the previous day, and Reid was flipping through the results. He had hoped it would provide some answers; instead, it only raised more questions.

The number of prenatal visits had been declining for 16 months. This was significant because prenatal care accounted for more than 60% of the clinics' business. Other types of visits, however, were holding steady. In fact, substance abusers had been coming in record numbers since the clinics began participating in the mayor's needle exchange program 3 months ago.

Russell placed the blame for the prenatal decline squarely on the city. "Two years ago, Marksville cut funding for prenatal outreach and advocacy programs to low income communities. Without supplementary outreach, pregnant women are less inclined to visit the clinics," she wrote.

The birth weight data were inconclusive. There was no difference between birth weights for clinic patients and birth weights for nonclinic patients from similar backgrounds. In fact, average birth weights were actually lower among clinic patients. Russell had concluded that the clinic program was too new to produce meaningful improvements.

On the positive side, inpatient referrals from the clinics had risen in the last few years, but Russell's comments about the reasons for the rise were speculative at best. HIV-related illnesses and violence-related injuries were a large part of the increase, but so were early detection of ailments such as cataracts and cancer. Reid made a note to ask for a follow-up study on this.

He put the report down and stared out his window. Blake had a responsibility to serve the uninsured, but it also had a responsibility to remain viable and self-sustaining. Which was the stronger force? It came down to finding the best way to provide high-quality care to the community and save the hospital from financial difficulties. The consequences of his decision ranged from another year of status quo management to totally redefining the role of the hospital in the community. He had less than a week to decide. What should Reid cut, and what should he keep?

9

Edgewood Lake Hospital

Leadership in a Rural Healthcare Facility During Challenging Economic Times

Brent C. Pottenger

Douglas Archer

Stephen Cheung

Robert C. Myrtle
University of Southern California

A CHALLENGE FOR AN INCOMING CEO

After 8 months of searching nationwide, the Edgewood Lake Hospital's board has just hired a new CEO, Shannon Johnson. She recently served as CFO of Rocky Hills Valley Hospital, a critical access facility in rural northern California. The previous CEO, Richard Fuchs, failed to make Edgewood Lake Hospital profitable and made several missteps by engaging in high-cost capital projects, including an elaborate wellness center that did not deliver expected profits. During the past 8 months, the interim CEO, Jenny Mayview, did little to rectify the messy situation.

This case is based on actual events. The organization, its location, and the names of people have been disguised.

Located in northern California, Edgewood Lake Hospital (ELH) is a 30-bed, independent, not-for-profit hospital. It provides inpatient and outpatient services for a close-knit, small community in a rural, forested, lakeside setting. Given challenging economic times, both inside and outside of the nation's healthcare system, the incoming CEO (Johnson) must provide strong leadership while figuring out how to make ELH profitable within 2 years (by 2011). Having experienced losses from 2006–2009, the board gave Johnson the challenge when hiring her. Finally, while plugging financial leaks and securing fiscal solvency for the organization, Johnson must also address the hospital's glaring physician recruitment problems, particularly in general surgery and primary care. If successful, the board hopes that Johnson can stabilize the hospital's executive leadership team and inspire increased staff productivity and performance in the process.

EDGEWOOD LAKE HOSPITAL HISTORY

Despite operating with financial losses since 2006, ELH has established itself as the rural region's leader for quality care. Members of the community hold the hospital in high regard, especially its exemplary team of experienced nurses who play active roles in the community, serving as leaders of multiple volunteer and church organizations. ELH opened in 1945 as the Edgewood Community Hospital, a 30-bed public facility. In order to capitalize on the hospital's beautiful lakeside setting, its board renamed the facility Edgewood Lake Hospital in 1985.

In 2003, then CEO Fuchs pursued a strategy of focusing on wellness and prevention instead of treatment and intervention. He initiated an enormous capital campaign to fund the development of a state-of-the-art wellness facility on the hospital's existing property. When presenting this plan to the hospital's board, Fuchs said:

> Healthcare in the 21st century will revolve around keeping people healthy, not reacting to illness and treating disease. With access to a healthy community space that provides nutrition classes, gym memberships, physical activity programs, and other social interactions, the Edgewood County community members will lead longer, healthier, and happier lives. As a healthcare facility, Edgewood Lake Hospital has a responsibility to the community to provide preventive and wellness services to people, while continuing to provide high-quality, traditional medical care.

After receiving board approval for a $1.2 million wellness center, Fuchs raised $120,000 in community donations to help fund the wellness center construction project. With so much community support behind this new venture, he expected the center to serve the community profitably for many years, especially as the population aged, retired, and spent more time (and money) focusing on health maintenance.

In 2006, Fuchs proudly opened the Edgewood Lake Wellness Center at a well-attended ribbon-cutting ceremony. "Edgewood Lake Wellness Center will provide the entire Edgewood County community with a place to be well, feel well, and get well," proclaimed Fuchs during his opening ceremony speech. Two years later, in Summer 2008, the board voted to dismiss Fuchs after ELH posted large losses in both 2007 and 2008. Fuchs had mobilized the community behind his wellness idea; however, at the end of the day, the wellness center's operations failed to prove profitable. Fuchs also failed to address the hospital's core operational problems of (1) poor financial performance, including extensive losses on Medicare patients; (2) low physician recruitment, especially in general surgery and primary care; and (3) strong community competition from Creekside Trails, a 45-bed, for-profit hospital located 35 miles away on the other side of Lake Edgewood that opened in 1995 with an emphasis on cardiology care.

CURRENT STATE OF RURAL HOSPITALS

Rural hospitals are often the sole provider of healthcare services for residents in rural communities. However, rural hospitals must overcome the complex public policies that often cater to larger, metropolitan hospitals. They must also surmount the effects of local economies and shortages of health professionals.

The current state of rural hospitals is dismal. Although about 25% of Americans live in rural areas, only about 10% of physicians actually practice in rural areas. Citizens in these rural areas have longer drive times to their nearest hospitals and consequently have difficult times accessing hospital services. This leads to residents delaying their routine visits, which exacerbates their illnesses.

DEMOGRAPHICS AND POPULATION DATA

Rural residents tend to have lower household incomes than the nation's average. In Edgewood County, the estimated median household income in 2007 was $44,238, compared to $59,948 for the national average. Residents living in rural areas tend to be older than the national average median age. In Edgewood County, the median age is 40.8 years, while the national average is 33.3 years. The demographics in Edgewood County reflect those of residents in other rural areas.

The population of Edgewood County is 5,135. With a larger percentage of older residents, the need for timely, efficient, and comprehensive chronic condition care is paramount. However, in this small county, similar to others across the nation, there is a lack of specialty physicians. As a result, primary care providers often must provide care that is out of their scope of practice, out of their comfort level, or both. Moreover, rural hospitals may not offer the same level of services to the public, which forces these hospitals to send their patients to other larger hospitals in metropolitan cities. This increases the travel time for patients who access care in rural settings.

To alleviate the longer travel times and difficulties accessing care for elderly patients, ELH created the Mobile Health Service Unit (MHSU), a large utility vehicle that services residents all the way out to the perimeter of Edgewood County. Equipped with basic equipment to perform physical assessments and other primary care services, this mobile unit solves the problem of geographic limitations for many of ELH's most needy patients.

NATIONAL HEALTHCARE POLICY

Rural hospitals are most affected by public policy changes due to their small sizes. For example, ELH is only a 30-bed facility. If a new public policy dictates that the hospital increase its fixed nursing ratio, ELH will encounter challenges due to the difficulty in attracting talented providers to rural areas. Other public policy and accreditation agencies are increasing the regulations on quality, privacy, efficiency, costs, and services. These regulations affect all hospitals throughout the United States, but larger hospital systems are better equipped than rural hospitals to adjust their practices to meet these new requirements because they have more resources at their disposal. In addition, larger hospital systems can control the political climate by lobbying and by leveraging economies of scale.

GOVERNMENT REIMBURSEMENT

Government reimbursement rates across the nation are declining, while the demands for quality and compliance regulations are increasing—a challenging combination for management, indeed. Hospitals across the nation must be able to bill Medicare correctly by investing in knowledgeable staff, as well as by implementing ongoing training programs and extensive information technology software to facilitate accurate coding and record keeping. Large hospital systems are more likely to have the necessary resources to keep up with increasing quality and compliance demands from Medicare. Across the board, small rural hospitals have many fewer coders and internal auditors than large hospitals do. With all of these demands on rural hospitals, they may not be able to allocate the same percentage of resources to maintain compliance with Medicare's standards. The result is more fines and denied claims for rural hospitals. In response to these pressures, many rural facilities across the nation have secured the designation critical access hospital (CAH) to receive better reimbursement rates from Medicare. A CAH designation changes hospital reimbursement from diagnosis-related groups (DRGs) to cost-based reimbursement, which provides rural facilities with budgeting stability. To qualify for the program, hospitals must be located at least 35 miles from the next nearest hospital, operate fewer than 25 beds, have an average length of stay (ALOS) under 96 days, and offer emergency services 24 hours a day, 7 days a week. Currently, ELH is not enrolled in the CAH program.

QUALITY

As the demand for quality services grows nationally, costs will initially rise as hospitals increase staffing, refine procedures, and create new workflows and best practices. ELH already has a great track record of quality. For instance, ELH scored 100% for delivering discharge instructions and 100% for providing smoking cessation counseling for congestive heart failure (CHF) cases, compared to the U.S. averages of 69% and 89%, respectively.

NATIONAL HEALTHCARE OBJECTIVES

There is increasing pressure from Medicare to ensure that all hospitals and physician offices are connected via electronic medical records (EMR). Furthermore, new ICD-10 coding will require a new set of computer systems to process the codes. Rural hospitals will continue to struggle with financing such large EMR systems. With the small size and relative simplicity of hospital operations and services as compared to larger hospitals, the benefits of EMR may not outweigh the costs. Small hospitals and single physician groups will have to invest in ICD-10 coding software and learn new rules and regulations regarding the coding. With limited staff on hand, learning new billing requirements will take a heavy toll on existing staff.

AN ORGANIZATION IN TRANSITION

Shannon Johnson's experience working at Rocky Hills Valley Hospital— a 24-bed rural facility like ELH—gave her some perspective regarding the main issues that are affecting ELH's operations, including: (1) the current state of rural hospitals; (2) demographics and population dynamics;

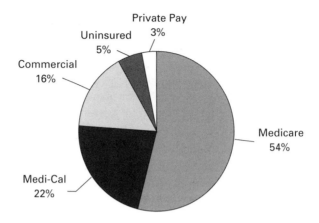

Exhibit 1. Edgewood Lake Hospital payer mix.

(3) national health policy; (4) government reimbursement; and (5) quality care. In addition, she understands that many other rural hospitals have survived by joining healthcare systems.

ELH's financial situation is bleak. The past 2 years of operations have resulted in a significant loss for the organization. Over half of the patients in the community are Medicare beneficiaries. Since the Balanced Budget Act of 1997, government-sponsored healthcare programs such as Medicare have drastically reduced reimbursement rates (ELH's payer mix is presented in Exhibit 1). In addition to challenges with its payer mix, ELH is also experiencing a rise in uncompensated care because of the socioeconomic demographics within Edgewood County, which are consistently below average in relation to the rest of the state of California.

Staffing inefficiencies have negatively affected operating costs, compounding ELH's financial problems. Currently, ELH is operating at nearly 8 full-time equivalents (FTEs) per occupied bed, which is nearly 40% higher than the industry benchmark of 5.2 FTEs. In addition, the new collective bargaining agreement with the area Hospital Workers Union Local 189 resulted in higher salaries for the RN (registered nurse) job class. Physician staffing has created an additional manpower cost. Two vacancies on the medical staff have forced the hospital to employ *locum tenens* physicians, resulting in lost revenue and at a significant cost to the organization.

Aside from declining reimbursement, a challenging payer mix, and increasing operating costs, which are all relatively uncontrollable elements, poor executive management represents the most disappointing contributor to the failures of ELH. The prepared 2008 budget in relation to the actual figures for 2007 and year-to-date for 2008 illustrate this management blunder (see Table 1). It is clear based on the projected net income for 2008 that

Table 1. Edgewood Lake Hospital Financials

	2007 Actual	Jun-08 YTD	Dec-08 Actual	2008 Budget
Inpatient Revenue	86,968,734	38,579,068	76,694,069	89,822,682
Outpatient Revenue	90,024,084	50,466,104	101,733,548	89,889,713
Gross Patient Revenue	176,992,818	89,045,172	178,427,617	179,712,395
Revenue from Wellness Center	698,435	398,987	704,532	732,997
Revenue Deductions	(109,167,181)	(55,364,031)	(109,552,632)	(107,407,333)
Charity Care	(3,020,986)	(1,471,287)	(2,863,373)	(1,440,001)
Other Revenue from Operations	1,438,726	544,697	1,116,269	1,188,552
Net Operating Revenue	66,941,812	33,153,538	67,832,413	72,786,610
Salary Expense	25,083,781	13,187,143	26,596,301	24,970,955
Employee Benefits	8,650,023	4,384,706	6,925,576	10,016,599
Physician Fees	3,812,265	2,401,619	5,242,532	3,732,940
Professional Fees	2,641,380	1,299,983	2,572,612	2,897,930
Supplies	7,185,118	3,556,264	7,104,929	7,457,775
Purchased Services	5,508,030	3,626,660	7,337,465	6,543,781
Insurance	745,358	401,183	798,446	772,193
Utilities	1,287,189	797,589	1,403,369	1,345,270
Rentals	359,438	182,529	405,820	352,479
Depreciation	3,510,991	1,897,875	3,906,404	3,648,059
Interest Expense	1,260,038	794,130	1,515,552	1,439,000
Management Fee	3,018,165	1,808,941	3,723,525	3,391,489
Licenses and Taxes	116,276	98,791	186,340	112,256
Bad Debt	2,872,678	1,781,388	4,106,819	3,221,136
Other Operating Expense	2,148,975	779,992	1,551,847	2,113,982
Total Operating Expense	68,199,705	36,638,793	72,887,542	72,015,844
Non Operating Income	388,403	219,578	239,333	369,444
Net Income	(869,490)	(3,265,677)	(4,815,796)	1,140,210
Pt Days (excl nursery)	9,937.00	3,755.00	7,380.00	10,300.00
IP Revenue per Pt Day	8,752.01	10,274.05	10,392.15	8,720.65
Average Daily Census	27.20	20.60	20.16	28.20
Net Operating Revenue per Pt day	3,275.63	3,779.23	3,909.73	3,496.44
Discharges (excl nursery)	2,591.00	1,159.00	2,360.00	2,641.00
Net Revenue per discharge	12,562.69	12,244.18	12,226.18	13,636.26
Salaries Cost/Pt Day	3,275.63	3,779.23	3,909.73	3,496.44
Supplies Cost/Pt Day	188.51	277.10	305.34	181.14
Length of Stay	3.80	3.20	3.13	3.90
FTEs/Occupied bed	6.56	7.74	7.80	6.21
Other visits	99,548.00	52,444.00	105,006.00	101,040.00
Surgeries	3,611.00	1,672.00	3,309.00	2,587.00
ER Visits	17,849.00	8,934.00	17,597.00	18,328.00

hospital leadership was "asleep at the wheel." Instead of realizing a surplus of over $1 million, the facility lost nearly $5 million. This is a tremendous discrepancy for a hospital with roughly $70 million in net operating revenue.

On the positive side, ELH enjoys strong community support and a regional reputation for superior quality. The competitor hospital, Creekside Trails, is an aggressive for-profit hospital that is known in the community for performing cardiac procedures excessively. Despite this notoriety, the hospital is only 15 years old and its facilities are superior to ELH's. Creekside Trails and ELH are located 35 miles apart on opposite ends of the lake, and they service fairly distinct patient populations. Because Creekside Trails offers more specialty services, ELH has noticed increased competition for patients in recent years.

In order for ELH to rise up from the ashes, new revenue must be injected into the organization. A solution to this problem is recruiting additional medical staff to alleviate the *locum tenens* costs and increase patient volumes. Physician recruitment has not been easy for the hospital. The rural environment is not appealing to most physicians and the lack of a medical foundation, or large medical group that offers an employment relationship, forces a new physician to bear the financial risk of starting up a new practice in a sparsely populated area. In California, hospitals are not allowed to employ physicians directly, and although a hospital can offer an income guarantee for 1–3 years, it is illegal to directly employ the physician. ELH's payer mix also impacts physicians and, when combined with the risk of startup, makes recruitment nearly impossible.

ELH has a strong and loyal customer base that supports the facility. Outmigration data demonstrates that the hospital captures 84% of the patients who need services within the scope of the facility, leaving only 16% of patients who seek care elsewhere. Each year, the hospital organizes a health and wellness fair, and the recent addition of the wellness center has increased the community image of the facility. The wellness center provides access to weight management and nutrition classes, aerobics, yoga, and a workout center. Future plans include an indoor heated swimming pool, sauna, and spa. In preparation for designing and opening the new facility, the hospital launched a capital campaign to raise funds for renovating the existing office complex that would be the future site of the wellness center. This campaign resulted in $120,000 in donations, further illustrating local support for and interest in the success of ELH.

The hospital has incredibly low turnover—6% in 2008—despite the difficulty in recruitment. In 2008, the hospital participated in an employee satisfaction survey and celebrated scores that placed them in the 96th percentile of similar-sized organizations. Luckily, the facility has a strong middle management team with significant tenure that is responsible for maintaining morale and commitment to patient care in spite of challenging times and lack of executive leadership. However, a tide of uncertainty is rising as the employees and the medical staff attempt to understand how the hospital ended up in such a dire financial position. The bullish style of the interim CEO demolished morale, and staff productivity dropped precipitously as a direct result. The entire community is anxious for new leadership to turn the ELH around.

THE LEADERSHIP CHALLENGE

At ELH's most recent board meeting, the senior management team and board members all agreed that Johnson, the new CEO, is the right fit for the facility as well as for the community. A graduate from a major university and a CPA, Johnson is bright and personable with a strong, diverse financial background. (Exhibit 2 presents an organization chart of ELH.) In an interview with the local Edgewood County newspaper, *The Edge*, Johnson discussed why she felt ready for this new challenge and step in her career:

> Working in a rural setting taught me so many things about managing the operations of small hospitals. I got to have my hands in everything, from engineering to nursing management to human resources. I look forward to combining my extensive financial background with my improved operational management skills to provide strong leadership at Edgewood Lake Hospital.

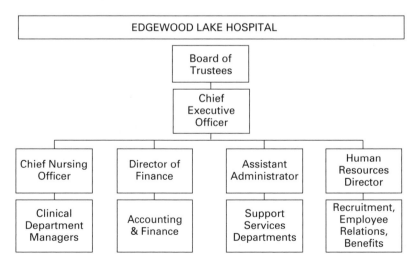

Exhibit 2. Edgewood Lake Hospital organization chart.

After 5 years as CFO at Rocky Hills Valley Hospital, Johnson feels she is prepared to excel in her new leadership role as CEO of ELH. However, after interviewing the interim CEO, Jenny Mayview, meeting with board members, and enjoying brief conversations with hospital physicians, nurses, and staff, Johnson is not quite sure how best to turn the tides in the right direction at ELH. What about the hospital's bleeding financials and challenging payer mix—what can she do to address these issues? Should she cut back on the wellness center budget? Should she shut down the wellness center so that this space can be used for more profitable services? If either of these options were pursued, how would the community react after investing so much money and energy into the new facility? What can she do to better recruit and retain physicians? All of these questions swirl through Johnson's mind as she runs on a treadmill inside the Edgewood Lake Wellness Center after her first official day on the job as CEO. When questioned about physician recruitment earlier in the day during a senior management team "huddle," Johnson said that she tackled these challenges in her previous position:

> Luckily, at Rocky Hills Valley Hospital, I managed and led our hospital's efforts to recruit physicians in general surgery, as well as in primary care. It takes a special type of doctor to work in a small, rural setting; but, with some years under my belt, I feel confident that I can help improve the recruitment situation here at Edgewood Lake Hospital. But, I do recognize that Edgewood County is a new region for me, so I am actively reflecting, talking to people, and searching for effective ways to build a more sustainable physician staff at our facility.

Clearly, challenges lie ahead for her. Drawing on her hands-on experiences, Johnson has made concerted efforts to transition effectively into her CEO role through collaboration, openness, transparency, and creativity. She wants to find new solutions to old problems. She also wants to understand what Fuchs, her predecessor, did wrong.

Thus, the leadership challenge is clear: What should Johnson do? How should she prioritize her action items? What creative solutions could she implement to turn ELH around that previous executives had not tried? How does Johnson not "rock the boat" too much and achieve balance between instituting change and respecting existing relationships and cultural dynamics in the organization? Operating under difficult economic times, Johnson certainly faces quite a leadership test; however, with the right decisions, she has the opportunity to make a lasting positive impact on her entire organization and in the community that the hospital serves.

10

Mueller-O'Keefe Memorial Home and Retirement Village

Strategic Planning in a Continuing Care Retirement Community

William E. Aaronson
Temple University, Philadelphia, Pennsylvania

CASE OVERVIEW

Steve Cantwell was preparing for the next meeting of the long-range planning committee of the board of directors of the Mueller-O'Keefe Memorial Home and Retirement Village. Cantwell was a consultant with a major independent long-term care consulting firm who had been given the task of directing this project. It had been a difficult task from the beginning. Although he had dealt with similar situations in the past, this project presented some unique challenges.

The consulting firm for which Cantwell worked dealt almost exclusively with not-for-profit long-term care providers. The majority of clients were church sponsored or affiliated. Although well intentioned, governing

This case and related notes are taken from the long-term care management case study collection found in *Cases in Long-Term Care Management: Building the Continuum*, by Donna Lind Infeld and John Kress, published in 1989 by AUPHA Press and used by permission.

board members of these types of providers were not always well informed about the current challenges and opportunities within the long-term care environment.

The Mueller-O'Keefe Home was one such church-related client. The home was affiliated with the Evangelical Free Church. All members of the board of directors except one were church members. The church district executive was an ex officio board member. Although the board consisted of church members, the home was not sponsored by the church. The board was self-perpetuating and independent but chose to maintain close ties with the church.

During a retreat, the board of directors had determined that they would require outside consulting services. They recognized their personal limitations when it came to the development, selection, and implementation of alternative courses of action. Through a subcommittee, the long-range planning committee, the consulting firm for which Cantwell worked was retained. The consulting firm was to assist the home in developing a long-range plan that included identification of new services and a capital development plan.

Cantwell felt comfortable working with this board. All members whom he had met were dedicated to and concerned about the home. A few of the members were actually looking forward to entering the retirement village when the time would come for their own postretirement moves.

Cantwell was approaching this latest meeting with a great deal of concern. The meeting was to serve as a working session in which his report would be discussed and the feasibility of the action recommendations would be considered. He had spent considerable time researching the market, analyzing the organization, and developing alternatives that he believed fit both the home's mission and the organization's abilities. His report was well prepared and appeared to be congruent with the board's perception of the home's mission. However, despite endless interviews with board members, staff, residents, competitors, and community representatives, and after extensive research on the alternatives, he wondered whether the board would approve and respond to his recommendations. He knew that *he* had every reason to be confident in his counsel, or did he?

HISTORY AND DEVELOPMENT OF THE HOME

The Mueller-O'Keefe Memorial Home was founded in 1905, when Dr. Robert Mueller bequeathed a large brick farmhouse and 90 acres of ground to a benevolent organization of members of the Evangelical Free Church. The purpose of the bequest was to establish a home for aged church members. The Evangelical Free Church "Old Folks Home," as it was called, became well established in the local community. The home is located in a rural setting in a small city in Ohio. Two wings were added to the original farmhouse in the 1930s as a result of an increasing number of requests for admission.

The home continued to care exclusively for members of the Evangelical Free Church until 1951. Because of the fine reputation of the home, and in response to some financial difficulties, Mr. Patrick O'Keefe, a prominent local industrialist, established a 25-year endowment. O'Keefe was Roman Catholic. The purpose of the endowment was to ensure financial stability, to allow expansion of facilities, and to encourage the home to open admissions to non–Free Church members. The endowment principal became fully available to the home last year.

The 1950s brought additional changes. The board began to recognize that residents of the home were requiring more nursing care. The home never had an empty bed. When a resident died, the bed was quickly filled. When residents moved into the home, however, they were generally in poorer health than entering residents had been in the past. Plans were initiated to build a nursing care wing onto the Old Folks Home. A 100-bed addition was built in the early 1960s, which brought the total complement to 140 beds.

Another major innovation for the Mueller-O'Keefe Home occurred in the 1960s. The first retirement cottage was built in 1962, initially as a house for the administrator, whose presence at the home was increasingly required. He retired soon after the house was built, and he was allowed to remain there. When it became known that the grounds could be used for retirement living, retired couples began to apply for lots where they could build houses to their liking. The retirement "cottages" (single-family, ranch-style houses) would become the property of the home on completion. The original residents were offered life care contracts in return for the donation of the constructed cottage to the home. This experiment with life care contracts was short-lived as a result of early recognition of the future potential for financial liability.

One current resident of the nursing home is the last such person to hold a life care contract. She is 96, and the cost of her care long ago exceeded the value of her property. The home continues to honor her contract, however, by providing free care. In the mid-1960s the first "continuing care" contract was written. Contingent liability for care was to be limited to the construction cost or resale value of the cottages. Residents would be given preference for admission to nursing care.

A row of eight apartments was added in the early 1970s. These apartments are similar in appearance to single-story townhouses. In the late 1970s, the first attempt to plan within the retirement village took place. An architect was hired to design a state-of-the-art quadriplex, similar to cottage construction taking place at other retirement communities. However, when the building was completed, it did not fit with the predominant design of the community—it resembled an Aspen ski lodge. The home had difficulty selling the cottages. This reinforced the board's belief that "seat of the pants" decisions generally resulted in better outcomes, a belief that many of the board members continued to hold. Haphazard land development had created its own problems, however, primarily involving efficient land use and sewage disposal.

In the 1970s the ratio of nursing care to residential care in the Old Folks Home changed rapidly. In 1970, only 53 beds were certified for nursing care. By 1977, all of the beds (100) in the nursing care building were certified. In 1985, two additional beds were added, bringing the total nursing care beds to 102. These new beds were to be held in reserve for the use of the retirement village residents. Personal care beds remained fixed at 40. They have continued to be located in the Mueller farmhouse. The buildings were modest, especially when compared to competing long-term care facilities.

By the 1980s the home's staff began to recognize that many of the home's residents had developed Alzheimer's disease or related dementias. Individuals in early and middle stages of the disease were particularly difficult to manage in a congregate living arrangement because of behavioral manifestations that the staff observed to be annoying to other residents. Therefore, a separate unit for confused, ambulatory residents was initiated. The Alzheimer's unit quickly developed a reputation for providing exceptional care. The administrator, Mr. Tom Clark, reported that the board was particularly interested in expanding this unit. However, he personally was uncertain about this option. Although it would certainly bring publicity and possibly additional sources of funding, it might also result in the home developing an image as a mental health facility, which might have negative consequences on future admissions.

According to Clark, the home had maintained a reputation for excellent basic care throughout its history. The Evangelical Free Church is a service-oriented denomination that draws its social philosophy from New Testament teachings. Church members are traditionally conscientious objectors and, like the Quakers and the Amish, are excused from military service when a national draft is in effect. Outward expressions of Christian values among administration, staff, and residents were very evident to Cantwell. According to Clark, this atmosphere, rather than the physical environment and other amenities, had been the key factor attracting residents to the home.

According to the board chairman, Mr. Polk, two important consequences had resulted. Many current residents of the retirement village and nursing care facilities had parents, grandparents, aunts, uncles, and siblings who were or had been residents of the home. Every resident of the home had heard of it by word of mouth and usually was intimately aware of it when making postretirement decisions. Second, the home had been frequently remembered in the wills of residents or relatives of residents who were pleased with the care received.

By the end of last May, the home's investment assets, held in the form of securities, were valued at approximately $3.5 million. Another $230,000 was held in a low interest savings account. Net fixed assets were valued at $1.7 million, for a fund balance of $5.6 million. The home did not have any long-term or short-term debt. This very positive financial picture, combined with an ever-growing demand for the services of the home, convinced the board of directors that some future-oriented growth strategies were required. The Long-Range Planning Committee was charged with the responsibility of developing alternative uses of the available funds.

Mr. O'Donnell, Long-Range Planning Committee chairman, stated that the committee immediately ran into problems. First, the board was not solidly behind any planning efforts. The home's growth in the past had been essentially unplanned. "Seat of the pants" decision making appeared to have worked well. Few free-standing nursing homes or retirement centers were as financially healthy as the home. Also, the debacle of the "ski lodge" cottage was seen as the result of the only planning endeavor ever undertaken.

Second, many board members were opposed to incurring long-term debt for any reason. Polk, who in the 1930s had seen what overextension of credit could do to a business, was especially opposed. It soon became apparent that, without debt, the home's options were severely limited.

Third, the home did not have a formally adopted mission statement. There was disagreement within the board as to whether one was necessary, because they had managed for 90 years without one. However, it did not seem likely that the board would agree on any plans because they were divided on issues related to the basic mission (who was to be served and how) and church relations. Because Mueller-O'Keefe is a church-affiliated home, a common mission was recognized as important by the board chairman and by some members of the committee who were trying to focus on acceptable growth options.

THE CONSULTANT'S ANALYSES

In the midst of these impending changes and conflicting opinions, a consulting firm was hired. The first meeting that Cantwell had with the Long-Range Planning Committee revealed several things. The initial proposal he submitted would have to be modified in response to some committee members' concerns. The chairman of the board, Mr. Polk, had objected to some of the terminology in particular. They would prefer to be called a home, not a facility. The committee requested that statistics and charts be kept to a minimum. They preferred to be given recommendations in common language. Finally, Cantwell had noted with some concern that the administrator, Tom Clark, was exceptionally quiet throughout the meeting. Despite the key role he would play in the planning process and in the implementation of any plans, his interactions and responses were subdued.

Cantwell was given a free hand by the committee to develop the long-range plan. The consulting contract stated that this plan would be developed through a process that ended with the presentation to the committee of several alternative strategies. Useful decision criteria were also to be developed. It was made clear to the board and the committee, however, that they were to make the final strategic choice. The consultants were to provide the professional expertise in areas of market analysis and internal organizational review. That knowledge, in conjunction with an in-depth analysis of the organization, was to result in the proposal of strategic alternatives that would be feasible and consistent with the organization's abilities.

Cantwell observed that the Long-Range Planning Committee was determined to take a passive role in the process. Polk, although not a member of the committee, took the most active role. Clark confided to Cantwell that, although Polk appeared to dominate the board and the committee, he was actually very democratic. He believed that if other members would exert themselves, Polk would yield to the will of the majority. Clark stated that he could see no reason why Polk's philosophy would be any different under these circumstances.

Polk had some very definite ideas about what should or should not be done. He viewed the rather substantial endowment and the excellent financial position of the home to be the result of his prudent financial management. Polk also served as the treasurer, which can be equated with the position of chief financial officer, for the home. In addition, he was the vice president for finance of a family-owned furniture business. His financial acumen was developed through a 45-year career with the furniture company. Experience taught him to be wary of debt of any kind.

In reviewing 4 years' worth of balance sheets (see Table 1), Cantwell noted that the accounts payable balance was identical ($10,360) at the close of each period. When questioned, Polk said that it was a fictitious amount. All bills had been paid on receipt. Consequently, the actual balance on the books in accounts payable at the end of the accounting period was zero. The state Medicaid program auditors, however, would not accept a zero balance.

Cantwell had initiated the planning process knowing that implementation of any plan would be problematic. Any program development, no

Table 1. Comparative balance sheets (in dollars)

	This year	Last year	2 years ago	3 years ago
Assets				
Current				
Cash	231,149	192,013	127,747	77,899
Accounts receivable	159,223	157,975	145,189	190,092
Inventory	400	400	400	400
Prepaid insurance	29,015	10,921	13,632	5,511
Total	419,787	361,309	286,968	273,902
Noncurrent				
Agent account	1,557,386	1,307,386	748,473	642,707
Trust account	1,901,122	1,651,122	1,388,735	1,193,165
Total	3,458,508	2,958,508	2,137,208	1,835,872
Fixed assets				
Land	10,284	10,284	10,284	10,284
Buildings	1,702,214	1,699,214	1,671,621	1,666,787
Water/sewer	204,747	204,747	204,747	178,885
Vehicles	105,532	104,846	54,356	54,356
Equipment	437,171	422,663	386,970	363,487
Cottages	303,452	254,050	230,224	150,494
Total	2,763,400	2,695,804	2,558,202	2,424,293
Depreciation	(1,073,784)	(1,052,207)	(998,329)	(953,807)
Net fixed assets	1,689,616	1,643,597	1,559,873	1,470,486
Total assets	5,567,911	4,963,414	3,984,049	3,580,260
Liabilities				
Accounts payable	10,360	10,360	10,360	10,360
Payroll	39,410	47,037	33,384	29,513
Taxes payable	5,368	5,171	4,912	4,441
Total	55,138	62,568	48,656	44,314
Reserves				
Resident care	(57,505)	(54,137)	(47,388)	(41,451)
Memorials	30,239	30,105	27,920	26,819
Resident expenses	(6,679)	1,372	(703)	0
Total	(33,945)	(22,660)	(20,171)	(14,632)
Fund balance	5,546,718	4,923,506	3,955,564	3,550,578
Total liabilities and fund balance	5,567,911	4,963,414	3,984,049	3,580,260

matter how modest, would result in debt being incurred. Furthermore, because of lack of depth in administration, organizational and management development would be required regardless of which direction was taken. The process was initiated with an organizational review, an analysis of current residents, a demographic analysis, and a financial review. A competitor analysis was also conducted, which included tours of and interviews at competing retirement communities and nursing homes. Staff from the Area Agency on Aging and the health systems agency were interviewed as well. Finally, residents, staff, and board members were selected for more extensive interviews.

Based on the findings from the first part of the study, sessions were to be conducted with the Long-Range Planning Committee in which the working papers would be discussed. These sessions would serve as the basis for preparation of the final document. The results of the working documents are summarized in the following sections.

Organizational Review

The board of directors had final responsibility for the operations of the home. The daily operational responsibilities for all facilities and programs were delegated to the administrator, Mr. Clark. Responsibility for the financial management of the home remained with the board chairman, Mr. Polk. The financial analyst and the bookkeeper, although reporting to Clark on paper, actually reported directly to Polk. Clark did have mid-level managers who were responsible for operations within the nursing unit, but he took full responsibility for the retirement village.

According to Polk, the board allowed Clark considerable latitude in running the home. The previous board chairman (Polk's predecessor) had allowed the previous administrator (Clark's predecessor) very little room for decision making. The home experienced some financial difficulties under the former chairman and administrator. Consequently, about 10 years ago, that board chairman was asked to resign. Later that year, the administrator was asked to resign as well. Polk was then selected as the new chairman and hired Clark as the administrator. Polk and Clark have been in their current positions approximately 10 years. They were both members of the same Evangelical Free Church congregation and had known each other for a considerably longer period of time. Substantial trust between the two men was apparent.

Cantwell observed that Clark exhibited little imagination in dealing with the home's operations. He also observed that Clark did an excellent job with the day-to-day management of the home. Employees were productive and contented with their work. Residents were generally well satisfied with their care. The home enjoyed an excellent reputation for the provision of high-quality basic care. Clark fostered the kind of work environment that made this possible. He did not, however, appear to have a thorough understanding of the current long-term care environment, in particular, the concept of a continuum of care. Clark did not seem to recognize the need to bridge the gap between total independence and total dependence of retirement village residents. He stated that he could not understand why the retirement village residents were becoming more vociferous in their demands for services.

Cantwell observed that financially the home was generally well managed. Polk appeared to be a prudent and well-intentioned individual who had managed to reverse previous financial problems without the benefit of a high-powered financial management staff. However, Polk also appeared to lack an understanding of the distinctions between financial management of a not-for-profit health care facility and that of a small, for-profit business. This was particularly apparent to Cantwell in the way that accounts were defined and segregated. The home actually had two equity accounts—capital contributions and retained earnings—which Cantwell combined into one account, the fund balance, for purposes of the financial review. Fund accounting techniques were not evident. All accounts were integrated despite restrictions placed on certain funds. The distinct financial management needs of the continuing care facility were also not recognized by the home's financial manager. Planning for future financial stability was difficult as a consequence.

Resident Profile

The home provided services at three levels of care. Each level of care had a distinct resident profile.

The retirement village housed residents living in 36 units. Twenty-four of the units were single-family homes. The residents tended to be atypical of those residing in other continuing care retirement communities. The average resident age on admission was 70.0 years, compared with a national average of 76 years. The average current age was 75.7 years, compared with mature communities, where the average age approximates 82 years (see Table 2). Thus, the retirement village had a relatively young resident population. Close to one half of the residents were members of the Evangelical Free Church (see Table 3). Residents also tended to originate from distances farther from the home than is typical (see Table 4).

The nursing and personal care units were more typical of other church-related nursing homes. The average age on admission (81 years) and the average current age (86 years) were comparable to national averages. Approximately 30% of nursing care and 25% of residential care residents were members of the Evangelical Free Church. This was similar to

Table 2. Average age of in-house residents as of December of last year versus national data (in years)

Level of care	Age at admission	National age at admission	Current age	National average age
Nursing care[a]	81.0	N/A	86.0	N/A
Personal care	82.0	N/A	86.0	N/A
Retirement village[b]	70.0	76	75.7	82

Source: American Association of Homes for the Aging. [1987]. *Continuing care retirement communities: An industry in action.* Washington, DC: Author.

[a]The age distribution of nursing home residents is skewed as a result of the NF/MR program (facilities for persons with mental retardation). According to the American College of Health Care Administrators Ready Reference Service, the current age is similar to the national experience, but the average length of stay at the Mueller-O'Keefe Home is approximately 3 years longer than the national average.

[b]82 years is the resident average age for those retirement communities that opened between 1963 and 1973.

the experience of other denominational homes. More residents had entered from areas outside of the typical 10-mile radius from the home, however, than would be expected of homes in areas of similar population density.

Despite the home's lack of promotional efforts, the nursing and residential care units and the retirement village remained full. Although 43% of the current residents' care was paid through the Medicaid program (see Table 5), 90% had entered as self-pay residents. According to Clark, the high rate of conversion from self-pay to Medicaid was most likely due to the long lengths of stay in nursing care (4.5 years compared to a national average of just over 2 years). Clark further stated that Medicaid, as a percentage of payer mix, would be higher if the home's private pay rates were equivalent to those of other nursing homes in the area: "Many of our residents are not well off. We want to give them the best care we can at the lowest rates so that we don't use up their assets any faster than necessary."

Table 3. Religious preference by level of care

	Level of care					
	Nursing care		Personal care		Retirement village	
Religious preference	Number	Percent	Number	Percent	Number	Percent
Evangelical Free Church	29	29.0	8	24.2	16	47.2
Methodist	27	27.0	13	39.4	5	14.7
Other Christian	40	40.0	12	36.4	8	23.4
None	4	4.0	0	0.0	5	14.7
Total	100	100.0	33	100.0	34	100.0

Table 4. Resident origin by level of care—in-house residents: December 31, last year

	Level of care					
	Nursing care		Personal care		Retirement village	
Prior residence	Number	Percent	Number	Percent	Number	Percent
Home county	68	66.7	26	76.5	15	44.1
Contiguous counties	20	19.6	6	17.6	3	8.8
Other	14	13.7	2	5.9	16	47.1
Total	102	100.0	34	100.0	34	100.0

Financial Review

The home appeared to be on firm financial footing. Results of the financial statement analyses are presented in Table 6. Declining net revenues were noted 2 and 3 years ago. According to Polk, this trend resulted from the board's decisions not to raise rates during each of those years. A rate increase was put into effect, however, at the end of last year, which resulted in an increase in net revenue during the opening months of this year.

The home had adopted a rate policy for nursing care that was considered to be unique in the nursing home industry. Private rates were to be set no higher than Medicaid rates for the same patient services classification. This was directly related both to the basic care philosophy and to the social philosophy of the Evangelical Free Church. Clark stated that this policy actually resulted in the home having to refund money to the state's Medicaid program last year when the cost reports were analyzed and the state auditors realized that the rate-setting commission had increased Medicaid rates to the home, but the private rates had not been increased by the board. Federal law does not permit Medicaid rates to exceed self-pay rates.

The retirement village residents, although not guaranteed care according to their contracts, were guaranteed a partial payment source for care based on their entrance fees. Entrance fees were to be depreciated over

Table 5. Nursing care utilization profile by payer classification

	Self-pay		Medicaid	
	Patient days	Percent	Patient days	Percent
Last year	21,731	59.5	14,773	40.5
2 years ago	20,407	57.7	15,383	42.3
3 years ago	22,102	60.6	14,368	39.4

Table 6. Comparative statement of revenues and expenses annualized (in dollars)

	This year	Last year	2 years ago
Operating revenues			
Resident care fees			
Personal care	324,408	312,927	319,186
Self-pay nursing facility	1,094,658	1,020,978	978,382
Medicaid nursing facility	729,772	683,162	698,229
Other operating revenues	50,070	47,131	35,880
Total	2,198,908	2,064,198	2,031,677
Operating expenses			
Employee compensation	1,720,057	1,702,209	1,636,782
Supplies	112,010	107,723	108,080
Maintenance	78,940	69,510	64,694
Utilities	97,295	91,753	91,059
Professional development	4,107	6,204	4,383
Professional services	36,785	35,652	34,757
Insurance	37,099	35,074	17,608
Miscellaneous	4,282	4,625	3,174
Total	2,090,575	2,052,750	1,960,537
Depreciation	73,470	62,704	44,522
Total expenses	2,164,045	2,115,454	2,005,059
Gain (loss) from operations	34,863	(51,256)	26,618
Nonoperating revenue	131,400	72,619	72,705
Net income for period	166,263	21,363	99,323

a 12-year period, with the undepreciated balance available to pay for nursing care if the resident should permanently transfer to the nursing home. Cantwell became quite concerned when he could not track the entrance fees. Consequently, he could not accurately calculate the home's potential liabilities for care. The resident care reserve fund appeared to cover only residents who had actually transferred to nursing care. When questioned, Polk became defensive about this procedure. He stated that fees were deposited directly into one of the trust accounts. Resident care was provided according to the contracts and no problems had occurred to date.

The agent and trust accounts were administered by a local bank. There had been dramatic growth in these accounts in recent years. There were two sources for growth. First, donations had increased. The second and more important source of fund growth, however, was related to the increase in value of the portfolio holdings. The holdings were revalued to current market levels at the end of each period. Although the portfolio was diversified, the account balances were sensitive to changes in financial markets.

Environmental Analysis

There were two competing continuing care retirement communities in the home's primary service area. Mueller-O'Keefe's entrance and maintenance fees are lower than the others' (see Table 7). There were also nine other nursing homes in competition for residents at that level of care (see Table 8). The most significant finding was that the home's rates at all levels of care were the lowest in the county. Cantwell noted with some concern the differences in monthly maintenance fees among the retirement communities. He had discussed this informally with Clark on first reviewing the internal rate structure. Clark recognized that the fees were nowhere near adequate to cover costs. However, he stated that the board was more concerned about those living in the retirement village who could not afford the $120 per month that other communities charged. Clark thought that $120 was outrageous and that the other communities could not justify that amount. Cantwell also noted that the home's physical plant was more modest than those of the competitors' facilities.

The demographic analysis revealed several things that explained, to some extent, the competitive advantage of the home. First, there were few vacant beds in the county. Even those patients capable of self-pay for extended periods of time were having difficulty finding a nursing home bed. The home was located in an area characterized by a rapidly expanding elderly population. Housing values and elderly income, however, were below the state and national averages. Also, a higher percentage than expected of the oldest old lived alone—a situation that resulted in heavy demand for nursing home care. In the adjacent city, close to 50% of those

Table 7. Continuing care retirement community fees (in dollars)

Community	Entrance fees		Maintenance fees (monthly)
Mueller-O'Keefe (church-related)	Cottages:	55,000	20
	Apartments:	25,000	20
The Woods (church-related)	Cottages:	70,500	130
	Apartments:	47,500	130
Luther Village (church-related)	Cottages:	60,000	120

Table 8.   Licensed nursing homes—primary service area

Facility	Beds		Nursing care rates (per diem, in dollars)
	Nursing care	Personal care	
Mueller-O'Keefe (church-related)	102	40	Semiprivate: 46 Private: 47–49
Andover Manor (for-profit)	221	0	Semiprivate: 57–59 Private: 59–64
Clifton Home (for-profit)	49	0	Semiprivate: 50
County Home (government)	51	0	Semiprivate: 50–60
The Court (for-profit)	160	0	Semiprivate: 71–74
Greywood Memorial (for-profit)	37	17	Semiprivate: 49
The Woods (church-related)	100	45	Semiprivate: 51 Private: 51
Luther Village (church-related)	88	0	Semiprivate: 58–60 Private: 61
Methodist Home (church-related)	150	0	Semiprivate: 58–65 Private: 68
Advent Home (church-related)	97	0	Semiprivate: 53–56 Private: 61
Total	1,055	102	

older than age 75 lived alone, compared to approximately one third on a national basis. The demographic and economic profiles also explained the slow growth that was experienced by the retirement village.

Interviews

The committee interviewed several key participants. Following are their ideas, compliments, and concerns, in their own words:

Mr. Clark, Administrator "The retirement village residents are taking an increasing amount of my time. Without an assistant administrator, it is becoming more difficult to deal with problems caused by increasing age and decreasing independence. They pay a $20 per month maintenance fee. I can't provide all of the services that they expect on that amount.

"We emphasize excellent basic care in the nursing home. We intend to be the highest quality, lowest cost home in the county. Our philosophy of care is based on Christian principles. I don't want to deplete our residents' hard-earned savings. We figure that they will be on Medicaid soon enough, so why hurry the process. That is why we don't set self-pay rates above the Medicaid rate. We also aren't tempted to treat residents any differently based on payer status.

"Relations with the church have not always been smooth. The ladies' auxiliary, consisting largely of area church members, has made significant contributions, both financially and in volunteer time. Some pastors, however, have been reluctant to become involved in the activities that we sponsor for the ladies' auxiliary, such as an annual barbecue and periodic breakfast meetings. We would like to have more involvement from the church.

"In the past, funds were severely limited. Construction was not always the highest quality. Maintenance costs are going up as a consequence. We may need to replace certain facilities in the future. The farmhouse may not be considered safe for residents at some point. Because of the historical significance of the building, however, we would want to continue to utilize it."

Mrs. Hancock, Director of Nursing "Care requirements are increasing across the board. We have had to increase our R.N. staff as a consequence. Of particular concern are the retirement village residents. A few of them should be in nursing care now. We end up providing free care on an emergency basis when they can't get to their personal physicians.

"We don't know enough about their care requirements. This may be more of a problem in the future, especially if people are older when they first enter the retirement village or the personal care facility. We should be more aware of the medical care that they are receiving from their personal physicians. I don't have the time to make the contacts myself, even if the residents gave me permission to make contact."

Ms. Webb, Director of Social Services "People seeking admissions are generally older and sicker at each level of care. Nursing home beds are filled as soon as they are vacated. Most residents come from home or from other nursing homes. I seldom have a bed when the hospital social worker calls. She calls me anyway to see if I might have a bed, because the nursing home beds in this area are generally in short supply. The hospital has added its own skilled nursing care unit, but this isn't adequate to provide care for the many discharges who will require long-term care, rather than post-acute extended care.

"People only leave the retirement village when they absolutely cannot care for themselves and then go directly to nursing care. We are supposed to have two beds in reserve for the retirement village. It doesn't, however, always work out. Personal care would be better than remaining in independent living, but the residents don't care for the accommodations there."

Mr. Polk, Chairman, Board of Directors "The local congregation of the Evangelical Free Church, to which I belong, has generously supported the home. Most board and ladies' auxiliary members also belong to my congregation. I'm not sure how much benefit increased church involvement would have, because other congregations have not been as financially generous.

"We're not sure how we should set our priorities. In particular, we would like to know how we can best use our available funds. I don't think it is appropriate, however, to jeopardize our residents' security by incurring debt. I know of homes that have had financial difficulties as a result of overextending debt. If the board decides to finance growth through debt, I may need to reconsider my position on the board.

"I've suggested several mission statements, but the board has not decided which, if any, to adopt. Many believe that a mission statement might be too rigid. Obviously, our policies reflect the Christian mission of service on which this home was founded. We just don't have it written down."

Mr. O'Donnell, Chairman, Long-Range Planning Committee "We need your help in planning for the future. We don't know enough about the different approaches to growth. We do know that if we grow, it has to be slow and planned. I don't like debt, but if we need it to meet our goals, then we should do it. That's why we hired you. We also need to agree on our mission. We know that we want to serve the elderly and especially Evangelical Free Church elderly, but we also don't want to discriminate against those of other denominations.

"Our buildings may need to be replaced in the future and we need to be prepared for that. Also, growth in the retirement village needs to be better planned."

Mrs. Ruth, Board Member "We need to have closer ties to the Evangelical Free Church. It is not so much the financial support that they give, but the anchor that the church provides. That is, the church is where we go to ensure that what we are doing is consistent with Christian social teaching and allows us to share our experience with others who have similar concerns."

Mrs. Jones, Nursing Home Ombudswoman, Area Agency on Aging "I hear only positive things. This is the only nursing home in my territory from which I have received no complaints since I was hired into this position 2 years ago."

Mr. and Mrs. Miller, Retirement Village Residents "We love the single-family homes and the community spirit here. Nursing care is excellent. We know that if we really need care, the nursing home will provide good care. We are growing older and may need help with daily activities, such as shopping, food preparation, and cleaning. It's just not available, except from neighbors.

"The personal care facility is inadequate. There are a few nice rooms, but not many. That's why people wait so long before deciding to go to personal or nursing care. The home needs to have a better personal care facility and maybe provide more services in the home."

THE WORKING SESSION

Cantwell entered the final working session feeling confident in his recommendations, but uncertain about what the board's responses might be. Although committee members had talked freely during the interviews, they had been relatively quiet in the working sessions in which the analyses were presented. Cantwell did not know whether that was a positive sign or not. He had managed to elicit responses from Polk on relatively minor points related to financial position. Cantwell assumed that he had done a thorough and professional job and took their silence to mean concurrence with his analyses. Cantwell presented the following options:

1. Basic option—no facility expansion
    a. Upgrade the financial management system, especially the management of entrance fees and contingent liabilities for retirement village residents.
    b. Provide service contract options for retirement village residents that encourage continued independence. Such services may include transportation, on-site medical care, and housecleaning. Optional contracts would result in higher monthly fees to residents.

2. Expand and modernize current facilities
    a. Enlarge the Alzheimer's unit. This option would take advantage of the home's experience and allow for increased care of persons with later stages of the disease. It would also expand bed capacity and may ease problems with the waiting list.
    b. Expand and modernize the personal care unit. This is one of the most rapidly growing programs among continuing care retirement communities. The current units are inadequate. Bathing facilities in particular need to be upgraded. An enhanced personal care unit may also make retirement living more attractive and result in growth in the retirement village. Replacement of the personal care rooms in the farmhouse may become necessary if the facility cannot continue to meet safety codes.

c. Develop a master plan for the retirement village. Growth has been unplanned to date. Future growth should be planned, including roads and sewage treatment plant improvements. Prospective residents should be given fewer options with new houses. The current system has discouraged sales in the past, especially to older persons who are not willing to expend the effort necessary to retain and supervise a builder.

In order to pursue this option, the board would need to hire an architect to lay out alternatives and estimate costs. Financing arrangements will depend on the options selected. A total marketing effort should be undertaken to support any program development effort.

3. Program initiatives

Provide adult day care for persons with Alzheimer's disease. This has been identified as a need by the Area Agency on Aging and the health systems agency. It could be done on-site and would complement the residential Alzheimer's unit. It would involve minimal investment.

As at previous meetings, few questions were raised. Polk disagreed that the current financial management system was inadequate. The other options appeared to be acceptable. Following this meeting the recommendations were to be presented to the board for approval and action.

At the conclusion of the meeting, Cantwell became uneasy. As he left for home, he wondered what went wrong. How could he further help the committee to decide or to take action? He could not help but think about Polk's faith in "seat of the pants" decisions. He had done the best job he could. He hoped to be able to assist the board in implementing the selected strategies. The waiting had begun.

11

Caregivers

Randi Priluck
Pace University, New York, New York

Beginning in 1997, Caregivers, a nonprofit agency that provides care to patients in need, faced a series of cutbacks in state funding that led to a deficit in its budget. The CEO of the agency, Don Arnold, was concerned that Caregivers would be unable to continue its mission of caring for older adults in need if the agency did not find a way to raise revenue.

In March 1998, Arnold set up the New Business Group to explore ways for the agency to convert some of the services that it currently offered for free to a profit-based system for those who could afford to pay. Included in the group, which met every Tuesday at 9:30 A.M., were Arnold, Beverly Slater (chief operating officer), Roslyn Warner (director of marketing mid-development), Gilda Newburgh (director of housing), Colleen Confit (marketing manager), Pamela Tilden (housing manager), and Emily Furley (social services manager).

A number of new business areas were explored. It was critical for Caregivers to assess the potential of these areas of business, set goals and objectives, and implement a plan of action. The expenses for the agency were divided among three basic areas: home care, housing, and social services (see Table 1).

Used by permission from *2000 Annual Advances in Business Cases*, the Society for Case Research (SCR). All rights reserved to the author and SCR. Copyright © 2001 by Randi Priluck.

This case was prepared by Randi Priluck of Pace University, New York, and is intended to be used as a basis for class discussion. The views represented here are those of the author and do not necessarily reflect the views of the Society for Case Research. The author's views are based on her own professional judgments. The names of the organizations, individuals, and locations have been disguised to preserve the organizations' request for anonymity.

Table 1. Caregivers agency budgeted revenue and expenses ($ in thousands)

	Amount	%
Revenue		
Social services	$31,037	58
Home care	13,882	26
Housing	5,807	11
Philanthropic	2,342	4
Total	$53,068	
Expenses		
Home care	$41,630	78
Housing	8,084	15
Social services	3,350	6
Total	$53,064	

Source: Caregivers Strategic Plan, 1998.

Staff within the organization did not fully support top management's efforts to require clients to pay for services. This was particularly true of social workers. Social workers were trained as advocates of people in need and did not recognize the difference between a client in need and one who could pay for services. They often did not recommend Caregivers to their clients for home-care services; they would recommend lower-priced alternatives instead.

THE ORGANIZATION

Caregivers' mission was to care for the needy in instances when they could not care for themselves. The agency operated exclusively in the Boston metropolitan area and offered a variety of services related to the mission. One main focus of the agency's effort was caring for the elderly, and this area was expected to grow because of the aging population in the United States (see Table 2). By 2040, more than 20% of the U.S. population will be 65 years of age or older.

DIVISIONS

The agency consisted of three divisions: Home Care, Housing, and Social Services. Each of the divisions operated independently with its

Table 2. Population by age (in thousands)

Year	Age 65–74		Age 75–84		Age 85+	
	Number	%	Number	%	Number	%
1990	18,045	7.3	10,012	4.0	3,021	1.2
2000	18,551	6.7	12,438	4.5	4,333	1.6
2010	20,978	7.0	13,157	4.4	5,969	2.0
2020	30,910	9.5	15,480	4.7	6,959	2.1
2030	37,984	10.9	23,348	6.7	8,843	2.5
2040	33,968	9.1	29,206	7.9	13,840	3.7
2050	34,628	8.8	26,588	6.8	18,893	4.8

Source: U.S. Bureau of Census, 1993, 2000–2050 projected data, middle-series assumptions.

own budget. The director of home care was responsible for both licensed and certified home-care programs as well as private-pay home care. The housing director ran senior centers and residences for older adults, and the director of social services managed the programs for the older adults in need.

Home Care

The Home Care division was a licensed home health care agency. It trained home health aides, homemakers, and housekeepers and placed them in positions. Home health aides were specially trained to assist older clients with personal care such as bathing, dressing, and toileting. They also served as companions for their older clients. Homemakers were trained to act as caregivers for children in the homes of incapacitated parents. Housekeepers cleaned and performed other household tasks for people incapable of doing so.

Within the Home Care division, services were provided through government contracts and Visiting Nurse Services (VNS), which billed Medicare or Medicaid. Alternatively, Caregivers billed the client directly, a payment system known as "private pay," which served about 10% of the home care business. Nationally, the private-pay home care market was smaller than the Medicare and Medicaid home care markets (see Table 3). Because Caregivers was a licensed agency, not a certified agency, it could not bill Medicare or Medicaid directly for services. Therefore, Caregivers had to align itself with a certified home health care agency that could bill in this manner (as did VNS).

In 1996, Caregivers had entered into a strategic alliance with VNS to provide home health aides in eastern Massachusetts exclusively, and by

Table 3.   National home-care market

Home-care market agency receipts	1997
Medicare	65.2%
Medicaid	9.6%
Private pay*	7.0%
Private insurance	6.6%
HMOs, PPOs, state and local government, and bad debt	11.6%

Source: Standard and Poor's industry surveys, 1997.
*The National Home Care Association places the private-pay market at 30%.

1998 the VNS business represented 90% of the home health aides dispatched. Because approximately 26% of the agency's revenues were generated by VNS contracts, the agency was highly committed to this business and was very careful not to jeopardize it. One issue was whether, and to what extent, Caregivers could compete with VNS, particularly in Brookline, Massachusetts, where Caregivers did contract work for VNS. Some staff members of the agency were very concerned about attempting to increase private-pay services while trying to maintain VNS contracts.

Housing

Caregivers operated five buildings in Framingham, Massachusetts (a town 30 minutes from downtown Boston), which altogether housed 1,000 older adults. Most of the buildings offered subsidized housing, and only one of the buildings, known as F3, rented at market value. Residents were charged $800 for one-bedroom apartments that had a very basic decor. In addition, Caregivers operated a senior center two blocks from F3 that served 7,000 older adults and provided many services, including a social program and meals. As of July 1998, 14 units were vacant in F3, and Gilda Newburgh had devised a plan to provide assisted living in those 14 units. Assisted living is a care plan for elderly residents that includes three meals daily, day and evening social programs, personal care, and medication management. The cost to the resident for assisted living was $3,000 a month. Attempts to use promotional efforts to fill vacancies in F3 at market value had been limited prior to the decision to provide assisted living.

Social Services

The Social Services division was primarily responsible for the care of individuals in need. The division managed a number of programs. The Community Guardian program assisted people who did not have families to care for them. A Caregivers social worker acted as the person's guardian in legal and care matters. There was also a Case Management program, which helped individuals who needed assistance with their care but did not require total guardianship. Finally, the Financial Management program assisted clients with paying their bills.

Social Services also managed Elderlink, an information and referral database that contained information on a variety of eldercare services in the Boston area, including home health care, senior centers, meal programs, assisted-living facilities, and nursing homes. Elderlink was part of a national network of information providers that was used by Statler Referral, a firm that provided the employees of Fortune 500 companies with a national system of information and referral on aging. Employees of these firms could call a national number and be connected directly to Caregivers' Elderlink service. A Caregivers social worker would provide information to help the employee care for an elderly relative in the Boston area. Referrals from Statler, however, had been dwindling lately.

[handwritten margin note: joint partnership, and get funding from referrals]

ALTERNATIVE PLANS OF ACTION

The New Business Group consisted of managers from each of the three divisions: Housing, Social Services, and Home Care. Through a series of brainstorming sessions, the New Business Group identified a number of potential businesses that would build on Caregivers' skills in the three divisional areas. However, the managers were unsure how to allocate resources among their ideas and which businesses were the most viable. They chose three areas to explore more fully: real estate development, real estate property management, and private-pay home care.

Real Estate Development

The New Business Group proposed the development of a 200-unit assisted-living facility somewhere in the Boston area and determined the costs for providing services to such a facility (see Table 4). Though Caregivers did not any expertise in real estate development, top management felt that its expertise in providing services and its nonprofit status would attract a developer who needed Caregivers' assistance with the particulars of providing assisted-living services to the elderly. As of July 1998, top management had met with a few developers, but Caregivers was not happy with the quality of the sites and did not feel comfortable lending the Caregivers name to a poorly located facility.

Table 4. Service Costs for Assisted-Living Facilities of 100 and 200 Units

Cost Category	100 Units	200 Units
Food	$ 547,500	$1,095,000
Linens	100,000	200,000
Household supplies	54,750	109,500
Recreational supplies	15,000	30,000
Office supplies	6,000	9,000
Printing, duplication	6,000	9,000
Postage	24,000	48,000
Telephone	15,000	30,000
Marketing materials	50,000	75,000
Contracts machines	10,000	10,000
Transportation	68,000	68,000
Emergency response system	100,000	200,000
Consultants	36,500	54,750
Insurance, professional	35,000	40,000
Legal	20,000	20,000
Audits	20,000	20,000
Information services	47,758	72,419
Human resources	95,517	144,839
Finance	98,928	150,012
Administration	98,928	150,912
Management	252,000	504,000
Total	$1,700,881	$3,039,532

Source: Caregivers internal documents, 1998.

Real Estate Property Management

The New Business Group determined that older inner-city residents would not be likely to leave their apartments as they aged because many of the day-to-day maintenance issues in a rental unit, co-op, or condominium were handled by the building management. Caregivers' management, however, saw an opportunity to market eldercare services to building managers who had large percentages of elderly residents in their buildings. The marketing department began to identify buildings built prior to 1965 in the Boston area with 300 or more apartments. Letters and brochures were sent to building managers emphasizing the dangers of leaving older residents without care. For instance, an older person might leave the gas stove on and start a fire, hoard garbage in the early stages of dementia, or forget to pay maintenance fees. On the phone, many managers expressed interest in the problem. They felt that they could use some assistance with their older residents but did not see spending up front to avoid potential accidents. They felt that caring for older adults was the responsibility of the family. A few meetings were set up with larger complexes, but in such instances, co-op and condo boards were reluctant to spend money on this matter.

The New Business Group developed the Property Management program, which consisted of two services: an on-site model and a consultation model. The on-site model was designed for large buildings (more than 400 total residents) with at least 30% of elderly residents. Caregivers would conduct a survey to determine where the elderly residents lived and would then place on the premises a part-time social worker who would provide social programs and assistance to the elderly residents. The social worker would also intervene in difficult cases and assist building employees in identifying problem situations. The price would be $2,800 per month for the building. The consultation model provided many of the same services, but operated out of Caregivers' offices and did not include a part-time social worker on the premises. The price would be $1,000 a month.

Private-Pay Home Care

Private-pay home care clients pay for their own home care rather than relying on Medicare or Medicaid for payment. Caregivers' license allowed the agency to provide home health aides to those who could afford to pay out of pocket for the service.

In July 1998, the exact size of the private-pay market in the Boston area was unknown, but national information on older adults with disabilities was available (see Table 5), as was information on the older population in the Boston area (see Table 6).

Competition was intense in the private-pay home care market. One important competitor was the "gray market" for home care services. Since home care services for older adults were often an ongoing expense, many adult children chose to hire home care workers who were untrained and did not demand that their employers pay Social Security tax. Aside from the gray market, a number of other agencies competed for the private-pay business (see Table 7).

The New Business Group discussed their concerns regarding how to furnish home health aides under a private-pay system, when Caregivers

Table 5.   Percent of elderly with functional limitations

Functional Limitation	Age 75–84	Age 85+
Walking	18.8	34.9
Getting outside	22.3	44.8
Bathing or showering	11.3	30.6
Transferring	11.6	21.9
Dressing	7.0	16.1
Toileting	5.7	14.2
Average	23.5	40.4

Source: U.S. Bureau of the Census, Survey of Income and Program Participation, Functional Limitations and Disability File, 1991, non-institutional persons.

also provided aides through VNS. As of July 1998, most of Caregivers' aides were working under VNS contracts and could not be switched to a private-pay case. Caregivers' management considered not pursuing the private-pay market because of the fear of losing the VNS contract. They also considered pursuing private-pay in areas that VNS did not serve.

The target market for home care services is the elderly population 75 years and older with one or more difficulties in the activities of daily living and incomes higher than $35,000 per year.

The New Business Group discovered some difficulties in marketing the private-pay home care business. First, home health aides were paid $6.50 an

Table 6.   Older adults by income, selected Massachusetts counties

Income	Age 75–84	Age 85+
Under $5,000	11,013	13,938
$5,000–$9,999	32,477	49,706
$10,000–$14,999	24,539	24,354
$15,000–$24,999	39,353	25,708
$25,000–$34,999	28,410	14,670
$35,000–$49,999	26,546	11,009
$50,000–$74,999	22,294	8,549
$75,000–$99,999	8,746	3,055
$100,000+	8,286	2,823

Source: U.S. Bureau of the Census: Norfolk, Suffolk, Middlesex, Bristol, Essex, and Plymouth counties.

Table 7. Competitor data

Home care agencies	Number of private-pay cases	Weekday rate per hour
U.S. Home Care	400	$15.00
All Metro	150	$13.75
Caring Hand	150	$9.50
Allen	100	$14.00
COHME	100	$14.00
Select	100	N/A
Partners in Care	100+	$14.00

Source: 1998 Caregivers competitor survey, completed in-house.

hour, which did not provide much incentive for them to deliver exceptional service. Second, there were no home health aides available exclusively for private-pay cases, and sometimes an aide could not be found to service a particular case. Finally, most of the clients wanted service in the morning from 9 A.M. to 12 noon, but aides were often already working on morning jobs and only had afternoon hours available. Not only were clients not able to receive care when they wanted it, but aides did not receive a full day's worth of hours and often got only morning work.

There were, however, some positive aspects of Caregivers' services that would appeal to the target market. Caregivers always sent a nurse to a client's home to assess the case prior to dispatching an aide (this was a requirement under its license). Caregivers also provided health and drug screening of aides, background checks, and training. If an aide was sick or unable to provide service on a particular day, a replacement was sent. A 24-hour telephone assistance line was available for home health aides to call in emergencies.

Caregivers charged an individual client $12.75 an hour for home care services during the week and $14 an hour for weekend service. The gray-market rate was between $9 and $11 an hour for care. The New Business Group determined that Caregivers earned 75 cents of profit on every hour of care they delivered. In other words, it cost $12 an hour to provide service to clients during the week and Caregivers charged $12.75. The median number of hours per case was 20.

Caregivers had also identified a number of possible niche markets within the larger home care market:

- *Specialty diseases:* The niche of specialty diseases was considered because people with certain diseases require a significant amount of care. Though aides were already trained to provide Alzheimer's care, other diseases would require additional training.

- *Skilled nursing:* Skilled nursing was another potential niche market. Pursuing this market would require that Caregivers hire more nurses and obtain a special license to offer such services in order to be able to bill Medicare and Medicaid directly. The size of that market was substantial, as shown in Table 3.

- *Difficult cases:* Over time, Caregivers had developed a reputation for being able to handle difficult cases. These cases, which had been rejected by other agencies because the client was disruptive and disrespectful to the aide, often ended up at Caregivers. Caregivers was better able to handle such cases because of the special training that was provided by the agency and the support that the aides received from the home office. However, it was more expensive to service a difficult case because it required more managerial time to arrange for proper care.

- *Long distance:* Another possible niche market was the long-distance market, which consisted of adult children who lived more than an hour's drive from Boston but who had an elderly relative to care for in the Boston area. It was believed that adult children who were not available to care for a parent would be a better target market because they would need to purchase more home care hours to make sure that the parent was well cared for. They might also be willing to pay a premium for such services. Though the actual size of the long-distance market was unknown, the number of adults over the age of 75 living in the Boston area was more than 300,000.

CONCLUSION

With the fall approaching and a board meeting scheduled for early October, Don Arnold needed to nail down a plan of action for the agency. He looked at the data on the home care market, considered developing an assisted-living facility, and thought about bringing services to existing buildings. Which would be the most profitable enterprise to pursue, and how could that be done without alienating VNS or staff members?

PART III

Management, Medical Staff, and Governing Body

12

Governance Challenges at Good Hands Healthcare (A)

Amy J. Hillman
Marilyn Seymann

Richard Ivey School of Business
The University of Western Ontario

Ivey

In mid-2000, the board of directors of Good Hands Healthcare (Good Hands), a $3 billion company trading on the New York Stock Exchange, was pondering its current situation. It had become increasingly discouraged by the downward spiral of Good Hands' stock and financial performance and by the continuing explanations of the situation by the company's chief executive officer (CEO), George Jackson. Jackson, who had been Good Hands' CEO for the past 30 years, had attributed the slide of Good Hands' performance to "external factors beyond their control."

Professors Amy J. Hillman and Marilyn Seymann prepared this case solely to provide material for class discussion. The authors do not intend to illustrate either effective or ineffective handling of a managerial situation. The authors may have disguised certain names and other identifying information to protect confidentiality.

The health-care industry was indeed subject to a great deal of environmental factors, not the least of which was the reliance on government reimbursement for services. One of the major issues facing the industry was significant reductions in federal funding of health and eldercare. In addition, the industry had experienced an increasing number of lawsuits filed by patients' families and attention by the media to incidents of poor care, especially of the elderly. Good Hands, one of the largest U.S. nursing home providers, was no exception to these lawsuits and, along with other industry players, was experiencing escalating patient care liability costs.

The board of directors wondered, however, why Good Hands' major competitors, HealthUS, ElderCare and Aged Services, Inc., were able to increase their profitability and market share at the same time that Good Hands' was slipping. After all, wasn't the whole industry affected by the same "external factors"? Was there something else to explain Good Hands' recent troubles beyond these industry threats?

In addition to questions regarding management's assessment of the firm's performance woes, the board of directors of Good Hands was concerned with the absence of a succession plan within the company. While Jackson was recognized as an industry leader, would he be able to stop the current downward spiral and perform a turnaround of the firm? And, if not, who would be able to step into his shoes? The lack of a succession plan at Good Hands coupled with no formal internal effort to develop leadership for the future cast an ominous shadow over the future of the company.

The board knew it didn't have a lot of time to waste. Good Hands was sliding precipitously towards bankruptcy. In fact, several of its competitors had already filed Chapter 11, and as a result of their restructuring, they were more nimble than Good Hands to weather the industry threats. The board set its sight on its next meeting, in two months, to address these important issues. All of the board members knew this meeting would be a critical turning point for the future of Good Hands.

THE COMPANY

Good Hands Healthcare was founded as a small nursing home business in 1970, in Brownsville, Texas. Through rapid expansion, the company went public in 1978 and now represented more than 400 facilities in 25 states. Good Hands operated facilities in three areas of operations: 285 nursing homes, 74 assisted living and outpatient facilities, and 47 care units for people with Alzheimer's disease. George Jackson, the current CEO, had founded the business and had served as its president/CEO and chairman of the board for 30 years.

While originally founded as a nursing home company, Good Hands diversified into assisted living and outpatient facilities in the early 1990s and later, in 1995, into care facilities for people with Alzheimer's disease. Nursing home facilities now provided residents with long-term care, including daily skilled nursing and nutritional services, along with the social and recreational services that accompany a long-term residence facility. Pharmacy and medical supplies were also provided to residents. Good Hands saw themselves as an "extension of patients' families." The Good Hands culture had long emphasized that employees treat each resident as they would their own family and that each Good Hands facility was akin to a family community. For example, in 1999, Good Hands began redesigning several of its facilities to reflect the newest trend in nursing homes, home-centric design.

Similarly, assisted living and facilities for people with Alzheimer's disease, while emphasizing a different mix of traditional services, also promoted a communal experience and a loving, caregiving environment. Assisted living centers were targeted at those elderly whose health did not necessitate daily nursing per se, but who were less able to safely live an independent lifestyle. These facilities resembled apartment complexes with a collection of small efficiency-like living spaces where residents could bring their own furniture and belongings. Access in and out of these facilities was not restricted; residents could come and go as they please. Meals were typically offered in communal dining halls or in-suite, while social activities included a full range of classes and excursions outside of the facility. The advantage of these living facilities was that a full-time nursing staff was always on hand should a resident require assistance. Residents were monitored throughout the day. This level of service was in stark contrast to that received by the elderly who lived alone in single-family residences. In addition to the availability of professional nursing help, assisted living centers provided many elderly with social interaction with other residents and the staff, something that was often lacking for elderly living at home.

The facilities for people with Alzheimer's disease, on the other hand, were centers meant to specifically meet the needs of the elderly suffering from the dementia and other indications of Alzheimer's disease. These patients required much more intensive supervision than both the assisted living or nursing home residents and Good Hands' facilities allowed for specialized treatment of these needs. Good Hands saw the need for more specialized care for people with Alzheimer's disease beyond the typical nursing home environment and was rolling out more such facilities as a part of its expansion plan.

By the end of 1999, more than 85 per cent of Good Hands' net operating revenues came from nursing home facilities, with 10 per cent and five per cent coming from assisted living and facilities for people with Alzheimer's disease, respectively. Occupancy of its 406 facilities in 1999 was 86 per cent, with Medicare patients representing 21 per cent of total patient days and 43 per cent of revenue.

Good Hands' facilities were staffed by more than 61,000 employee caregivers. Typically, 30 per cent to 34 percent of the staff at a given facility were certified, skilled nursing professionals. The remainder were typically staff paid little more than minimum-wage, such as custodians and housekeepers ($7 per hour), aides ($9 per hour) and office personnel, cooks and maintenance workers ($12 per hour). More than 98 per cent of Good Hands' employees were female with an average of a high-school education for non-certified staff. Turnover among Good Hands' employees averaged 80 per cent a year for non-certified staff, and 47 per cent for certified staff, and the company encountered periodic difficulty attracting and retaining registered and licensed nurses, certified nurses' aides and other facility personnel. Approximately 21 per cent of the employees in more than 150 facilities were represented by various labor unions, the largest of which was the AFL-CIO. While relations with these unions had been generally good (Good Hands had not experienced any work stoppages as a result), the unions had commonly targeted Good Hands because of its visible position as one of the largest companies in the U.S. eldercare industry.

Good Hands' financial position had deteriorated in the last three years (see Exhibit 1). Most notably, for each of the previous three years, Good Hands had experienced declining sales growth and net income. In 1999, this loss was 10.3 per cent in sales from the previous year and a loss of $143.7 million in net income. Its competitors' experiences in recent years were much more robust. HealthUS grew sales from 1998 to 1999 by 44.2 per cent despite a drop of 33 per cent in net income, while ElderCare's one-year sales growth was 5.7 per cent with a 90.7 per cent increase in net income. Aged Services, Inc. posted an eight per cent loss in sales over the previous year, but had a total net income of more than $1 billion.

As a result of Good Hands' declining performance, the company was in a critical cash position, with cash at the end of 1999 of only $21 million. The funds needed to sustain its business were provided largely through revolving credit that increased overall short-term borrowing to $173 million. Total debt, on and off balance sheet, had grown by early 2000 to nearly $1 billion, and, along with it, the cost of debt for Good Hands had also risen considerably. This put Good Hands at a substantial disadvantage vis-à-vis its major competitors, HealthUS and Aged Services, Inc., who as a result of coming out of Chapter 11 bankruptcy had restructured their debt and were much less encumbered than Good Hands.

THE ELDERCARE INDUSTRY

Health care and general care for the elderly was a highly regulated industry and a fragmented industry with a significant number of "mom and

CONSOLIDATED BALANCE SHEETS
($000s)
(for years ending December 31)

ASSETS	1999	1998
Current Assets:		
Cash and cash equivalents	$ 21,086	$ 67,984
Accounts receivables—patient, less allowance for doubtful accounts	248,443	190,504
Accounts receivables—nonpatient, less allowance for doubtful accounts	48,005	30,890
Notes receivables, less allowance for doubtful notes	2,799	16,930
Operating supplies	34,320	44,534
Deferred income taxes	70,057	25,666
Prepaid expenses and other	17,654	18,643
Total current assets	$ 442,364	$ 395,151
Property and equipment, net	901,649	910,065
Other assets:		
Goodwill, net	201,111	265,443
Deferred income taxes	38,744	10
Other, less allowance for doubtful accounts and notes	123,338	23,393
Total other assets	363,193	255,802
	$ 1,732,206	$ 1,561,018
LIABILITIES AND STOCKHOLDERS' EQUITY		
Current Liabilities:		
Accounts payable	$ 109,420	$ 89,040
Accrued wages and related liabilities	134,002	78,094
Accrued interest	26,550	19,448
Other accrued liabilities	60,628	163,292
Short-term debt and current portion of long-term debt	240,513	28,990
Total current liabilities	$ 571,113	$ 378,864
Long-term debt	438,039	335,605
Deferred income taxes payable	-	-
Other liabilities and deferred items	170,374	325,432
Total Liabilities	$ 1,154,526	$ 1,039,901
Stockholders' equity:		
Preferred stock, shares authorized: 20,000,000	-	-
Common stock, shares issued: 1999—112,808,705;	11,844	11,038
1998—120,382,356		
Additional paid-in capital	776,981	775,637
Accumulated deficit	(81,081)	(139,429)
Accumulated other comprehensive income	953	1,054
Treasury stock, at cost: 1999—18,954,450 shares;	(131,057)	(127,183)
1998—16,807,800 shares		
Total stockholders' equity	577,680	521,117
Total liabilities and stockholders' equity	1,732,206	1,561,018

Exhibit 1. Consolidated balance sheets and consolidated statements of operations, for years ending December 31.

(continued)

pop" facilities. While Good Hands Healthcare was one of the largest companies in the industry, and they had the largest share of the nursing home market, this only represented 3.8 per cent of the market. It was estimated that in the also very fragmented assisted-living industry, the top 25 players accounted for only two per cent to five per cent of the market. The leader

Consolidated Statements of Operations
($000s)
(for years ending December 31)

	1999	1998	1997
Net operating revenues	2,764,034	2,801,339	3,346,556
Interest income	2,650	4,335	10,708
Total revenues	2,766,684	2,805,674	3,357,264
Costs and expenses:			
Operating and administrative:			
Wages and related	1,886,990	1,846,363	1,914,452
Provision for insurance and related items	72,456	117,215	177,407
Other	645,889	708,183	936,246
Interest	121,990	53,105	19,349
Depreciation and amortization	100,061	109,076	107,780
Asset impairments, workforce reductions and other unusual items	43,033	38,602	89,578
Total costs and expenses	2,870,419	2,872,544	3,244,813
Net income/(loss) before benefit from income taxes, extraordinary charge and cumulative effect of change in accounting	(103,735)	(66,870)	112,451
Income taxes	31,121	26,138	(25,936)
Net income/(loss) before extraordinary charge and cumulative effect of change in accounting	(72,615)	(40,732)	86,515
Special charges related to settlements of regulatory claims and disputes	(82,510)	(1,865)	-
Extraordinary charge, net income tax benefit	11,420	653	1,985
Cumulative effect of change in accounting designation			550
Net Income/(Loss)	(143,705)	(41,944)	89,050
Basic and diluted loss per share of common stock:			
Before extraordinary charge and cumulative effect of change in accounting	(0.70)	(0.39)	0.83
Extraordinary charge	(0.68)	(0.01)	0.02
Cumulative effect of change in accounting			(0.04)
Net income/(loss)	(1.38)	(0.40)	0.86
Shares used to compute per share amounts	103,864	103,574	103,762

Exhibit 1. *(continued)*

in the home health-care industry, Sullivan Services, similarly had only four per cent of the market.

Increasing life expectancies and aging baby boomers were driving U.S. revenues for long-term health care. U.S. revenues for long-term health care were estimated to total $225.8 billion by 2003, versus $149.4 billion in 1998. Revenues for nursing homes were expected to rise to $115.4 billion in 2003, versus $87.3 billion in 1998 when home-care revenues were expected to rise to $48.7 billion from $33.2 billion.

Despite the healthy forecasts for growth in revenue, the 1995 National Nursing Home Survey suggested that elderly Americans were reducing their use of nursing home care. The changes from 1985 to 1995 per thousand elderly are illustrative. In 1985, 219.4 per thousand elderly aged 65 to 74 used nursing homes, whereas by 1995, this number dropped to 198.6 per thousand. For ages 75 to 85 this number dropped from 57.5 per thousand to 45.9 per thousand, and for ages 85 and older, from 12.5 to 10.1 per thousand. The gap left by decreasing nursing home use was being filled by alternatives, such as assisted living and home health care.

Health-care service providers were subject to various federal, state and local health-care statutes and regulations. State licenses were required to operate health-care facilities and to participate in government health care funding programs, such as Medicaid and Medicare. Medicaid was operated by individual states, funded by the federal government and designed to provide health care to the indigent. Medicare, on the other hand, was a health insurance program for the elderly and other disabled people and was operated by the federal government. Increasingly, the government and general public had been concerned with not only improving the quality of care provided but, paradoxically, also with cutting overall expenses.

Payments for services provided by companies such as Good Hands typically were funded by the states, via Medicaid; the government, under Medicare and other programs, such as the Department of Veterans Affairs; and from private payers, such as insurance companies and managed care providers. For the past three years, Good Hands' percentage from each source has varied from 52 per cent to 55 per cent from Medicaid, representing 70 per cent of patient days; from 21 per cent to 26 per cent from Medicare, or 11 per cent of patient days; and 19 per cent to 23 per cent from private and other payers, or 17 per cent to 18 per cent of patient days.

Most of the state Medicaid programs operated on a cost-based reimbursement system, with some states including efficiency incentives subject to certain cost limits. Cost reimbursement in these programs typically covered the administrative, general, property and equipment costs in addition to the direct and indirect allowable costs the company incurred in providing routine patient services. State Medicaid programs varied in the level of allowable costs reimbursed to operators.

In 1999, health-care reform measures, resulting from concern over the rising cost of Medicaid and Medicare programs, were passed, requiring nursing facilities to continue to provide care to Medicaid residents as well as those who might qualify for Medicaid in the future, even if the facility decided to withdraw from the program. In addition, cuts were made to the payments made for acute nursing care, initially put in place by the 1997 Balanced Budget Act. In 1997, efforts to balance the federal budget led Congress to cut reimbursements for Medicare patients. The 1999 cuts only added more problems for the industry, and, to make matters worse, further cuts were anticipated for 2000.

In addition to the reliance of the industry on government revenues, government regulations also strictly enforced quality standards for patient care. Government authorities periodically inspected facilities to ensure compliance with standards set for continued licensing and Medicare and Medicaid participation. Deficiencies could result in the imposition of fines, temporary suspension of new patient admissions into the facility, decertification from Medicare or Medicaid and, in extreme circumstances, revocation of a facility's license.

General liability and professional liability costs of the long-term care industry had become quite expensive in recent years. The past decade had seen a tremendous increase in the number and size of claims and lawsuits against the industry. The Florida Healthcare Association estimated that in Florida alone, in 1999, seven out of every 10 facilities had open claims against them, and nine out of 10 faced potential new lawsuits. Not only were there more claims, but they were growing in size. The 1999 average litigation claim in Florida was $279,000, a 250 per cent increase over the year prior.

This growing number and size of claims led to dramatically more expensive liability costs. For example, liability insurance per bed in 1999 ranged between $100 and $200 annually, but this number was estimated to grow by 100 per cent to 200 per cent per year. In some states, these numbers were considerably higher: in Texas, this rate was $2,000 to $3,000 per bed per year, and in Florida, it could reach as high as $7,000 per bed per year. Primarily as a result of these increases, insurance companies were ceasing to insure long-term care companies or were limiting their liability insurance severely. Substantially increased premiums and increased liability retention levels for reduced coverage were the norm when insurance coverage was available.

Other important industry trends included an overbuilding of nursing facilities in states that had eliminated the certificate of need process for new construction; the growing availability of eldercare delivered to the home; rapid expansion of assisted living facilities; and the expansion of acute care hospitals into long-term care.

GOOD HANDS' CEO AND MANAGEMENT TEAM

George Jackson, president, CEO and chairman of Good Hands Healthcare, founded the company and helped build the firm over its 30-year history. In early 2000, Jackson was 62 years of age and frequently discussed with the board his desire to work past the age of 65. A well-loved and admired industry expert, Jackson received his bachelor's degree in business administration from the University of Texas at Austin. Prior to founding Good Hands Healthcare, Jackson had worked in the banking industry for 12 years.

Jackson was a charismatic figure, handsome and personable. From Good Hands' beginning, he saw the company as an extension of himself, often blurring the line between the profession and the person. This created issues with his top management team and board in that he often perceived questioning of his strategies as a lack of confidence in his personal abilities. His top management team soon learned that it was prudent from a career perspective to play a supportive role to Jackson's vision. In early 2000, this cadre of Jackson's top management team represented a variety of people he had personally chosen for their positions.

A primary concern of Good Hands' board was the lack of succession planning within the firm. In mid-1999, the board raised its concern with Jackson and recommended he consider not only developing a formal succession plan, but that he consider bringing in some new leadership from outside the firm and industry to jump-start the company and try to turn around the situation so that Good Hands could regain its leadership position.

At the next meeting, the board received a complex chart of all the CEO's direct reports and their proposed successors. Each was accompanied by an appropriate development plan. Noticeably absent from this plan, however, was the CEO's succession plan. When the board queried Jackson about this, he stated he intended to keep working "as long as possible" and that if the proverbial bus ran him over, he was confident the current team, with help from the board, could run the company while a search was conducted for a successor.

One of Jackson's other responses to the succession plan discussion was to argue for substantial year-end bonuses for his top management team, despite the deteriorating financial conditions of the firm. His argument was that these individuals were underpaid given industry standards and that large bonuses were needed to retain them. He hinted that a large increase in his own compensation would also be appropriate although he did not go so far as to threaten to quit.

Chief Financial Officer (CFO) Bob Wayman (age 61) joined Good Hands in 1976. Wayman had experience with a Wall Street investment company prior to joining Good Hands. He had a bachelor's degree and a master's degree in business administration from Minnesota State University. A highly competent but extremely competitive person, especially with Chief Legal Counsel David Baker, the board was concerned that Wayman lacked the personality to be an effective leader. Wayman frequently commented that the numbers were the heart of the business. On multiple occasions, the board had questioned Wayman's ability to strategically manage the balance sheet to reflect the needs of the cash flow situation. The board questioned whether he was "old school" cautious since he refused to discuss any use of derivatives or any of the other financial instruments available to smooth out the peaks and valleys in the reimbursement stream. In addition, when asked questions by the board on routine financial issues, he tended to be defensive and often treated the question as if it were stupid. Another issue that arose with some frequency was that he did not see his role as reporting to the board's Audit

Committee and often circumvented the committee to resolve an issue with the CEO without bringing it to the board's attention. However, the marked lack of financial expertise among the rest of the senior management team had made him indispensable to the CEO, especially in his dealings with Wall Street.

Chief Operating Officer (COO) James O'Malley (age 64) joined Good Hands in 1987 after working for a competitor in the health-care industry for eight years. Since that time, O'Malley had risen up the ranks of Good Hands through the operations division and, in 1990, was appointed both COO and a member of the board of directors. While O'Malley was well liked and respected throughout the company, he was nearing retirement and was not likely to continue employment with Good Hands for more than another year or two. O'Malley was also well liked by the board but had been questioned frequently about his resistance to making changes to the operating model. His responses were typically a stream of explanations and excuses, mostly attributable, in his estimation, to "causes outside his control." However, given the quality-of-care issues and the difficulty finding more experienced people in the industry, the board had not pursued any aggressive questioning of his effectiveness.

Chief Legal Counsel (CLC) David Baker (age 54) was a close confidant of Jackson. The two of them were social acquaintances before Jackson persuaded Baker to leave his law firm to become in-house counsel for Good Hands in 1989. Baker often played the role of smoothing over the CEO's behavior when it was questioned by the board, and he was quick to defend Jackson's actions. While Baker was an accomplished attorney and had valuable expertise in the health-care arena, he lacked any management experience beyond the legal areas of the business. The board commonly regarded him as "a thorn in their side" and often questioned his handling of legal matters. His exclusive use of only one outside law firm, regardless of the matter, had caused many late-night discussions among board members. The board's concern over his competence had been discussed with the CEO in several executive sessions and had become a point of contention between the board and the CEO, who ardently defended his friend. Baker had also been the key person to structure all of the employment contracts of the senior management team and was, therefore, held in high regard by his peers in the company.

GOOD HANDS' BOARD

Good Hands Healthcare's board was composed of 10 members total: eight outside members with varied lengths of tenure and two inside members, Good Hands' CEO and Chair George Jackson and COO James O'Malley.

Five of the board members had been on the board since it was founded and were handpicked by Jackson. The three newer members joined the board within months of each other in 1998 when the existing board realized that there were too few members to effectively handle all of the board committees. When there were only five independent directors, they found they were all attending every committee meeting and, as a result, they were either devoting too much or not enough time to the issues at hand. Not wanting to be remiss, they decided that the addition of three new members, each with the ability to chair one of the committees, would be the appropriate number. They hired a search firm and recruited three directors within one year of beginning the search.

Since adding the last three members to the board, no new directors had been added. The board discussed frequently the need for "new ideas and diversity" but had made no progress in replacing the more senior directors.

Howard Learned was the dean of the School of Business at Minnesota State University. He was 62 years old and had been on the board for nine terms of three years each. He was a professor of business when the CFO of the company was in business school getting an MBA. When the company went public and was recruiting a board, the CFO thought of his old professor. Learned brought good experience and knowledge to the board and added the prestige of having a business school dean on the board. Learned had chaired a number of committees over his board tenure, but, perhaps most importantly, he had chaired the Compensation Committee for the past 20 years. He also had served on the local board of a national bank.

Steven Scales was 60 years old, from a small town near the corporate headquarters and was the managing partner of a small law firm. He was known to the former CEO through years of golfing together, and his wife and the CEO's wife had been longtime friends. Steven Scales' legal knowledge had been essential in keeping Good Hands in regulatory compliance as they grew. Scales had chaired the Governance Committee, the Nominating Committee and the Audit Committee over his terms as a director. He did not serve on any other public board but was active on many civic boards in his community.

Norm Current, age 61, was a banker from Brownsville, Texas, where the corporation was founded. Although the corporate headquarters had since relocated, Current decided to stay on and maintained an excellent contact base among employees and legislators. He had chaired the Compensation and Audit Committees during his tenure and was a close, personal friend of the CEO. His behavior in board meetings had been very unpredictable and he tended to be somewhat volatile. He either contributed very little or contributed on issues he felt strongly about in an aggressive fashion, using terms that were sometimes inappropriate in the board setting. Current served on a variety of local civic boards and on the board of the community hospital.

Don Anson is 63 years old, an attorney and a former U.S. congressman. He had been friends with Jackson since college. They frequently went on fishing trips, hunting trips and vacations together with their wives. His national clout had been an important factor in getting things done in Washington in a highly regulated industry. He had chaired the Nominating Committee for most of the years he was on the board and also had chaired the Compensation Committee for several years. He was active in national politics and, since his retirement from Congress, served on the boards of various political organizations.

Frank Fowler, age 61, was an investment banker whose company did the earliest financing of Good Hands. Fowler's company also took the company public and held a significant portion of Good Hands' stock. He and Jackson had been hunting buddies for many years. Fowler was probably the board member who was the closest business advisor/confidant of the CEO. He served on the boards of various companies that his company had financed.

The three newer members of the board had been recruited by executive search firms and had no prior relationship with anyone on the board or on the management team.

Gerry Comco, age 62, was the retired CEO of a telecommunications company and lived in Boca Raton, Florida. He had been recruited during the time when the board was discussing a change to its strategy and wanted additional "out of industry" perspective. Comco was aggressive and outspoken, respected and liked by the rest of the board. He had recently been named chair of the Governance Committee and undertook a thorough review of the committee charters, calendars and board composition. Prior to leaving his company, he had served on its board of directors.

Mark Andrews was 58 years old, and was the senior vice-president (SVP) of a global company. This was his first experience on a public board but his professional background made him an excellent board member. He was well liked and spoke up about the most important issues. He had particular expertise in operations and could make some significant contributions as the company expanded its operating model beyond nursing home operations. He was the chairman of the Compensation Committee and had initiated an exhaustive review of the company's compensation policies and philosophy upon accepting the chairmanship. He served on the board of one of the subsidiaries of his company and was a competitive athlete.

Greg Simon, age 59, was a consultant, a former banker and presidential appointee to the board of a national regulatory agency. He was also an expert in the areas of corporate governance, strategy and risk. He had been asked to chair the Nominating Committee shortly after joining the board.

In this capacity he had initiated a formal process for evaluating the board and CEO. He sat on the boards of four public companies.

THE DECISION

Good Hands' board of directors knew the company was at a crossroads. Was the industry environment really the cause of Good Hands' sliding financial performance? What strategies would be necessary to stop the slide and regain Good Hands' dominant position? How would Good Hands weather the changing regulatory climate and reimbursement cuts? These were among many questions that the board knew had to be addressed to keep the company afloat and to ensure its survival as a viable entity in the future.

But, perhaps more pragmatically, was Jackson still the best CEO to lead Good Hands? Did he have the management team in place that could help chart a new course for the future? If not, who would take Jackson's place?

The board saw three primary alternatives. First, they could keep Jackson on as CEO and see how Good Hands fared in the coming months. But, could they continue to do so in light of the company's precarious financial position? Jackson had grown the company to its heights but also had presided over its recent decline. Had conditions changed so much that a new leader was needed? Most pragmatically, keeping Jackson in place would be the lowest cost option due to the nature of his employment contract. In 1997, the board (then consisting of Learned, Scales, Current, Anson and Fowler) had approved an employment contract for Jackson that would grant him in excess of $25 million (including severance, salary, options, benefits, etc.) if he were removed from his position as CEO (see Exhibit 2).

Second, the board could ask for Jackson's resignation and undertake a search for his replacement. Asking Jackson, the company's founder and leader for more than 30 years, to step down would be no easy task. If he left Good Hands, what would be the effect on the culture? How would the company make up for the loss of his experience and guidance? How would the board handle his severance payments when the company was already short on cash? Would they find a suitable replacement within Good Hands' top management team or would they need to look outside the company and/or industry? On the one hand, promoting from within would minimize additional losses in the top management team who may resign if they are overlooked for promotion. And, continuity in experience, strategy, etc. would be achieved by promotion within. On the other hand, was the board satisfied that any of the current top management team could

1. Proscription of responsibilities, duties and location of performance	Specifies Executive's obligations under the agreement
2. Duration	5 years, automatically renewed annually
3. Compensation and benefits treatment	Total package is composed of base salary, long- and short-term incentives and benefits (1999 approximately $3 million total)
4. Hold harmless/indemnification	Provides financial protection to the Executive for costs incurred in event of legal action and/or judgment against Executive as Director, Officer, employee or agent of the Corporation

5. Termination protection	Specifies protection provided in event of termination
	• Causes (defined) . . . payment of all accrued bonuses and vested long-term incentives
	• Without cause . . . payments equal to remaining term plus one year times salary, short-term bonuses and FMV of long-term incentives in event of:
	   – Diminution
	   – Office Move
	   – Change in control . . . single trigger; includes Excise tax
	   – Material breach by Good Hands
	• Disability/death . . . same as without cause
	• Benefit extension/credits and accelerated vesting of long-term incentives/equity in case of w/out cause term.
	• Lump sum payment option (trust arrangement)

6. Non-compete, non-solicitation and confidentiality	2 years
7. Attorney's fees	Reimbursement of all costs associated with legal actions taken to enforce/ interpret agreement, if Executive prevails
8. Arbitration	Requires arbitration to settle all contractual disputes

Exhibit 2. Key provisions of George Jackson's employment contract.

tackle the job and work well with them? Going outside could bring in some fresh perspectives that may be much needed as well as one potentially improving Good Hands' competitiveness via the insights into other companies' best practices and operating models.

Finally, the board saw a compromise position. Could they ask Jackson to give up his position as CEO yet stay on as chairman of the board? This option would be much easier than a total resignation and overcome the loss of his expertise, etc. Under this option, the board expected to keep Jackson's current compensation package, which totaled just over $3 million annually, intact but they would not be liable for any additional compensation because such a move would not trigger any additional severance under the terms of his agreement. But even at this generous pay package for a reduction in duties, would Jackson accept this? How much could a new CEO accomplish with Jackson still around and leading the board? And, what message would this send to Wall Street?

The board members knew the answers to these questions were not going to come easily. But, they felt they had to resolve the issues and resolve them quickly. They set their sights on their next board meeting in two months' time to make a succession decision on which alternative was the best to adopt.

13

The Day After

Richard L. Johnson
Physician Management Resources, Inc.,
Clarendon Hills, Illinois

Charlie Jones opened his eyes and looked at the clock, which stood at 7:40 A.M., then gazed up at the ceiling asking himself if he had just had a nightmare or if he really had been—terminated . . . let go . . . fired . . . relieved of his administrative responsibilities—whatever it was that Russell Adams, the board chairman, had said to him at 8:13 P.M. last night. It was then he had been informed that his services as the chief executive of Riley Memorial Hospital were no longer needed.

Automatically, after 23 years as the chief executive, his thoughts turned to the hospital. For the first time in more than 2 decades he realized that his day's activities no longer included the hospital, but were concerned with what he wanted to do for Charlie Jones. Getting out of bed, he realized that he could dress leisurely this morning and not have to hurry to get to work—there was, for him, no work to go to.

As he adjusted the hot water faucet in the shower, he began to ask himself why this had happened. Mentally reviewing various aspects of the hospital operation, he knew that the cost at Riley per patient day was next to the lowest of the seven hospitals in the area, so productivity was not a factor. The physical plant certainly was in A-1 condition. During the past 4 years, $3.5 million had been spent on bringing the mechanical and electrical systems up to date, and he had paid for those improvements out of

Adapted and reprinted with permission from "The Day After," by Richard L. Johnson, in *Hospital & Health Services Administration*, 30, no. 6 (November/December 1989): 106–117.

operating surpluses. No board member, that he could recall, had ever taken exception to this.

Certainly he and the board had been concerned that the average occupancy had fallen to the mid-60s in the last 18 months. This had forced the hospital to lay off 134 people to keep the hospital from going into the red. That had caused some problems with a few trustees; several physicians had gone to them and complained about the closing of two specialized nursing units and the commingling of their patients with those on the general medical and surgical floors. On balance, he concluded that the board had understood the necessity for taking these steps and that there had been general support for doing so.

As he stepped out of the shower, he directed his thoughts toward his relationships with the board and the medical staff and asked himself how the two had changed. What immediately came to mind was his inability to control the number of matters of importance that he had had to bring to the board. Because of the speed with which matters were changing in the external environment, he had lost the ability to time decision making with the pace at which the board could comfortably handle the items.

As he dressed, he realized that his greatest concern about the governing board was its lack of understanding of the medical staff and individual physician relationships to the hospital. He had known for well over a year that this was the most likely arena to give him problems. As the surplus of physicians had grown, coupled with the downturn in use of physicians and hospitals by the public, he had watched the medical staff become fearful of their economic futures. He had been particularly surprised by some of the older, well-established practitioners, who had been telling him that they had been experiencing a downturn in the number of patients they were seeing. He had instinctively known that this would inevitably lead to difficulties with these physicians because the hospital would be economically forced to compete for revenues on the same turf as the physicians on the medical staff. What bothered him the most was that he had seen this conflict coming, had tried to prepare the governing board for dealing with this kind of situation, but had had little success because of resistance from the four physicians on the governing board.

Pausing to look out the window, he let his eyes follow the path of the youngsters on their way to school as he recalled the difficulties he had encountered in a recent board meeting when he had attempted to review a proposed contract submitted by a health maintenance organization. Rather than reviewing the contract, as he had expected, the physicians had taken the position that the hospital's responsibility was to be supportive of private practitioners engaged in fee-for-service medicine and that the hospital should not be a party to any payment scheme that deviated from what was already in place. He remembered thinking, at the time, that the four physician board members probably regarded his actions as the first step in an attempt to take over the medical staff. After the board meeting, he had walked with the board chairman out to the parking lot, where they talked for almost an hour about what had happened, and the chairman had assured him that he knew those physicians and that they could be counted on to keep the hospital's needs and interests above those of the medical staff. Although he only half-believed what Russell Adams said, Charlie mentally conceded that this might indeed be true, given time and the changing events going on in the hospital field.

Charlie sat down to breakfast, staring out of the window, lost in thought. Thinking back over the last 6 months, he began to appreciate that his naming of Bill Handy as chief operating officer and turning over all of the internal operations to him, an action that had been fully endorsed by the board, had really never been understood or accepted by many of the physicians. They considered Charlie's role to consist primarily of serving the interests of the medical staff. The fact that he had little familiarity with the parking problem of physicians, which had surfaced at a general medical staff meeting, had led to comments being made in the corridors by physicians that Charlie Jones really didn't care whether Riley Memorial had a medical staff or not.

As he finished his cup of coffee, Charlie thought about the straw that broke the camel's back. All too vividly the events of the last 3 weeks rushed through his mind. On Monday, 3 weeks ago, Bill Handy told Charlie that he had received a call from a local real estate broker, with whom he was friendly, stating that the hospital's three radiologists had purchased a 2-acre site across the street from the hospital and were planning to build an ambulatory imaging center. Hearing this, Charlie had reached into a file drawer in his desk and quickly scanned the hospital's contract with the radiologists. Although there was no provision preventing them from investing in this kind of activity, the contract did specify that their full-time professional services were to be devoted to the hospital. The contract further specified that only the chief executive of the hospital could make any exceptions.

Armed with the contract, Charlie had gone to the radiology department and looked up Dr. Ralph Kemper, the chief, whom he'd known for the last 15 years. Sitting in Ralph's office drinking coffee together, he had asked him about the broker's information. Dr. Kemper, without hesitation, said that it was true, that they had the schematics in hand from the architect, and had a preliminary understanding with the largest local bank about a loan. When Charlie asked about the hospital's contract, Ralph indicated that the three radiologists had agreed they would not divert ambulatory patients from using the hospital and went on to add that the three planned to staff it on their days off and bring in one additional radiologist, who would be completing his residency in 3 months. They did not plan on bringing him into their partnership that served the hospital but planned to employ him by the new company, "Imaging Center, Inc.," the vehicle they'd created to undertake this venture.

Charlie finished his cup of coffee and left Ralph's office with a sinking feeling in the pit of his stomach that the wheels were now set in motion for a confrontation that could not be avoided. He knew that the three radiologists were regarded by their colleagues as the best in the city, and that any attempt made by the hospital to enforce its contract with them would create a real storm with the entire medical staff. Yet, to do nothing would lead to a significant loss in revenue; in spite of the assurances of the radiologists, it was clear that building an imaging center across the street from the hospital was no coincidence. Charlie knew he was caught in the middle without any workable alternatives. He remembered he had listed possibilities in his mind:

- Go along and do nothing.

- Threaten to terminate their contract.

- Have the board hold a session with them.

- Bring it up at the joint conference committee meeting.

- Find an alternative radiology group and give notice of cancellation of contract.

As he had mulled over the list, Charlie realized that the board would be willing to hold a meeting with the radiologists, but when the chips were down they would not force the issue. Instead, they somehow would expect the hospital management to develop a program that would compensate for lost revenues. At that point Charlie had smiled to himself; the safest way out for him was to make no waves and get along by going along. If he followed the course, it would be about 3 years before the impact would be felt in the financial statement of the hospital; in the meantime he could look around for another CEO position at his leisure and be out long before the hospital faced serious financial problems. He quickly rejected this notion, saying to himself that this was not in the hospital's best interests, yet he knew that he would be exposed if he took any other course. Although he hadn't anticipated his dismissal, he realized he had known that something like this was bound to occur, sooner or later. In fact, he had raised the question of a long-term contract for his services with the executive committee of the governing board 6 months earlier.

Charlie had pointed out at that meeting that the hospital field was undergoing rapid change that was adversely affecting the financial picture and that he could foresee a time ahead when he would be coming to the board with recommendations that would be highly unpopular with the medical staff but would be necessary to the financial viability of the hospital. His comments were politely received and it was indicated that this would be studied. He had heard nothing further on the subject and had found himself reluctant to again raise the issue.

As he looked back from his perspective of this morning, Charlie realized that he should have been much more forceful about a contract, but he'd been afraid that if he had brought up the subject a second time, he would have been turned down and then forced to decide whether to stay or to look seriously for another hospital. Had he looked around and received an offer from another hospital, he knew that one of the conditions of employment would be a contract. He knew this was becoming routine in CEO positions filled in the last couple of years. He also knew that CEOs with long tenure, such as he had, were seldom able to achieve the same results. Boards usually had to go through replacing one CEO for another in order to learn that competent executives were no longer willing to take chances with boards seeing issues realistically and were therefore seeking to protect themselves financially for taking on a job that had become increasingly risky in the last few years.

As he reviewed the contract situation, Charlie recalled two other instances in the past 3 years when he'd thought about the desirability of having a contract. The first had taken place during consideration of the hospital's constructing a medical office building 5 miles away in a newly developing area of the city. At that time he had discussed the idea with the medical executive committee, who had agreed with him about the timing and location of such a facility but had taken the position that this was a physician activity and the hospital should not be involved. They had been so adamant that Charlie had backed off without pursuing it. To this day he regretted not having gone ahead with the project.

The other incident had occurred about a year ago when Charlie had wanted to develop three off-site primary care centers. Again he had discussed it with the medical executive committee, as well as the executive committee of the governing board. Both groups had seen the desirability of this program, but as before, the physicians had taken the position that the hospital should not be involved. They had added a wrinkle to their argument that had led the board to agree with their position. The physicians claimed that, if the hospital went ahead, this would be the corporate practice of medicine. Charlie thought to himself, if I had a contract I would have pushed harder in both of those situations. Thinking back over those two instances, he realized that the physicians wanted to keep the hospital as an economic neutral in the health field and certainly did not want competition from hospitals in addition to what they already encountered from their own colleagues.

The difference between those two situations and this last problem with the radiologists was that this latest incident no longer kept the hospital neutral. As Charlie saw it, it would lead to a significant drop in radiology revenue, and therefore was a step beyond what had previously been the case. If he had had a contract, he would not have been forced to accept the political pressure so readily, but would have had more organizational flexibility to protect the best interests of the hospital. Looking to the future, he knew that his successor, whoever it might be, would need a contract if the hospital was to remain financially viable.

Grudgingly, Charlie had to admit to himself that, on "the day after," he sure wished he had had a contract. Knowing the board members as he did, he figured that they probably would give him 3 months' severance pay and the title to the hospital car he drove and wish him well.

At 54 years of age, he knew he had to find a position. He didn't have enough money saved to retire, nor did he want to, but he was concerned that his age would be a barrier to employment. Thinking about retirement, he suddenly realized that when the hospital had altered its pension plan 6 years ago, vesting had been an important issue but had ultimately been resolved by establishing a 10-year period and that prior employment in the hospital would not be counted. Thinking back on those discussions, he knew that, as of today, he would receive no pension benefits even though he had been at the hospital for 23 years. Ruefully, he admitted to himself that he had looked out for the interests of the hospital for a long time but he surely had ignored his own.

As he thought about the radiology problem that had brought everything to a head, he realized that physicians today were concerned with the growing surplus and the decline in the use of medical services by the public. They would take whatever steps they could to protect their incomes, even at the expense of the hospital. He admitted to himself that, if he were in their shoes, he would do the same.

After breakfast, Charlie decided to go for a walk and think about his own future. As he put on his jacket, he couldn't help but wonder what lay ahead for him and Myra, his wife. At his age, he speculated that he might not be too saleable in the marketplace, given the difficulties of managing a hospital in the last few years; he wasn't too sure that he wanted to go back to a hospital. He had been thinking for the last year or so that he ought to go into some kind of business for himself. As he thought about that possibility, he knew that any step in a new direction would require remortgaging his house; and, at his age, with one son still in college, he wasn't sure that taking such a risk was advisable. If the business failed, he would have nothing for the rest of his life. Turning the corner and starting to walk down the next block, he wondered what other kinds of work he might consider. Given his knowledge of a hospital, he wondered if he should go into consulting. This would be a field where he would be able to help others gain from his experiences and he'd also earn an excellent income. He thought he might look into that possibility, even though he wasn't sure how one goes about getting clients.

Another idea occurred to him—what about becoming president of an HMO? This was certainly a growing field that would need leadership. He knew the health field, had served for 6 years on the board of the Blue Cross plan, and always had an interest in prepayment. As he thought on, he concluded that claims management wouldn't be much different from the way accounts receivable are handled in the hospital, and marketing should be easy if the plan offers a good package of benefits.

Once again his thoughts turned to the events of the last few days. He knew that what had taken place was not a reflection on his administrative skills; he ran a good hospital and he knew it, but he had just gotten trapped by circumstances. When he had recommended to the board that they terminate the radiologists' contract by giving the required 90-day notice, because they were dead set on moving ahead, the board had assured him that they were all in accord that this was the proper course to follow. He remembered that he'd carefully drafted the letter to the radiologists clearly indicating that this was a board decision and that, acting as their agent, he was transmitting the action to them by letter. As a courtesy, he had sent a copy of the letter to the president of the medical staff. Although he knew the letter would create a problem, he had not been prepared for the storm that ensued.

For the 3 days following the receipt of the letter, the radiologists spent the majority of each day buttonholing as many members of the medical staff as possible, telling the physicians that Charlie Jones was taking steps to move them off of their percentage arrangement with the hospital to a salary basis, and that this was the reason behind his opposition to their building a new facility across the street.

By the end of the week, the president of the medical staff had called a special meeting of that body to discuss the hospital's intrusion into the private practice of medicine, which was held the following Wednesday evening in the hospital's cafeteria. Charlie recalled the meeting vividly—it was one of the worst he had ever attended. It started off with the president reading the copy of the letter to the entire medical staff. Charlie remembered looking around the room and thinking to himself that this was the largest turnout in the history of the hospital. When the president finished, a dozen hands shot up in the audience. The first one to his feet was a physician who seldom admitted a patient but was an outspoken critic of the administration. He quickly pointed out that the radiologists had as much right as others on the staff to go into another business for themselves, even if it was the same one in which they were engaged in the hospital. He, for one, would refer all of his ambulatory patients to them for imaging.

From the other side of the room, another physician stood, was recognized by the chair, and said that the real trouble with the hospital was not the medical staff but the administration. He said that the physicians had been asking for a private dining room for 3 years and it was still only a hope, that not enough parking spaces were provided for doctors, and that in his eyes Charlie Jones wanted to run the medical staff just as he did the rest of the hospital. What was really needed, he said, was a motion to terminate the administrator. This was immediately seconded, passed by a substantial majority with only a scattering of nays. The meeting was adjourned shortly thereafter.

At the next meeting of the board, Charlie had been excused after the routine matters had been disposed of, and he had gone back to his office knowing that the physician board members were going to present the staff recommendation. Although he had mentally counted noses during the time between the special medical staff meeting and this board meeting, he had made no attempt to meet individually with selected board members because he had told himself that after 23 years of service, the board had long ago come to a decision about his abilities and that they would therefore vote accordingly, if the question of his continued employment came to a vote. As far as he could tell, of the 13 board members, the 4 physician board members would vote in accordance with the wishes of the staff, the two lay board members would automatically vote with them as they always did, and the others would be in Charlie's corner. He thought it would be tight, but that he would win. When at 8:13 P.M. Russ Adams came to his office and informed him that he had been terminated, Charlie had been shocked. He knew he'd heard incorrectly. However, Russ had repeated the statement when he had asked him again.

Returning from his walk, Charlie slowly hung up his coat and began to recount the board vote of the previous evening. Russ Adams had told him that the vote had been close and he had lost by only the narrowest of margins. He took this to mean the vote had been 7 to 6 for terminating his services. That meant that one vote he had counted on had swung against him. As Charlie reviewed the possible swing votes, he realized that it really didn't matter. What he hadn't fully appreciated up to now was that a bloc of votes, even if less than a majority, can be effective in swaying a group decision. When the governing board had decided to include four physicians of the medical staff in their group 8 years ago, Charlie had not objected because the size of the board had been increased from 9 to 13 at the same time. He'd concluded that, because the physicians would only be one third of the votes, he really didn't have to be concerned. Now, in retrospect, he knew that it really did make a major difference, as he had witnessed on innumerable occasions when the four had voted together. He could recall no instance in which the board vote had been against the position of the physicians when they all voted alike. When the physicians had voted 3 to 1 on issues, Charlie remembered several times when the board would vote with the one and not the three, but, when the physicians all stood together, the rest of the governing board had always gone along with their thinking.

Having picked up the daily newspaper on his way into the house from his walk, Charlie sat down in his rocking chair in the living room, determined to take his mind off the events of the previous day. Finishing the sports section, he casually turned to the help wanted pages and scanned the columns, wondering if he would shortly be reading them carefully every day. The ringing of the phone interrupted his thoughts. Answering it, he found himself talking with an old friend, the chief executive of a large hospital in an adjoining state. He had just heard about Charlie's termination from Bill Handy, the COO at Riley. Charlie's friend had gone through a similar experience not too many years before and had found it traumatic. Like Charlie, on the day after, he wished he'd had a contract. When he took his present position he had been firm on the necessity for one, and, looking back, he told Charlie that, as the CEO of a hospital, he thought it to be the only prudent course to follow. He told Charlie that, before he had a contract, he had never realized the advantages of having one. He considered the recommendations he now made to his board to be more open and frank because of it. He was comfortable in this because of the economic safeguards that protected him in the event he had to make a choice between telling it like it is and providing the politically palatable answer or recommendation. He then asked Charlie if Charlie intended to retain an attorney.

Charlie admitted the thought had crossed his mind, and he was considering calling the hospital attorney. They had worked together for more than 15 years and had a warm, personal relationship. Charlie's friend immediately reacted to this comment by pointing out that Charlie should not do that because the attorney represents the hospital as his client, and Charlie has to appreciate that he may well become an adversary of the hospital, so he needs to discuss the matter with an attorney who is not associated with the hospital or any of its governing board members. Charlie acknowledged this made sense and thanked his friend for calling.

As he put down the telephone, Charlie began to consider more seriously the question of whether or not to discuss what had happened with an outside attorney. He recalled hearing in corridor conversations at the last meeting of the state hospital association that three chief executives had recently reached settlements of several hundreds of thousands of dollars each, after encountering similar situations with similar results.

He wondered if they had experienced any difficulties in finding a new position because they had sought legal remedies. Charlie thought about how he would answer the question, "Have you taken, or are you contemplating, any legal action against your former employer?" Would such an admission rule him out of further consideration? He wasn't sure, however, that he was still marketable, having crossed the 50-year mark a while back, in which case he wouldn't have to worry about answering such a question.

Then there was the question of whether or not it was ethical to sue the hospital. Not long ago, Charlie had terminated 134 employees because of the decline in census and not one of them had threatened to take the hospital to court. Was his situation so different? Yet, didn't his 23 years count for something? The more he thought about it, the more he thought he should at least sit down with an attorney experienced in this field and get an opinion as to what course he should follow. Having dealt with attorneys for years, he appreciated that seeking counsel didn't mean he would sue the board, but that he really needed to understand his current situation. Never having been fired before, he thought he might benefit from such a conversation.

With that, Charlie began considering calling Russ Adams and suggesting that the board may have overreacted the previous evening and might want to reconsider the action they had taken. Because the vote had been so close, one person changing positions would be enough to reverse the decision. Yet, the more he considered doing this, the more he realized that neither he nor the board members would forget what had taken place, and that it would color any situation that might be encountered in the future. Furthermore, suppose no one did change his vote in his favor? Suppose one or more of those who had voted for him elected to change their votes? All things considered, Charlie concluded, the best for all concerned would be not to contact Russ Adams. For better or worse, what was done was done, and he realized he needed to get on with his life. But, he vowed, I am not going to make the same mistakes in the future that I have in the past.

14

Hartland Memorial Hospital

In-Box and Priority-Setting Exercise,
Part 1 (REVISED)

Kent V. Rondeau
University of Alberta, Edmonton, Canada

John E. Paul
University of North Carolina at Chapel Hill

Jonathon S. Rakich
Indiana University Southeast, New Albany, Indiana

INTRODUCTION

Hartland Memorial Hospital, established 85 years ago when wealthy benefactor Sir Reginald Hartland left an estate valued at more than $2 million, is a 285-bed, free-standing community general hospital located in Westfield, a ski resort community of 85,000 people. Ridgeview Hospital is the only other hospital in the area, situated some 18 miles away in the village of Easton. Hartland Memorial is a fully accredited institution that provides a full range of medical and surgical services. It has an excellent reputation for delivering high-quality medical care for the citizens of Westfield and the surrounding area.

YOU AND THE HOSPITAL

You are Elizabeth Parsons, B.S.N., M.S.N., Ph.D., Vice President for Nursing Services at Hartland Memorial. You accepted this position 17 months ago and have been instrumental in introducing a number of innovations in nursing practice and management. In particular, these innovations have included the establishment of job sharing, self-scheduling, and a compressed workweek for all general-duty nurses. In addition, you have developed a new performance appraisal system and are contemplating using it to create a merit pay system for the nursing staff.

Your administrative assistant is Wilma Smith, who handles your correspondence and schedules meetings and conferences. Each morning she opens the hard-copy mail and memos that you have received and puts them on your desk. She also places hard-copy phone messages on your desk, from those people who did not want to be routed to your voice mail. Although she has access to your e-mail, voice mail, and electronic calendar, she does not routinely monitor them. Wilma is only moderately comfortable with the current modes of communication, generally preferring the ways of the "pre-electronic" era.

Your second-in-command is Anne Armstrong, who is Assistant Director for Nursing Services. Anne has worked at Hartland Memorial for 7 years and is very competent. She has only recently returned to work, however, after spending some time in the hospital recovering from the suicide of her husband.

A list of the key personnel at Hartland Memorial is presented in Exhibit 1, and selected biographical sketches can be found in Exhibit 2. The hospital's organization chart is presented in Exhibit 3.

THE SITUATION

You have just returned from a greatly needed long weekend off. At your husband's insistence, the two of you left Thursday evening for a mountain resort and just got back last night. Long hours, high stress, and constantly being accessible by cell phone, voice mail, and e-mail have been taking their toll—you seem to have been "on call" continuously for months now. Compounding the demands of these "curses of the modern job" has been the time you have had to devote to meeting the needs of your school-age children, as well as tending to your parents' needs (a recent development) as they grow older. In particular, your mom seems increasingly incapable of taking care of your dad, for whom some other living arrangement may have

Name	Position
Allan Reid	President and CEO
Scott Little	Assistant to the President
Elizabeth Parsons	Vice President–Nursing Services
Anne Armstrong	Assistant Director–Nursing Services
Cynthia Nichols	Vice President–Human Resources
Clement Westaway, MD	President–Medical Staff
Janet Trist	Nursing Supervisor–3 East
Sylvia Godfrey	Weekend Supervisor
Jane Sawchuck	Clinical Nurse Specialist
Norm Sutter	Vice President–Finance
Marion Simpson	Auditing Clerk
Fran Nixon	Staff Relations Officer
George Cross	Nurses Union Representative
Bernard Stevens	Chairman of the Board
Wilma Smith	Administrative Assistant

Exhibit 1. List of key personnel at Hartland Memorial Hospital

to be found. Caught between responsibilities to your kids and parents (to say nothing about your spouse), you are truly in the "sandwich" generation.

The weekend away, however, was wonderful. You were out of cell phone range, and the inn where you stayed did not make their computer generally available to guests. In any case, your husband would have probably left you if you'd logged on or called in.

Sunday night after returning home you had planned to log on and assess the situation facing you at work, after three blessed days out of touch. The kids, however, needed your attention and the dog needed walking. Mom also called and spoke with you for over an hour about what to do about Dad. You never got to your voice mail, either.

It is now 7:45 A.M. on Monday morning, and you have just a little over 1 hour until your first meeting of the day with Norm Sutter, Vice President for Finance. You really have to get through your e-mail, voice mail, and the hard-copy items that Wilma left on your desk—letters, phone messages, etc.—and take some action before meeting with Norm. You know that the rest of the day will be a blur and you'll have no further opportunities to get caught up. Moreover, new items will be coming in and piling up constantly.

Elizabeth Parsons	A professionally trained and degreed registered nurse (B.S.N., M.S.N., Ph.D.). Age 45, with 20 years of progressive management and nursing experience. Married, two children, ages 10 and 12.
Allan Reid	CEO at Hartland Memorial Hospital for 2 years. Age 35, with 6 years' experience as an assistant administrator at a 100-bed rural hospital. M.H.A. degree. Married, two children.
Bernard Stevens	Colonel, U.S. Army Infantry (retired). Chairman of the Board for Hartland Memorial Hospital for the past 12 years. Age 70. Widower, four grown children.
Clement Westaway, MD	Medical degree from the University of Pennsylvania. Internist. Member of the Hartland medical staff for 30 years and president of medical staff for the past 10 years. Age 64. Divorced, two grown children.
Anne Armstrong	Assistant Director for Nursing Services at Hartland for the past 5 years. M.S.N. degree. Age 35. Recently widowed, two children.
Janet Trist	Nursing Supervisor. Interrupted career at age 26 to raise her children. Resumed working 2 years ago. R.N. (diploma program). Age 41. Married.
Wilma Smith	Administrative Assistant in her present position for the past 15 years. Has worked at Hartland for 28 years. Age 50. Single, no children.

Exhibit 2.   Brief biographical sketches of key players at Hartland Memorial Hospital

The refreshed feeling you had after the weekend out of town is rapidly slipping away . . .

On Friday, Wilma left on your desk a hard copy of your schedule for the day, which is shown in Exhibit 4. You know that it likely will be changing.

WHAT NEEDS TO BE DONE

Exhibit 6 shows the various e-mails, voice mails, and hard-copy letters and messages that Elizabeth finds waiting for her when she arrives Monday morning. Wilma doesn't arrive until 8:30 A.M., so Elizabeth has the office

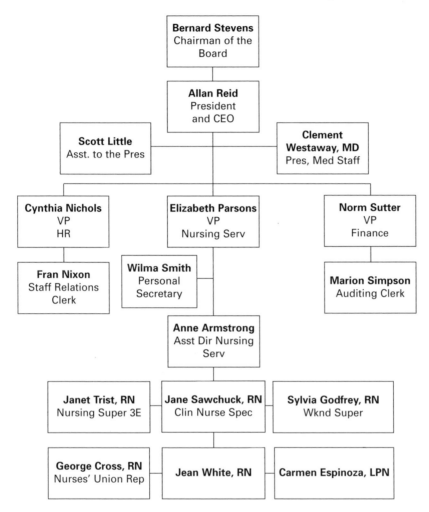

Exhibit 3. Hartland Memorial Hospital, partial organization chart.

to herself. Note that the Hartland Memorial IT system does a fairly good job of filtering out spam and junk mail. The occasional piece of spam does make it through, which Elizabeth immediately deletes. In addition, there are the e-newsletters to which Elizabeth subscribes from the Kaiser Family Foundation, the Commonwealth Fund, ACHE and so forth, but which she rarely has time to read. She tends to let these pile up in her in-box, which at times makes it difficult to find the critical items that she needs to

(as of 7:45 A.M.; left on your desk by Wilma, Friday afternoon at 5:00 P.M.)	
8:00 A.M.	
8:30	
9:00	Meeting with Norm Sutter
9:30	
10:00	Regular Monday morning meeting with nursing supervisors
10:30	
11:00	Meeting with Clement Westaway
11:30	
12:00 P.M.	Lunch with Anne Armstrong
12:30	"
1:00	Orientation talk to new nursing recruits
1:30	"
2:00	
2:30	Meeting of infection control committee
3:00	"
3:30	
4:00	Meeting with Allan Reid
4:30	"
5:00	
5:30	

Exhibit 4. Schedule of appointments, Monday, October 7

address immediately. (The newsletters and listserv items that came in over her mini-holiday are not included in the in-box items that follow.)

For each item, indicate on the worksheet, Hartland Memorial Hospital, In-Box Exercise (see Exhibit 5), the course of action you think Elizabeth should pursue. Be prepared to defend your underlying rationale. If delegating, identify who should be responsible for each item. *Work sequentially through each item.*

Because this case study may not contain all of the information or details needed to make a decision, please make any assumptions that you believe are necessary to justify your actions. Make notes of those assumptions on the worksheet.

Hartland Memorial Hospital, In-Box Exercise

Name _____ Sec/Team No. ____ Team Name _____

Item No.	Action Alternatives (check one)	Item Action Content (quick notes/ bullet points)
1. Scott Little (e-mail)	☐ Call immediately ☐ Note to call w/in 2–3 days ☐ Email immediately ☐ Email w/in day ☐ Meet with ASAP ☐ Forward to: _____ ☐ Note to meet w/in 2–3 days ☐ Other (specify:_____) ☐ No response needed	
2. Mable Westfield (letter)	☐ Call immediately ☐ Note to call w/in 2–3 days ☐ Email immediately ☐ Email w/in day ☐ Meet with ASAP ☐ Forward to: _____ ☐ Note to meet w/in 2–3 days ☐ Other (specify:_____) ☐ No response needed	
3. Mom (voice mail)	☐ Call immediately ☐ Note to call w/in 2–3 days ☐ Email immediately ☐ Email w/in day ☐ Meet with ASAP ☐ Forward to: _____ ☐ Note to meet w/in 2–3 days ☐ Other (specify:_____) ☐ No response needed	
4. Allan Reid (e-mail)	☐ Call immediately ☐ Note to call w/in 2–3 days ☐ Email immediately ☐ Email w/in day ☐ Meet with ASAP ☐ Forward to: _____ ☐ Note to meet w/in 2–3 days ☐ Other (specify:_____) ☐ No response needed	

Exhibit 5. Worksheet—*(continued)*

5. Sylvia Godfrey
   (e-mail)

   ☐ Call immediately
   ☐ Note to call w/in 2–3 days
   ☐ Email immediately
   ☐ Email w/in day
   ☐ Meet with ASAP
   ☐ Forward to: _____
   ☐ Note to meet w/in 2–3 days
   ☐ Other (specify: _____)
   ☐ No response needed

6. Janet Trist
   (e-mail)

   ☐ Call immediately
   ☐ Note to call w/in 2–3 days
   ☐ Email immediately
   ☐ Email w/in day
   ☐ Meet with ASAP
   ☐ Forward to: _____
   ☐ Note to meet w/in 2–3 days
   ☐ Other (specify: _____)
   ☐ No response needed

7. Westfield High School
   (letter)

   ☐ Call immediately
   ☐ Note to call w/in 2–3 days
   ☐ Email immediately
   ☐ Email w/in day
   ☐ Meet with ASAP
   ☐ Forward to: _____
   ☐ Note to meet w/in 2–3 days
   ☐ Other (specify: _____)
   ☐ No response needed

8. Marion Simpson
   (e-mail)

   ☐ Call immediately
   ☐ Note to call w/in 2–3 days
   ☐ Email immediately
   ☐ Email w/in day
   ☐ Meet with ASAP
   ☐ Forward to: _____
   ☐ Note to meet w/in 2–3 days
   ☐ Other (specify: _____)
   ☐ No response needed

9. Wilma
   (written note)

   ☐ Call immediately
   ☐ Note to call w/in 2–3 days
   ☐ Email immediately
   ☐ Email w/in day
   ☐ Meet with ASAP

Exhibit 5. Worksheet—*(continued)*

☐ Forward to: _____
☐ Note to meet w/in 2–3 days
☐ Other (specify:_____)
☐ No response needed

10. Cynthia Nichols
    (e-mail)

☐ Call immediately
☐ Note to call w/in 2–3 days
☐ Email immediately
☐ Email w/in day
☐ Meet with ASAP
☐ Forward to: _____
☐ Note to meet w/in 2–3 days
☐ Other (specify:_____)
☐ No response needed

11. Marion Simpson
    (memo)

☐ Call immediately
☐ Note to call w/in 2–3 days
☐ Email immediately
☐ Email w/in day
☐ Meet with ASAP
☐ Forward to: _____
☐ Note to meet w/in 2–3 days
☐ Other (specify:_____)
☐ No response needed

12. Norm Sutter
    (phone message)

☐ Call immediately
☐ Note to call w/in 2–3 days
☐ Email immediately
☐ Email w/in day
☐ Meet with ASAP
☐ Forward to: _____
☐ Note to meet w/in 2–3 days
☐ Other (specify:_____)
☐ No response needed

13. Scott Little
    (memo)

☐ Call immediately
☐ Note to call w/in 2–3 days
☐ Email immediately
☐ Email w/in day
☐ Meet with ASAP
☐ Forward to: _____
☐ Note to meet w/in 2–3 days
☐ Other (specify:_____)
☐ No response needed

Exhibit 5. Worksheet—*(continued)*

14. Wilma
(written note)

☐ Call immediately
☐ Note to call w/in 2–3 days
☐ Email immediately
☐ Email w/in day
☐ Meet with ASAP
☐ Forward to: _____
☐ Note to meet w/in 2–3 days
☐ Other (specify: _____)
☐ No response needed

15. Coach Bailey
(e-mail)

☐ Call immediately
☐ Note to call w/in 2–3 days
☐ Email immediately
☐ Email w/in day
☐ Meet with ASAP
☐ Forward to: _____
☐ Note to meet w/in 2–3 days
☐ Other (specify: _____)
☐ No response needed

16. Jane Sawchuck
(e-mail)

☐ Call immediately
☐ Note to call w/in 2–3 days
☐ Email immediately
☐ Email w/in day
☐ Meet with ASAP
☐ Forward to: _____
☐ Note to meet w/in 2–3 days
☐ Other (specify: _____)
☐ No response needed

17. Allan Reid
(e-mail)

☐ Call immediately
☐ Note to call w/in 2–3 days
☐ Email immediately
☐ Email w/in day
☐ Meet with ASAP
☐ Forward to: _____
☐ Note to meet w/in 2–3 days
☐ Other (specify: _____)
☐ No response needed

18. Scott Little
(e-mail)

☐ Call immediately
☐ Note to call w/in 2–3 days
☐ Email immediately
☐ Email w/in day
☐ Meet with ASAP

Exhibit 5.   Worksheet—*(continued)*

☐ Forward to: _____
☐ Note to meet w/in 2–3 days
☐ Other (specify:_____)
☐ No response needed

19. Bernard Stevens
    (phone message)

☐ Call immediately
☐ Note to call w/in 2–3 days
☐ Email immediately
☐ Email w/in day
☐ Meet with ASAP
☐ Forward to: _____
☐ Note to meet w/in 2–3 days
☐ Other (specify:_____)
☐ No response needed

20. Dr. Clement Westaway
    (e-mail)

☐ Call immediately
☐ Note to call w/in 2–3 days
☐ Email immediately
☐ Email w/in day
☐ Meet with ASAP
☐ Forward to: _____
☐ Note to meet w/in 2–3 days
☐ Other (specify:_____)
☐ No response needed

21. Cynthia Nichols
    (e-mail)

☐ Call immediately
☐ Note to call w/in 2–3 days
☐ Email immediately
☐ Email w/in day
☐ Meet with ASAP
☐ Forward to: _____
☐ Note to meet w/in 2–3 days
☐ Other (specify:_____)
☐ No response needed

22. What do you do now?
    Allan Reid
    (on the phone)

☐ Call immediately
☐ Note to call w/in 2–3 days
☐ Email immediately
☐ Email w/in day
☐ Meet with ASAP
☐ Forward to: _____
☐ Note to meet w/in 2–3 days
☐ Other (specify:_____)
☐ No response needed

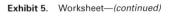

Exhibit 5. Worksheet—*(continued)*

Team Summary/Consensus:

1. Aside from the last item (#22), which are the <u>four</u> most critical items to address? (Indicate item numbers below.)

   _____

2. Think of reasons why these four items are the most critical. *What professional/personal values and priorities do they reflect?*

3. Total number of items marked:

   Call immediately _____   Note to call w/in 2–3 days _____

   E-mail immediately _____   E-mail w/in day _____

   Meet with ASAP _____   Forward to _____

   Note to meet w/in 2–3 days _____   Other: _____

   No response needed _____

4. Looking back on the work you have just laid out, is it feasible to accomplish in the time constraints faced by this administrator? What happens next? What techniques would your group suggest for Elizabeth to make it successfully through this day?

Notes/Comments:

_____
_____
_____

Exhibit 5. Worksheet

ITEM 1: E-MAIL

To: Elizabeth Parsons, VP–Nursing Services

From: Scott Little, Assistant to the President

Date: October 4   8:00 AM

Subject: Wandering patient—IMPORTANT!

On Thursday evening, Mrs. Grace O'Brien, a patient with diabetes and Alzheimer's disease, was missing from her room when her daughter came to visit her. It took the staff more than 3 hours to finally locate her. She was found naked and unconscious in the basement washroom of the Stuart Annex. Her daughter is extremely upset and is threatening to sue the hospital.

We don't need another lawsuit!!!

—Scott

ITEM 2: LETTER

September 26

President, Hartland Memorial Hospital

Eliz: Please note.
What actions are needed?
—Allan

Dear Sir,

I have been a patient in your hospital on three different occasions over the last 4 years. In the past I have been very satisfied with the nursing care that I have received; however, my last stay there has left much to be desired. For the most part I have found that many of your nurses are very rude and arrogant. A number of times when I asked these people for assistance, they would either refuse to help me, tell me they were too busy, or ignore me altogether.

I have great respect for Hartland Hospital and I trust that you would want to correct this problem. My late husband, Horace, was once a trustee at your hospital and would never have allowed this to happen.

Sincerely,

Mable Coleman Westfield

Mable Coleman Westfield

Exhibit 6. Elizabeth Parson's "In-Box" Monday, October 7, 7:30 A.M.—*(continued)*

ITEM 3:   VOICE MAIL MESSAGE

To: Elizabeth Parsons

From: Your mother

Date: Monday 7:30 AM

(Voice message left at 7:30 AM on office phone—you forgot to turn on your cell phone driving into work.)

"Elizabeth, this is Mom. I tried to get you before you left home this morning, but just missed you—Dad got up today upset and saying that 'he was a burden.' He's gone back to sleep now. What should I do??? Please call when you get a chance!"

ITEM 4:   E-MAIL

To: Elizabeth Parsons, VP–Nursing Services

From: Allan Reid, President/CEO

Date: October 4

Time: 2:10 P.M.

Subject: EOM

I have heard that a number of other hospitals have been very successful at motivating their staff by implementing employee recognition programs. These programs can go a long way toward increasing employee commitment and morale. I would like to institute an "Employee-of-the-Month" award here at Hartland. I have a few ideas and would like to discuss them with you.

—A.

Exhibit 6.   Elizabeth Parson's "In-Box" Monday, October 7, 7:30 A.M.—*(continued)*

ITEM 5:   E-MAIL

To: Elizabeth Parsons, VP–Nursing Services

From: Sylvia Godfrey, RN, Weekend Supervisor

Date: October 6

Time: 9:07 P.M.

Subject: Insufficient staffing

Again this weekend we had a number of nurses call in sick and we were subsequently short staffed. I had to call in nurses from the "availability list" that was provided by the Temp Placement Agency. I don't really think these nurses are any good because they are poorly trained and make too many errors. I am sick and tired of having to go through this **hassle every week!**

—Sylvia

ITEM 6:   E-MAIL

To: Elizabeth Parsons, VP–Nursing Services

From: Janet Trist, RN, Supervisor–3 East

Date: October 4

Time: 1:23 P.M.

Subject: Scheduling problems

I am really having a problem with this new self-scheduling system that we adopted last month. A number of my senior nurses are refusing to go along with it and are threatening to quit unless we go back to the old system. It's affecting the morale on my unit and making my life miserable. We need to discuss this right away.

—Janet

Exhibit 6.   Elizabeth Parson's "In-Box" Monday, October 7, 7:30 A.M.—*(continued)*

ITEM 7:   LETTER

WESTFIELD HIGH SCHOOL

September 28

Elizabeth Parsons
Vice President–Nursing Services
Hartland Memorial Hospital, Westfield

Dear Mrs. Parsons:

The Future Careers Club of Westfield High School would like to invite you to be the guest speaker at our November meeting. The meeting will be held on November 14 at 8:00 P.M. in the school auditorium. We would like you to discuss "The Changing Role of the Professional Nurse."

We believe that your presentation will be quite informative for us because several of our students are interested in pursuing a nursing career.

We hope that you will be able to accept this invitation. Please call our sponsor, Mrs. Bonnie Tartabull, to confirm at your earliest convenience. Thank you.

Sincerely,

Kathy Muller

Kathy Muller
President, Westfield High Future Careers Club

Exhibit 6.   Elizabeth Parson's "In-Box" Monday, October 7, 7:30 A.M.—*(continued)*

ITEM 8: E-MAIL

To: Elizabeth Parsons, VP–Nursing Services

From: Marion Simpson, Auditing

Date: October 4

Time: 9:45 A.M.

Subject: Hours of work for part-time nurses

Once again, many part-time nurses are working between 25 and 30 hours per week. If we permit this to continue, under the terms of the collective agreement, we must give full-time benefits to those involved.

The agreement states that full-time benefits must be given to those working in excess of 25 hours per week.

The actual number of hours worked per week for part-timers averaged 24.5 hours for the month of September.

—Marion Simpson

ITEM 9: WRITTEN NOTE FROM WILMA

To: Elizabeth Parsons

From: Scott Little, Assistant to the President

Time: 10:20 AM

Mr. Little called, but did not leave a message.

Exhibit 6. Elizabeth Parson's "In-Box" Monday, October 7, 7:30 A.M.—*(continued)*

ITEM 10:   E-MAIL

To: Elizabeth Parsons, Vice President–Nursing Services

From: Cynthia Nichols, Vice President–Human Resources

Date: October 2

Time: 4:45 P.M.

Subject: Sexual harassment charges

STRICTLY CONFIDENTIAL

We have just received a notification from a nurse employed here at Hartland alleging sexual harassment by one of our physicians on staff. The charges, if verified, are extremely serious. I would like to appoint you, along with Fran Nixon, from our staff relations department, and George Cross, union representative for the nurses' association, to form a committee to investigate these charges. I have been told that the individual claiming harassment has already begun legal action, so we need to proceed with haste.

—Cynthia Nichols, Vice President

ITEM 11:   MEMO

To: Elizabeth Parsons, Vice President–Nursing Services

From: Marion Simpson, Auditing

Date: October 3

Subject: Reimbursement for travel

Regarding your request for travel reimbursement for your upcoming conference, I regret to inform you that you have already used up this year's travel budget allocation and therefore will not be reimbursed from this account.

Marion Simpson

Exhibit 6. Elizabeth Parson's "In-Box" Monday, October 7, 7:30 A.M.—*(continued)*

ITEM 12: TELEPHONE MESSAGE

To: Elizabeth Parsons

From: Norm Sutter

Date: October 4

Time: 3:05 PM

Mr. Sutter called and asked if next year's budget projections for nursing have been finished. He needs these figures by Monday.

ITEM 13: MEMO

To: Elizabeth Parsons, VP–Nursing Services

From: Scott Little, Assistant to the President

Date: October 3

Subject: United Way Campaign

This is a follow up to our discussion of last week concerning the appointment of someone from your department to serve as a representative for our hospital's annual United Way Campaign. I need to have the name of your representative by Friday, October 4th.

—Scott

ITEM 14: WRITTEN NOTE FROM WILMA

To: Elizabeth Parsons

Date: October 4

Time: 2:12 PM

Mr. Stevens dropped in and was looking for you. He seemed quite upset and was muttering something about a lawsuit. He wants you to call him as soon as you get back from your trip.

—Wilma

Exhibit 6. Elizabeth Parson's "In-Box" Monday, October 7, 7:30 A.M.—*(continued)*

ITEM 15:   E-MAIL

To: Elizabeth Parsons, Vice President–Nursing Services

From: Coach Bailey

Date: October 4

Time: 4:45 P.M.

Subject: Snacks needed!!

Ms. Parsons—

Can you **please** bring the snacks for the team for Jimmy's softball game Monday night? Several other moms have already said they couldn't! Please confirm if this is OK.

Thanks so much!! You're the true "Super Mom"!

Regards, Coach Bailey

ITEM 16:   E-MAIL

To: Elizabeth Parsons, VP–Nursing Services

From: Jane Sawchuck, Clinical Nurse Specialist

Date: October 3

Subject: Nosocomial Infections

It has come to my attention that, again last month, we have recorded high levels of Staphylococcus and Pseudomonas in operating rooms B and C. It is becoming apparent that we need to review our standard procedures in this area before an epidemic breaks out.

—Jane

Exhibit 6.   Elizabeth Parson's "In-Box" Monday, October 7, 7:30 A.M.—*(continued)*

ITEM 17:   E-MAIL

To: Elizabeth Parsons

From: Allan Reid

Date: October 3

Time: 7:00 PM

Subject: Need a favor!

My niece, Jennifer, just graduated from nursing school and will be in town just one day, Monday, October 7. She is looking for a job in her field and I have asked her to talk to you. She is a delightful girl. Would you please see her?

—Allan

ITEM 18:   E-MAIL

To: Elizabeth Parsons, VP–Nursing Services

From: Scott Little, Assistant to the President

Date: October 4

Time: 7:34 AM

Subject: Nurse working illegally

Carmen Espinoza, the woman I talked to you about, was working illegally for us. She was using a stolen Social Security number. The Immigration and Naturalization Services (INS) contacted me yesterday, and a representative will be coming Monday afternoon to inquire about the matter.

Please give me a call right away.

—Scott

Exhibit 6.   Elizabeth Parson's "In-Box" Monday, October 7, 7:30 A.M.—*(continued)*

ITEM 19:   TELEPHONE MESSAGE

(Wilma intercepted the call and took a message; she put the note in front of you.)

To: Elizabeth Parsons

From: Bernard Stevens, Chairman of the Board

Date: October 7

Time: 8:55 AM

Mr. Stevens just called and says that he needs to meet with you and Allan Reid this morning at 10:00 AM

ITEM 20:   E-MAIL

To: Elizabeth Parsons, Vice President–Nursing Services

From: Dr. Clement Westaway, President–Medical Staff

Date: October 2

Time: 12:34 PM

Subject: Nurse–physician relations

Further to our discussion last week concerning the pressing need to improve communication between physicians and nurses at Hartland Memorial, I am hoping that the suggestions that I gave you will be successfully implemented by your staff. Remember, we are all trying to provide the best possible medical care for our patients.

—C.W., MD

Exhibit 6. Elizabeth Parson's "In-Box" Monday, October 7, 7:30 A.M.—*(continued)*

ITEM 21:   E-MAIL

To: Elizabeth Parsons, Vice President–Nursing Services

From: Cynthia Nichols, VP–Human Resources

Date: October 3

Time: 2:15 PM

Subject: Firing Ms. Jean White, R.N.

As we discussed yesterday, it is important to conduct the termination interview of nurse Jean White as soon as possible. Her last day of work at Hartland will be October 18 and, according to our collective agreement, she requires 2 weeks' notice. Please call me when the deed is done.

—Cynthia Nichols, VP–HR

Exhibit 6. Elizabeth Parson's "In-Box" Monday, October 7, 7:30 A.M.—*(continued)*

STOP!

Do not proceed to the next page until you have responded to all previous items (1–21) in the in-box.

ITEM 22:   TELEPHONE CALL (**LIVE**)

Time: 9:45 AM, Monday, October 7

Allan Reid calls and tells you that Mrs. Grace O'Brien, the patient with diabetes and Alzheimer's disease, is again missing from her room, apparently since late last night. He advises you that he was just informed of this by a local newspaper reporter who had gotten wind of the story. He instructs you to call Mrs. O'Brien's daughter to tell her of this recent development before she hears or reads about it in the media. Reid gives you no opportunity to respond, saying, "I have the reporter on the other line and have to go."

He then hangs up the telephone.

Exhibit 6.   Elizabeth Parson's "In-Box" Monday, October 7, 7:30 A.M.

15

The Bad Image
Radiology Department

Kurt Darr
The George Washington University, Washington, D.C.

HISTORY AND SETTING

MacMillan Hospital was established in a metropolitan area of the southeastern United States in the decade following the Civil War. It was named for Abner MacMillan, a successful lumber and hardware merchant whose business had prospered at war's end when there was a great need for rebuilding in his war-ravaged region. The hospital was originally located in a large, colonnaded antebellum home that was MacMillan's residence before his death. In addition to the house, MacMillan had donated the 40 acres on which it stood and $50,000—a large sum in the 1870s—for the charitable purposes to which the hospital was to be dedicated. Originally named for the city in which it was located, the board voted to change the name after MacMillan's death.

In the 125 years since MacMillan Hospital was established, it has undergone numerous building projects and renovations. By the late 1990s it was licensed for 350 beds, but operated only 250, which have an average occupancy rate of 75%. The parcel of land was large enough that construction and renovation could occur without the need to move the hospital. The original house had been restored and at present is occupied by the hospital's administrative offices.

MacMillan Hospital offers all primary and secondary acute care inpatient services. A few tertiary services are available: autologous bone marrow transplant services, neonatal intensive care, cardiac catheterization, and radiation oncology. Annual outpatient admissions exceed 50,000. Its busy emergency department has more than 25,000 admissions annually. The hospital has just over 1,000 full-time equivalent (FTE) employees. MacMillan has no bargaining units, but there are occasional rumors that union organizers have talked to employees.

MacMillan's service area has two hospitals of similar size that offer similar services. Many area physicians have privileges at all three hospitals. MacMillan has several advantages, however. It has enjoyed a good reputation in its service area and its competitors face natural barriers that include two rivers and a range of foothills. MacMillan's competitors are not served by public transportation; the road system favors it, as well. The service area has several physician-owned, freestanding centers that offer urgent care, imaging, and ambulatory surgical services. A small psychiatric care facility offers inpatient alcohol and drug detoxification services and rehabilitation. MacMillan and its competitors refer complex cases to the university hospital, which is 75 miles distant.

In terms of hospital-based physicians MacMillan has contracts with five different physician groups that independently provide anesthesiology, cardiology, emergency medicine, clinical and anatomical laboratory, and medical imaging (radiology) services. These concessionaires use equity-owner physicians as well as physician employees to provide services. As is true in most hospitals, these clinical departments at MacMillan are closed—which means that only physicians in the group or employed by the group may have privileges in them. Nonetheless, physicians must go through the usual credentialing process. Nonphysician staff in these five clinical areas are employed by the hospital, but their work is directly supervised and evaluated clinically by physicians in the group. This split between supervision and employment is common in health services delivery. The resulting matrix-type approach facilitates delivery of services by improving coordination and communication, but divides employee loyalty, blurs lines of authority and reporting, and violates Henri Fayol's principle of unity of command. MacMillan has been continuously accredited by The Joint Commission on Accreditation of Healthcare Organizations. The "deemed" status provided by Joint Commission accreditation is important for reimbursement of Medicare and Medicaid patients, which represent 35% of admissions.

BOARD OF TRUSTEES

MacMillan Hospital is governed by a 21-member board of trustees, who are true trustees because they are responsible for the trust originally established by Abner MacMillan. The board is self-perpetuating, which means that it nominates and selects replacement trustees. Trustees serve 3-year terms, and they may be renominated for two additional terms. One third of terms expire each year. The hospital CEO is an *ex officio* member of the board, but has no vote. Board committees include executive, professional staff organization (PSO), human resources, strategic planning, budget and fiscal, quality evaluation, and nominating. The executive committee meets monthly and is comprised of the chair of the board and the chairs of the seven committees. The board bylaws require that committees meet at least quarterly, but they are subject to call of the chairs.

The board chair is Harriet Buchanan, a retired schoolteacher and community leader. She recently started her second 3-year term as chair and is seen by other board members and management as dedicated, well intentioned, and reasonably effective. The board is comprised of interface stakeholders who are social and economic leaders in the community and who are of various ages and ethnic backgrounds. Three are physicians who are members of the active medical staff at MacMillan and not part of a contract group. The board has been active and successful in strategic planning and fundraising. It emphasizes the hospital's financial performance and uses that as a major basis for judging management's success. Implementation of board policy decisions (resolutions) is left to senior management and there is no review of day-to-day performance. The PSO committee makes recommendations through the executive committee after it reviews credentialing recommendations of the PSO, which have come to it through the PSO credentialing and executive committees.

THE PROFESSIONAL STAFF ORGANIZATION (PSO)

The professional staff at MacMillan Hospital are organized, self-governing, and quasi autonomous; like the overwhelming majority of hospital medical staffs, it has chosen not to be a separate corporation. Although legally subordinate to the board of trustees because its bylaws (and revisions), as well as PSO appointments and clinical privileges, must be approved by the board, the PSO sees itself as a partner in the full range of hospital activities. As is typical in private (nongovernmental) hospitals the PSO has bylaws that describe its organizational structure, including officers, committees, and policies. There are also PSO "Rules and Regulations" that include specific procedures and rules. In addition to the vice president for medical affairs (VP/MA) who is appointed by the CEO (with approval of the board) and is part of administration, the PSO elects a president who represents the PSO to administration and the board. PSO standing committees include executive, credentials, bylaws, technology, nominating, quality assurance, and medical records. The chairs of the standing committees serve on the executive committee, whose presiding officer is the president of the PSO.

There are 920 physicians on MacMillan's PSO, of whom 200 are active. In addition to physicians, the PSO bylaws allow doctors of podiatric medicine (DPM), certified registered nurse anesthetists (CRNAs), and certified nurse midwives (CNMs) to be members of the PSO. Podiatrists' privileges are determined individually. Privileges for the CRNAs and CNMs are determined as a group; they have a vote on the PSO, but may not hold office. The PSO bylaws define "active" as physicians who admit five or more inpatients per year. For purposes of defining active, three outpatient admissions are considered equal to one inpatient admission. Only active members of the PSO are allowed to hold office or chair committees. All members of the PSO may vote on general matters such as elections; the vote on matters such as amending the bylaws, however, is limited to active staff.

Hospitals commonly use *locum tenens* physicians to temporarily staff hospital-based physician clinical departments. The PSO bylaws at MacMillan allow appointment of *locum tenens* physicians and state in part:

> All appointments to the PSO shall be reviewed by the PSO department, which is to be the applicant physician's primary department.... The department chair shall make a recommendation to the credentials committee as to the appropriateness of the appointment and the suitability of the clinical privileges requested by the applicant, in consultation with such members of the department as are deemed appropriate. All appointments shall be subject to approval by the board of trustees.

Historically, this provision has been interpreted to include *locum tenens* appointments and temporary physicians have been processed consistent with this provision. Ultimately, as is universal practice for hospitals, the board at MacMillan approves all appointments to the PSO and the specific privileges of each individually credentialed member of the PSO, or the credentials held by groups such as the CRNAs.

ADMINISTRATION

MacMillan's chief executive is Jack Gargon, who was appointed 15 years ago. Gargon is 60 years old and holds a master's degree from an accredited health services administration program. He is a Fellow of the American College of Healthcare Executives and has more than 25 years of senior-level experience. A first task on assuming his duties at MacMillan was to reorganize the management hierarchy. One of the goals was to reduce the number of middle managers in anticipation of reduced reimbursement because of implementation of the federal diagnosis-related groups payment system. The resulting structure was much flatter and had fewer middle managers. The board was very pleased with the reorganization and other efficiencies Gargon implemented and concluded that he was a capable and technically proficient manager. Mr. Gargon's elimination of middle management, however, caused significant grumbling among surviving middle managers who had seen friends and colleagues fired. Satisfied that its internal operations were under control, the board increasingly turned its attention to external responsibilities. Gargon's reputation in the hospital is that of a capable and technically proficient manager who gives his management team wide latitude in decision making. He expects them to solve problems on their own and not to bother him unless his specific assistance or intervention is needed.

Gregory Halton is Gargon's vice president for clinical services (VP/CS). Halton is 27 years old and has been at MacMillan since he completed a postgraduate internship there 5 years ago. Prior to being promoted to VP/CS 2 years ago, he was responsible for strategic planning and marketing. He holds a bachelor of science in health services management and is working part-time on his master's degree; his areas of responsibility include medical imaging. Halton is seen by his hospital colleagues as enthusiastic, hardworking, and work-oriented. He can be stubborn, however, and occasionally peers have questioned his judgment.

The guidelines for managers who are responsible for clinical departments are general and unwritten, but reflect long-standing custom at MacMillan. Managers are expected to focus on the nonphysician staff and to leave the review of physicians' activities to the VP/MA and the PSO. The chief technologist in medical imaging, for example, reports to the clinical department head for clinical matters and to the VP/CS for administrative matters, which results in a matrix-type arrangement. The clinical chief and the responsible manager jointly do evaluations of the performance of support staff in clinical departments. Halton is administratively responsible for the Department of Medical Imaging, which until recently was known as the Department of Radiology.

The VP/MA position has been vacant for 6 months, despite efforts to recruit a replacement for the previous incumbent who retired.

MEDICAL IMAGING

The chief of medical imaging is Harold Goodview, M.D., a board-certified radiologist. Goodview is the majority stockholder in Good Views Medical Imaging, LLC, the professional corporation that has had an exclusive contract to provide radiographic services at MacMillan for the past 15 years. Goodview's wife and her family are minority stockholders. Two years ago, MacMillan and Good Views signed a 5-year extension of the basic contract. Good Views employs all the radiologists, including Goodview, who is both an employee and an owner.

The Department of Medical Imaging is extraordinarily busy and has a volume of more than 100,000 cases per year. There are 40 FTE radiologic technologists and 27 FTE file room clerks, secretaries, receptionists, and transporters. The technologists include radiographers, cardiovascular-interventional technologists, sonographers, radiation therapists, and magnetic resonance imaging technologists. Each area of activity has a lead technologist. There is a chief technologist for the entire department who functions as the department administrator. The department performs a wide range of radiographic studies including plain film studies, contrast studies, intravenous pyelograms, magnetic resonance imaging (MRI), computed tomography (CT), needle biopsies, drainages, nuclear medicine, ultrasound, and interventional procedures such as angiograms and stent placements.

The terms of the contract between MacMillan and Good Views are typical for the field. MacMillan provides and maintains all capital and noncapital equipment. It provides and maintains the space and all supplies and consumables, including disposables. MacMillan employs the nonphysician staff. The hospital is paid for its work by budgetarily apportioning part of the DRGs for Medicare and Medicaid patients and by billing other third-party payers and the small number of self-pay directly. Good Views has a contract billing service that does the billing for the professional fee charged by the radiologists. Part B pays for Medicare beneficiaries; Medicaid, other third-party payers, and self-pay patients are billed directly. Primarily because of the high volume, this basic arrangement has been very financially rewarding for both parties.

Relationships with administration have generally been business-like, if distant. Goodview prefers "dealing with the top" and calls Gargon whenever there is a problem that needs attention. Even when there was a VP/MA, Gargon rarely involved her in any departmental problems. Being bypassed in this manner greatly annoys Halton, but the pattern was established before he came to MacMillan. Halton has mentioned the problem to Gargon several times, but Gargon has taken no action. Believing this reflects a lack of support in terms of his role in medical imaging, Halton has been reluctant to challenge Goodview's actions directly. Consequently, Halton has been embarrassed numerous times when he learned about decisions affecting his responsibilities in medical imaging from the chief technologist. Halton's efforts to develop a more effective working relationship have been rebuffed by Goodview.

Historically, Goodview has had difficulty keeping radiologists employed in his company and, thus, in staffing the department. When Good Views Medical Imaging first obtained the exclusive concession to provide radiology services, the group had four equal partners. Over the years Goodview bought them out when they wanted to leave. His long-term employed radiologists have become fewer and fewer; currently there are only two, Drs. Banda and Leipzig. In addition, there are several *locum tenens* radiologists.

The chief radiographic technologist is Sally Lebeau, who has been employed in the department for 18 years, during half of which she has been the chief technologist. She is well regarded by her staff and is seen as fair and reasonable, especially given the fast-paced and intense working environment. Lebeau has tried to implement Deming's quality principles and the methods of continuous quality improvement, but neither Goodview nor the administration supported her efforts, and they have come to nought. Lebeau is concerned with what she perceives to be a decline in the quality of work in medical imaging. She has unsuccessfully tried to discuss it with Goodview on numerous occasions. In the past several years she has seen other developments that have raised concerns. First is that there are fewer radiologists in total in the department, despite increased volume. Second, the constant turnover of radiologists, because of all the *locum tenens* physicians, is very disruptive to the department's work. Third, Goodview does more and more of the work himself—both because of the radiologists staffing problems and because of what Lebeau thinks is an increasing obsession with money. Fourth, without the knowledge of senior administration, Goodview ordered a cable connection so that he could follow the stock market and trade technology stocks on line. He is often distracted from reading radiographs by stock market developments and his reaction to them, especially in the volatile technology stocks, in which he invests heavily.

Lebeau's concerns were such that she went to see Halton. When Lebeau described how she saw the four problems, Halton frankly told her that he could do little about the first three, nor did he think they were his responsibility. The number of *locum tenens* physicians and the quality issues would have to be dealt with by someone else—probably the PSO. Halton seemed incensed, however, that Goodview would be so bold as to order installation of Internet access without clearing it with administration. While Lebeau was in his office Halton called maintenance, which reports to the vice president for support services (VP/SS). The head of mainte-nance confirmed that there was a cable hook-up and the hospital was pay-ing the fee. While Lebeau waited, Halton called the VP/SS, Susan Williams. After a lengthy discussion in which Halton became quite agi-tated and began to shout, Williams finally agreed to have the cable disconnected the next day. This greatly pleased Halton, who said to Lebeau, "I've been trying to get Goodview's attention; I bet this'll do it. He'll have to come to me to resolve this problem—I'm sure that, over the long term, it will help us develop a better working relationship."

Lebeau was disappointed by Halton's response, especially his feeling that he had no role in quality. She thought that the cable issue was the least of the problems, even though it was clearly a distraction and Goodview was using hospital resources for his private purposes. When Lebeau returned to medical imaging, she saw several of the staff standing as though transfixed outside the room where the radiologists read the films. They were listening intently to a heated conversation Goodview was having with an online broker who Goodview alleged had failed to make a trade in time to avoid a significant loss. The language was foul and was becoming so loud that patients waiting for procedures could hear it. Lebeau quietly shut the door to the reading room and told the staff to go back to work.

The next day Goodview's Internet connection suddenly went dead, just as he was trying to execute a sell order on a rapidly falling technology stock. He reacted violently and threw the monitor on the floor breaking the screen and chipping the flooring. Upon calling the cable company Goodview was told that the hospital had ordered it disconnected. Goodview stormed over to "management house" to see Gargon, who was only partly successful in calming him before Goodview left his office. After talking to Halton, Gargon basically agreed with his action, but chided him for how he had handled it. In the weeks that followed, Goodview brooded about the loss of his cable connection; he frequently cursed out administration. Several times he stated that if he had a bomb he'd blow up "management house."

Goodview's agitation was increasingly reflected in his work. For example, he read mammograms as quickly as he could put them up on the view box. He found virtually none that required more than a few seconds of study. When Dr. Leipzig raised a question about the speed of his readings, Goodview said, "Reading mammograms is so simple that a one-eyed first-year medical student could do it." To check Goodview's readings, Leipzig reread 100 randomly selected mammograms and found several that he thought warranted follow-up studies, including repeat mammograms and fine needle aspirations. He ordered them without telling Goodview.

Concerned about the mammograms and similar problems, Leipzig followed Goodview's custom and went "to the top" to see Mr. Gargon. Gargon was initially noncommittal and told Leipzig that he would have to undertake his own investigation. Gargon called Halton and asked him to speak to Lebeau. When their meeting began Halton asked Lebeau for her comments on the information relayed from Leipzig. Her response was a torrent: poor staff morale, low patient satisfaction, high turnover among the radiologists, and Goodview's continuing bad behavior were causing a great deal of stress. Alarmed, Halton met with Gargon, but they were unsure how to proceed and the meeting produced no plan of action. The following week, Dr. Leipzig resigned, citing in his letter the continuing and significant quality problems in medical imaging. This meant that Drs. Banda and Goodview were the only nontemporary radiologists in the department. The other radiologists were *locum tenens*, who usually stayed only 1–3 months.

The controversy between administration and Goodview and questions about the quality of work in medical imaging were common knowledge in the hospital. Their extent and duration were such, however, that admitting and referring physicians in the community were increasingly concerned about the quality of imaging services their patients would get at MacMillan. Gargon and several board members, including Ms. Buchanan, had received calls from prominent active staff physicians who said that they had become uncomfortable referring their patients to MacMillan for radiographic work and that they would use one of the competing hospitals or a free-standing imaging center. In the short term fewer referrals would reduce hospital revenue from medical imaging; in the long term inpatient admissions would be affected, thus potentially affecting quality of care received by persons in the hospital's service area, but certainly causing a decline in hospital revenue.

Greatly concerned and prompted by a call from the board chair, Ms. Buchanan, Gargon scheduled a meeting with Goodview and Halton. As usual, Goodview arrived late. Looking at Halton he blurted out, "What are you doing here?" With little conviction, Halton replied that as the VP/CS he was administratively accountable for medical imaging and it was his responsibility to be present. Goodview proceeded to harangue Gargon about the poor support he was getting from administration, how the technologists were badly trained and disloyal to him, and the equipment was inadequate for a 21st-century radiology department. All the while he ignored Halton. Gargon began by expressing his concern that there were too few radiologists for the volume of procedures. Goodview said that radiologists were in great demand and that he was doing the best he could to recruit additional staff and in the meantime he, Banda, and the *locum tenens* radiologists could handle the workload. After 30 minutes of heated discussion, the meeting ended with no resolution.

After Goodview left, Gargon told Halton to contact physician search firms and determine whether Goodview was correct about the shortage of radiologists. A week later, in early July, Halton reported that the search firms had sent him information that radiologists were available in adequate numbers, but that they were being attracted to groups that paid better than Good Views was willing to pay. Goodview's salary offers were well known to search firms—one even called Goodview "a cheapskate." The search firms sent 10 résumés of radiologists who could be employed on a long-term basis by Good Views or who could be hired as *locum tenens*, if the salary offers were adequate.

Armed with this information, another meeting was held with Gargon, Halton, and Goodview. Goodview was adamant that he would not bring any more "traitors" such as Leipzig or other full-time radiologists into his company. He felt that all of his full-time radiologists had betrayed his trust and friendship over the years. He said, however, that he would consider more *locum tenens* appointments, but only if he really needed them. A week later, in mid-July, Goodview had done nothing about hiring more *locum tenens* radiologists. This prompted Halton to contact the search firms. He asked them to send applications from the 10 radiologists whose résumés they had been sent previously. Halton was sure this would force Goodview to take action. Applications received in administration were forwarded to Goodview, who stubbornly ignored them.

CONTRACT TERMINATION

When Gargon arrived at work on August 1 his secretary told him there had been a voice mail from the chair of the hospital board, which had been received at 5:30 A.M. Buchanan stated that she had slept little the night before because the problems in medical imaging were weighing on her mind. She ended her recording by stating that something had to be done and that she wanted Gargon to review the contract with Good Views to determine how to terminate it. By noon she had called twice to see if there was an answer to her request. Gargon had to put her off until early afternoon; by then he had checked with legal counsel and was able to speak to Buchanan in an informed manner. The relevant contract provision stated:

> Either party may, upon demonstration of adequate cause, terminate the contract with a 30-day notice. Cause is defined as either party's: inability to meet the clinical needs of the other; nonperformance of a significant provision of this contract; and actions that interfere with the ability of the other party to perform this contract.

After talking to Halton, who said, "It's about time!" Gargon called Buchanan and told her that legal counsel had informed him that there appeared to be adequate cause to terminate the contract. Buchanan instructed him to draft a letter advising Good Views Medical Imaging that its contract with MacMillan would be terminated as of September 1.

Consistent with board bylaws, Buchanan polled the executive committee, which approved the action. The letter, which was signed by Gargon, was hand delivered to Goodview the same day. Goodview was performing a fine needle biopsy and he asked a technologist to read the letter to him. Upon hearing the contents he became enraged. He shouted for Banda, who was on a coffee break, to "get in here and finish up this patient." The patient became very agitated and had to be reassured by the technologist before Banda could complete the procedure. Goodview stormed over to "management house" and burst into Gargon's office without being announced. Gargon's executive assistant was so concerned about Goodview's rage and the potential for violence that she called security and asked them to send two officers to the administrative suite immediately. Goodview left shortly thereafter, vowing to get the "meanest, nastiest lawyer in town."

Goodview's attorney petitioned the court for a temporary restraining order (TRO), arguing that contract termination would cause irreparable economic harm to Good Views Medical Imaging and would also irreparably harm Goodview's professional reputation. The TRO was granted despite arguments by MacMillan's lawyers that focused on the need to provide quality radiologic services and maintain the quality of patient care. The TRO prohibited MacMillan and its management from interfering in the role of Good Views Medical Imaging and its agents and employees in the medical imaging department of MacMillan. Less than a week after the TRO was granted, Goodview filed suit against MacMillan for breach of contract and defamation of character. Gargon and Halton were named personally as having "conspired to deprive Goodview of his business and professional livelihood and of causing irreparable harm to his professional reputation." In addition to economic damages for breach of contract, the lawsuit asked that the court award punitive damages based on the alleged conspiracy and bad faith on the parts of Gargon and Halton, as agents of the hospital. Given the urgency of the situation, MacMillan was successful in gaining an early trial date on the breach of contract and defamation lawsuit. Trial was scheduled for December 1st, even as the TRO remained in effect.

BREAST CANCER AWARENESS MONTH

As it had for the past 8 years, MacMillan Hospital's "Health-Promotion Promotion" program had designated October as breast cancer awareness month. The local radio and television stations aired public service announcements that urged women older than age 45 to go to MacMillan for a free screening mammogram. Special efforts were directed at MacMillan Hospital staff. The Health-Promotion Promotion used flyers, bulletin board notices, and public address announcements in the cafeteria to encourage women older than 45 to be screened. The extra workload seemed especially burdensome this year, both because of the continuing shortage of radiologists and the pending legal proceeding.

Cowed by the TRO and the pending lawsuit for breach of contract and defamation and concerned that there might be charges of harassment, which could result in being held in contempt of court or prompt another lawsuit, Gargon and Halton stayed as far away from medical imaging and Goodview as they could. Goodview was emboldened by the initial success of obtaining the TRO; he was even more critical of administration and his behavior became increasingly bizarre. Lebeau's stress level was so high that she sought medical attention and began taking a mild tranquilizer. To the technologists and other staff, the whole situation was overwhelming; morale sank even lower and there was talk of a mass resignation. Only the perseverance of Lebeau gave the staff some encouragement.

A MacMillan Hospital housekeeper, Amelia Tendo, presented herself at medical imaging early one morning in October for a screening mammogram. She said she had felt a small lump in her right breast and was concerned about it. Goodview read the mammogram in his usual fashion and diagnosed the lump as benign and "nothing more than a calcium deposit in an overly anxious female." Reassured, Tendo asked that a copy of the report be sent to her primary care physician.

THE FIRST TRIAL

In preparing for trial, attorneys for MacMillan and Goodview/Good Views took depositions (questions answered under oath) of the major parties in the case. Without exception, persons employed by the hospital, including radiologic technologists, stated in their depositions that Goodview's work in managing and providing radiologic services was well below acceptable limits and that his actions that effectively resulted in inadequate radiologist staffing had put and were putting patients at risk. Testimony such as this was necessary because the hospital had the burden of proving that the grounds for termination in the contract had been met. In addition, the hospital had retained two medical experts who stated, after reviewing Goodview's readings, diagnoses, and the depositions of the other witnesses, that Goodview's work fell below the standard of care.

Except for tepid support from Banda and the *locum tenens* radiologists, Goodview had few allies in the hospital. He did have an expert witness who stated that his work and GoodViews' performance of the contract were at an acceptable level and within the range of performance for departments of radiology nationwide.

The Bad Image Radiology Department

The trial commenced December 1st and lasted 5 days. The witn who appeared also had given depositions. Goodview could not res___ himself when he testified, and he proved to be his own worst enemy, even as he tried to present himself as a poor physician who was being bullied by an overwhelming bureaucracy. The jury found in favor of the hospital and against Goodview and Good Views Medical Imaging on both the breach of contract and the defamation claims. The findings caused the TRO to be vacated.

Hospital administration was jubilant and, with Good Views' contract terminating in 30 days, it immediately began efforts to find a new radiology group to staff medical imaging. Radiologists who had been part of Good Views were contacted. Dr. Leipzig indicated he was interested and he set about organizing a radiology group.

SECOND LAWSUIT

Ms. Tendo, who had had the screening mammogram done in October during breast cancer awareness month, continued to be concerned by the lump. When she performed her intermittent breast self examinations over the next several months it seemed to be getting larger. Whenever her anxiety rose, she recalled Dr. Goodview's reading and diagnosis that it was only a calcium deposit and was reassured. Six months later, in April she had become convinced that the lump was substantially larger and she scheduled an examination with her gynecologist. He immediately ordered a mammogram at a free-standing imaging center, which led to a fine needle aspiration. After other tests, the final diagnosis was cancer of the right breast with metastases to one lung, nearby lymph nodes, and liver. She died less than 3 months later. Within a year, Ms. Tendo's estate sued Dr. Goodview, Good Views Medical Imaging, and MacMillan Hospital for medical negligence.

Questions

1. Identify the issues in the case.

2. Prepare a time line of major events in the case. Determine the points at which intervention by hospital administration or the board might have prevented the problems in medical imaging from developing as they did. For each intervention point, outline the intervention that you think should have been undertaken.

3. What is the role of hospital executives in monitoring quality and intervening, as needed, in the delivery and/or quality of clinical services?

4. Identify the points at which hospital administration should have intervened to lessen the probability of Dr. Goodview's failure to diagnose Ms. Tendo's breast cancer.

5. What steps should be taken by MacMillan to resolve the lawsuit brought by Ms. Tendo's estate? Is an apology part of an appropriate response?

6. What actions, if any, should be taken against Messrs. Gargon and Halton? Who should take these actions?

16

Westmount Nursing Homes, Inc.

Implementing a Continuous Quality Improvement Initiative

Kent V. Rondeau
University of Alberta, Edmonton, Canada

Shirley Carpenter took a deep breath and looked at her watch. It was 3:40 P.M. and just 20 minutes were left to get ready for her meeting with the board. She knew there was going to be a difficult confrontation and believed that many board members would call into question her leadership skills and administrative judgment. She felt that her well-earned reputation as a brilliant strategist and dynamic change agent would be put to a severe test. She needed to find a way to calm the widespread fear that the total quality management (TQM) initiative she had worked so hard to implement at Westmount Nursing Homes was badly off the rails. She wondered what had gone wrong and how it could be saved.

BACKGROUND

Shirley Carpenter came to Westmount 22 months ago to assume the role of president and chief executive officer. Westmount Nursing Homes,

Used with permission from *Cases in Long-Term Care Management* by Donna Lind Infeld and John R. Kress. (Chicago: Health Administration Press, 1995, pp. 85–95.)

Incorporated is a for-profit chain of seven nursing homes located in a northeastern state. Since 1953, it had grown from a single 42-bed residential facility for affluent seniors, to a dynamic company comprised of four divisions: 1) the Facilities Division, managing skilled nursing homes; 2) the Home Care Division, operating homemaker and nursing services for seniors in their own homes; 3) the Commissary Services Division, operating a central kitchen preparing and distributing meals to four of its homes, two small local hospitals, and elderly people in their own homes; and 4) the Consulting Division, marketing management consulting and accounting services to a variety of clients in the long-term care industry. Westmount's statement of profit and loss for the past 3 years can be found in Table 1.

Westmount continues to search vigorously for opportunities to expand its core business. Last year it began a comprehensive day care program for seniors at five of its homes. Recently, discussions have been undertaken with Breton Funeral Homes to purchase its assets, including four family-owned funeral establishments. Westmount has also commenced negotiations with a regional chain of drug stores to lease them commercial space in its three largest homes. It also is exploring the establishment of a home care alliance with two other hospital-based home care programs in order to attract new managed care contracts and to improve referrals from existing contracts involving their parent hospitals.

Over the past 2 years, under the leadership of Shirley Carpenter, Westmount purchased two additional nursing homes, increasing its total

Table 1. Westmount Nursing Homes, Incorporated Statement of Revenue and Expense (years 200x–200z) (figures in thousands of dollars)

Year	200x	200y	200z
Facilities Division			
Revenue	15,640	18,622	26,453
Expenses	12,458	15,140	22,512
Profit margin (%)	20.3	18.7	14.9
Home Care Division			
Revenue	1,741	2,254	3,060
Expenses	1,360	1,752	2,493
Profit margin (%)	21.9	22.3	18.5
Commissary Services Division			
Revenue	1,382	1,940	2,188
Expenses	1,162	1,614	1,870
Profit margin (%)	15.9	16.8	14.5
Consulting Division			
Revenue	—	42	426
Expenses	—	16	230
Profit margin (%)	—	61.9	46.0

skilled nursing bed complement by almost 43%. A strategic planning process began last year. Out of this initiative came Westmount's formal declaration to pursue the goal of becoming the "home of choice" in the tri-state area. Its primary target market was identified as affluent seniors who desire a broad range of single access, high-quality health and social services. This strategy was based on the belief that to survive in a rapidly changing health care environment, customers require "one-stop shopping" for a wide variety of services outside of the acute care setting. Westmount firmly believes that future success will go to those proactive organizations that achieve a vertically and horizontally integrated delivery system.

SHIRLEY CARPENTER

Shirley Carpenter, R.N., M.B.A., came to Westmount Nursing Homes 2 years ago from Grasslands Community General Hospital, where she had been the vice president of nursing. Grasslands is a 325-bed acute care hospital located in a rapidly growing community in the Midwest. At Grasslands, Shirley was widely received as a dynamic and resourceful leader who was not afraid of making the difficult decisions that went with her job description. She was primarily responsible for Grasslands' radical redesign of its patient care delivery system toward a highly integrated patient-focused approach. The changes she had initiated saved the hospital more than $1.7 million per year on direct patient care services, while at the same time lowering hospital length of stay and improving patient outcomes. When the press got wind of Grasslands' successful reorganization, the hospital and Shirley received a great deal of local and national media attention. Grasslands became recognized as an innovative organization at the cutting edge of excellence in patient care delivery. It wasn't long before Shirley was being asked to speak at forums about a wide variety of health care issues. She also received additional recognition when she was selected as "one of the most outstanding young health care executives in the nation."

Although the changes Shirley had instituted were widely acclaimed as successful, she did have her detractors. Her direct, no-nonsense style was often seen as confrontational, and many found her to be intellectually intimidating. On several occasions she had openly chastised staff members with whom she took issue. Although she was greatly respected and even admired by her staff, people tended to give her a wide berth on most issues. Shirley demanded perfection from her staff but also held herself up to the very highest level of performance expectation. She once stated, "You've got to be visible and out front if you're going to navigate an organization toward progressive change. This requires that you stand behind your words and accept the consequences of your convictions. Complacency never got the job done. Too many people are attached to the status quo. You can't make an omelet without breaking a few eggs."

George Pearson had been the chief executive officer at Grasslands during Shirley Carpenter's tenure. George once stated that Shirley was "the daughter I never had." He had given her wide latitude and regularly deferred to her judgment in most areas related to running the hospital. Everyone had assumed that George had been grooming Shirley to take over the hospital upon his pending retirement. When he departed, the selection committee did the unexpected and chose another candidate. Shirley was devastated; 6 weeks later, she left Grasslands for Westmount Nursing Homes.

A NEW DIRECTION FOR WESTMOUNT

Shirley Carpenter's arrival at Westmount created a great deal of anticipation and excitement. Her reputation as a health care innovator and progressive change agent was now well established. Over the years, Westmount had languished through a series of rather bland administrators who lacked the vision that could move the organization forcefully into the 21st century.

The first year of Shirley's tenure at Westmount was marked by a number of bold initiatives on her part. Soon after arriving, she was able to dissipate the threat of loss of licensure and potential funding on two of its nursing homes that had been cited for a number of violations. Shirley also instituted a broad and sweeping reorganization at Westmount in creating the four operating divisions. In addition, after securing support from her board, Shirley began a very aggressive program of asset diversification because the firm had relied for too long on revenues from its affiliate homes. Declining reimbursement rates, coupled with full occupancy, meant that Westmount needed to broaden its base of revenue. This was partially achieved by expansion of its home care and food commissary services, and by establishing a consulting division to market management services to a variety of clients in the long-term care industry. In particular, the Consulting Division was thought to have significant growth potential due to a perceived lack of expertise by most local consultants on long-term care management issues. During this period, Westmount also purchased two additional homes with the option of acquiring three more. The firm spent more than $1.5 million on renovations to these facilities.

Within 18 months, Shirley had implemented a number of innovative programs at Westmount focused on providing augmented services to its seniors and, in addition, expanded employee services. Shirley formed and chaired a quality-of-work-life committee aimed at improving conditions for Westmount's employees and staff. Morale in all of the homes had suffered after years of neglect. At the time of Shirley's arrival, the turnover level of staff nurses and nursing assistants at Westmount was among the highest in the state. To reverse this, a recognition and performance-based pay system was implemented identifying and rewarding outstanding individual and group achievement. A career planning and inventory program was developed to assist employees in identifying their career goals and charting a path toward these goals. In addition, the staff education and development program was greatly expanded. All employees were openly encouraged and received financial support to acquire their high school equivalency or to seek further education and skills enhancement. Westmount also established a progressive literacy program to address the intractable problem of illiteracy in the work place. The quality-of-work-life committee estimated that about 35% of the workforce at Westmount had deficiencies in reading and writing. Shirley once stated, "Organizational excellence comes about only when people are sufficiently motivated and empowered to make a difference. The bedrock of staff empowerment is knowledge and education. This requires a significant investment in the intellectual potential of each employee. Our people are our most important asset."

THE TOTAL QUALITY MANAGEMENT INITIATIVE

Three months after arriving at Westmount, Shirley initiated a strategic planning retreat to identify Westmount's preferred future. One conclusion emerging from the retreat was that there was a need to find a way to better address quality-of-care issues in delivering services to seniors. Shirley latched on to the notion that TQM would be the vehicle through which Westmount could achieve the cultural transformation articulated in its vision statement, which included a statement that "Westmount Nursing Homes, Incorporated believes in striving for excellence in everything we do."

Shirley quickly became immersed in the burgeoning literature on TQM. Her interest in and passion for its possibilities grew. In fact, she was so determined to become an expert in its theory and application that she began to explore the possibility of focusing her doctoral dissertation in this area.

Her faculty advisor and mentor was Dr. Daylon Quinby, a sage yet crusty academic, now nearing retirement. Shirley asked the venerable professor if he would "lead the quality improvement journey at Westmount." Dr. Quinby readily agreed, and was soon found wandering around the grounds at all hours observing people at work or showing up quite unannounced at management committee meetings. Several staff members found Dr. Quinby to be "an odd old duck" whose presence was somewhat annoying, if not unnerving. Most people did not know why he was there; some speculated that it was management's way of spying on them.

One of Dr. Quinby's first activities was to evaluate the organizational culture in the seven nursing homes. Findings from the cultural audit, used to assess readiness to pursue organizational change, indicated that much work would be required to transform Westmount. In particular, the professor found that prevailing work practices at Westmount were, in many respects, antithetical to the philosophy of TQM. Dr. Quinby announced the findings of the cultural audit at the semiannual general meeting of board, management, and staff. He stated in his address that "if Westmount is to successfully implement total quality management, no less than a total and unequivocable repudiation of current work place values and norms needs to be achieved." Quinby further stated that "the management in the homes consistently demonstrates patterns of practice that are overly autocratic, rigid, and dysfunctional. All too often, management treats its employees like little children. Employees respond by behaving as if management believes they cannot be trusted. An overly confrontational atmosphere, based on suspicion bordering on paranoia, has created an element of fear surrounding and pervading work in many of the homes." Dr. Quinby cited several examples from incidents he had observed. Needless to say, the conclusions he rendered were not well received by a number of members of the staff and managers.

Soon after the cultural audit feedback sessions, Shirley Carpenter and 12 senior managers embarked on a 10-day educational retreat to learn the tools and techniques of TQM and the leadership skills needed to successfully navigate the cultural transformation it required. Although the retreat was located on a resort island in the Caribbean, Shirley impressed on her managers that the time spent was not a paid holiday, but an opportunity to acquire new leadership and management skills. When the news broke that management had gone to a resort for a "working retreat," many employees openly questioned why they needed to "go so far away to learn how to manage better at home."

When the senior managers returned from the retreat, many could scarcely contain their enthusiasm and set about immediately to apply the principles they had learned. A quality council was quickly formed, chaired jointly by Shirley Carpenter and Dr. Quinby. The quality council was charged with leading and directing the TQM transformation at Westmount. Its membership consisted of the directors of the seven homes and the divisional directors of home care, commissary services, and consulting services, along with senior representatives from human resources and strategic planning. Within 2 weeks, executives in each of the homes and divisions were busy holding educational seminars for their middle managers and supervisors on the philosophy, tools, and techniques of TQM.

Not long afterward, under the supervision of the quality council, the first quality improvement (QI) team was formed. Led by Shirley Carpenter and facilitated by Dr. Quinby, a seven-member multifunctional team of service providers suggested innovative ways to dramatically reduce the waiting period for nursing response to requests from bedridden residents. Within 2 months, 23 QI teams examined quality-related problems ranging from improving resident food to designing a new commercial exercise video program for seniors. Table 2 provides a list of these early quality improvement projects at Westmount.

Initial interest and excitement generated by many employees for the TQM initiative at Westmount convinced Shirley that she was on to some-

Table 2. Westmount Nursing Homes, Incorporated Quality Improvement Projects

QI Program	Responsibility
1. Client satisfaction survey	Headquarters
2. Family satisfaction survey	Headquarters
3. Nursing response times	Facilities
4. Seniors' exercise video	Headquarters
5. Staff retention study	Facilities
6. Guest relations study	Headquarters
7. Medication errors	Facilities
8. Suggestion system design	Headquarters
9. Resident fall study	Facilities
10. Wandering patients study	Facilities
11. Employee recognition program	Headquarters
12. Patient accounts	Headquarters
13. Food quality	Facilities
14. Food preparation	Headquarters
15. Pet therapy	Headquarters
16. Job redesign	Headquarters
17. Physician reimbursement	Headquarters
18. Physician satisfaction	Headquarters
19. Ethical review	Facilities
20. Grounds beautification	Facilities
21. Resident transportation	Facilities
22. Self-scheduling	Facilities
23. New ventures	Headquarters

thing big. Many of her junior managers, however, were privately expressing fear that the changes, which now were transforming Westmount's once
placid culture, were happening all too fast. Vice President of Finance Norm
Taylor's opinion was shared by many other managers at Westmount: "It's a
proven fact that people in the long-term care industry really can't absorb
organizational change as easily as those working in acute care settings.
People here just have too much respect for tradition and past practice."

For her part, Shirley was strongly convinced that these changes could
not occur fast enough. Shirley stated, "I don't believe in waiting around
and hoping that something good comes your way. That just never happens. I like to create success right away. One small victory produces
another, and soon you've won the war. The fact is people like to associate
with winners."

THE WESTMOUNT BOARD RESPONDS

The board of Westmount was never really very enthusiastic about Shirley's
TQM makeover. Explained to them as a tool to enhance productivity and
create a long-term competitive advantage in Westmount's chosen markets,
the board reluctantly gave its approval "to implement a TQM program, as
long as it wasn't too costly." The chairperson of the board was Dr. Ann
Howard, age 57, a highly respected family physician with a specialty in
geriatric medicine who was a long-time board member. Dr. Howard was
not convinced that TQM could work at Westmount, and stated, "Total
quality management might be all right for building cars, but I just can't
understand how it can work in a nursing home. Anyway, I read somewhere
that this TQM stuff is just an expensive fad, and that over 80% of health
care organizations who have tried to implement it have failed. Can we
really afford to try something with such a spotty track record? Perhaps
Shirley should be spending her time and the organization's money on
proven management methods."

Shirley knew that the turnaround at Westmount would not happen
overnight. She chalked up the board's indifference to ignorance, and
resolved that she would not be deterred from her quest to transform
Westmount. "Give me 3 years and you won't recognize this place," she was
heard to have said.

LABOR CONTRACT NEGOTIATIONS

Several months after the TQM initiative had begun, Westmount began
contract negotiations with the local chapter of the United Federation of

Nurses, representing Westmount's 214 registered nurses and nurse assistants. Shirley believed in taking a hands-on approach to dealing with the unions, and insisted on conducting all negotiations personally. In the beginning, management at Westmount felt that contract discussions would be straightforward and would proceed with little of the rancor that had characterized much of their collective bargaining in the past. In the earliest months of the TQM initiative, Westmount had witnessed a remarkable improvement in work place morale. It was hoped that improved morale would pay an important "peace dividend" with the organization, winning important concessions from the union.

In fact, all three of the unions representing nonmanagement employees at Westmount believed that the active participation of their membership in TQM demonstrated their steadfast commitment to finding new ways of working responsibly with management. For many years, the fractious nature of their contract negotiations had left both sides bitter after they had concluded.

From the union's vantage point, negotiations were aimed at improving the collective agreement by obtaining significant wage gains and achieving formal union representation on the Westmount board. Two issues were of particular significance during contract talks. First, the union sought to replace the merit pay plan for registered nurses with an across-the-board pay increase for all nurses. Most people felt the merit pay plan, conceived to reward top performers, was not working very well. Many viewed it as a complicated and subjective protocol that caused a great deal of confusion and bitterness in its application. Second, the union sought protection against what it felt was management's abhorrent practice of substituting RNs with certified nursing assistants (CNAs) and other personal care workers. The union claimed that management was using lower-paid nursing auxiliaries for tasks that legally should be done by RNs.

Early in the contract negotiations it became apparent that they would be very difficult indeed. In its opening address at the negotiation table, the union stated that its "price of compliance" with Westmount's total quality program was significant wage increases for its membership. Shirley countered by offering to provide job security and suggesting the formation of a committee to study questions of nursing labor deployment. She also stated that she was in favor of allowing union representation on the board. This was consistent with her idea of incorporating more vibrant forms of employee participation in the work place. Shirley insisted, however, that the merit pay plan must remain in place. As its architect, she felt a deep personal commitment to its consummation. Shirley stated, "You've got to have a way of rewarding those people who consistently perform above the call of duty. That's what quality service is all about. Pay is a great way to motivate people. To ignore the impact money has on the performance of employees is to remove a very powerful weapon from your arsenal." After several heated meetings, the negotiations seemed to be at an impasse.

THE BOARD STEPS IN

It was soon apparent to the Westmount board that contract negotiations with the nurses' union were not going well. The executive committee of the board met with Shirley to determine an appropriate strategy to help reach an agreement. After much heated discussion, they decided that management should take a more direct approach in dealing with the union. Dr. Howard summed up the attitude of the board in saying, "You can't allow a union to ruin the financial viability of your enterprise. The truth is 80% of our costs are direct expenditures for labor. If we are ever to reverse our fiscal problems around here, we need to get control of our labor costs. These people have to realize we're all in this thing together." The board also gave a thumb's down to the idea of allowing union representation on the board. Dr. Howard remarked, "You know, this move to democratize the work place is just a bunch of rampant socialism. You give these people an inch and they take a mile."

When Shirley returned to the bargaining table, she brought along Dr. Quinby to assist in discussions. Unfortunately, he was not able to expedite breaking the impasse. His abrasive and abrupt manner further alienated the union and created additional tensions at the table. With no new offer made by either side, no resolution on any of the major outstanding issues could be achieved. Shirley suspended negotiations by claiming that the union was being inflexible while "holding the residents of the homes ransom for a few extra pennies."

THE FLASH POINT

At this point the executive committee of the board began to make direct overtures to union representatives requesting an informal meeting to "determine if there were not avenues of mutual interest that could be explored." Dr. Howard and two other board members met in private with the union negotiators and suggested the possibility of major staff cuts if the union did not agree to make significant wage concessions. The union representatives countered by insinuating that the Westmount management was bargaining in bad faith. Robert Sawyer, the chief negotiator, said, "We will not be bullied into signing a collective agreement that does not have the best interests of our membership at heart. We have showed our willingness to bargain in good conscience by engaging in activities aimed at improving productivity. The participation of our members in these efforts is often unpaid and obviously unappreciated." The meeting ended with the union threatening to boycott further participation by its membership in future quality improvement activities. According to Robert Sawyer, "If we are going to be treated with such contempt, I can only recommend to my membership that we suspend our active participation in this program immediately."

As Shirley prepared for the 4 P.M. board meeting she was frustrated and angry that persons and events had conspired against her. She had always felt pride in her ability to control any agenda. Her record of achievement was one of soaring accomplishments. She wondered how she could regain control of her board and move ahead with the important reforms she had initiated.

17

District Hospital

A Lesson in Governance

Cynthia Levin
Kaiser Permanente Medical Group

Kurt Darr
The George Washington University, Washington, D.C.

HISTORY

Barclay Memorial Hospital (BMH) has enjoyed a reputation for excellent medical care in an affluent community for more than 50 years. In the mid-1940s the community was mainly agricultural, but it was becoming urbanized. Hospitals in the area were operating at capacity. Community members and physicians proposed a solution: Form a hospital district that would be supported by the community through a tax. Voters approved the district in 1945 by a 5-to-1 margin. Its first decision was the selection of a 15-acre construction site. In 1947, the voters approved a $7.3 million bond issue to finance construction and operation of a 300-bed hospital. The tax district spans seven townships that elect five district community members to a governing board for the district hospital's four entities, which include the hospital, a joint venture operating an urgent-care center and a hospice, and the hospital foundation.

Used by permission of the authors. Copyright © 2004 by Cynthia Levin and Kurt Darr.

THE PHO

About 10 years ago, the district hospital board and the CEO devised a strategic plan to form a physician–hospital organization (PHO) with Valley Physician Group (VPG). VPG was formed in 1951 when a group of physicians agreed that they could provide better care to their patients by sharing resources and ideas. Over the years, VPG expanded as more physicians and physician groups joined. Currently, VPG is composed of more than 140 physicians in 28 medical specialties and subspecialties. VPG provides services to 325,000 patients and delivers 2,500 babies each year. It employs 600 full-time equivalent (FTE) staff, and enjoys gross revenue of $120 million.

Joining with VPG to form a PHO required that BMH change its legal classification from a public (governmental) hospital to a private, not-for-profit hospital. The new governing board was responsible for the PHO, which included the Barclay Hospital and the VPG. Within 2 years, it became apparent that the PHO was going bankrupt because of poor management and a lack of focused leadership. In-fighting among VPG and non-VPG physicians began as the hospital deteriorated financially and employee morale plummeted. With the help of consultant Gregory Schilling, the district board, which had not disbanded, fought against the PHO's governing board and successfully brought the hospital back under the district's control. As a tax district (governmental) hospital, BMH has several advantages: it is a public hospital and a political subdivision of the state, which gives it certain legal advantages; board members are elected by voters in the tax district; financial surpluses are put back into the hospital; and it has authority to levy a tax on homeowners in the district. Schilling was asked to become the new CEO immediately following the dissolution of the PHO (see Exhibit 1).

MARKET POSITION

Currently, BMH is licensed for 400 beds, but last year operated only 275 beds with an average daily census of 249 patients. This number reflects a decrease in volumes in many service lines. Discharges totaled 26,731. The average length of stay for all inpatients was 3.4 days. This has increased somewhat due to changes in the law allowing new mothers to stay in the hospital longer than 24 hours for normal deliveries. Deliveries last year were at an all-time high with 3,216 and will most likely increase because BMH is the desirable maternity hospital in the area. The nurses are particularly attentive and the nursing units have only private, newly renovated patient rooms. Outpatient visits totaled 232,363, which should continue to

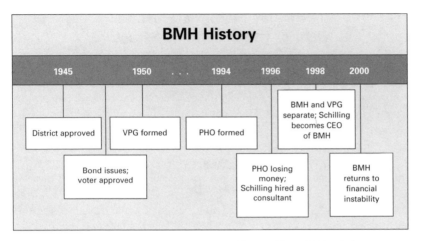

Exhibit 1. Timeline of major events in the history of Barclay Memorial Hospital.

rise as technology allows for less invasive treatments. Surgeries totaled 6,201. Projections show a potential for increases in occupancy if more surgeons admit at BMH and the processes for delivery of services become more efficient, which, in turn, would make them more profitable. Transplant surgery, however, should be generating more revenue. Orthopedics is another service that could be expanded; it has only 60% of the estimated market. Total full-time and part-time employees were 2,705, giving the hospital a higher than average FTE ratio compared to other hospitals in the area, which, in turn, is reflected in the high percentage of revenue used for salaries and benefits. There are 654 physicians on staff, reflecting a decade-long downward trend. The number of hospital volunteers also has decreased from 890 last year. The operating budget was $200 million for the last fiscal year. Managing to budget has been difficult. A hiring freeze mid-year showed some positive results, but after three months some nursing departments were concerned that nurse–patient ratios were too low (see Exhibit 2).

THE DISTRICT BOARD

The BMH district board has five members that are elected by residents in the district to serve three-year terms. The CEO is hired by the district board and is a voting member of the board. The chairman of the district board, Dr. Larry Harvey, is an orthopedic surgeon with privileges at the hospital. His responsibility and authority within the hospital have raised

Barclay Memorial Hospital
District Organizational Structure

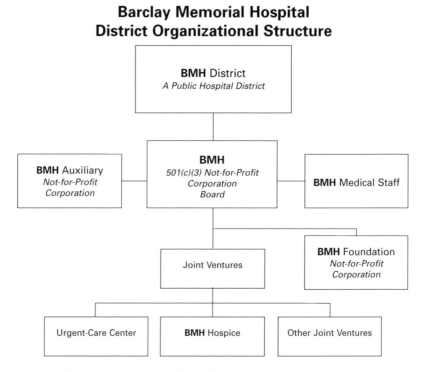

Exhibit 2. Organizational structure of the BMH District.

questions of conflicts of interest. He used this power to disregard requests from the operating room supervisor that he arrive on time for his cases. His patients waited unnecessarily for their procedures; highly paid staff were also idle. Harvey threatened to have the orthopedic surgery department manager fired because she tried to control excessive use of supplies and pressed him to keep to his schedule. According to the estimates of demand shown in marketing reports, the orthopedic surgery service should be producing a profit; instead, it has continued to lose money. When the subject was broached by Schilling, Harvey threatened to admit his patients to a competing hospital. He would often become emotional in meetings, accusing Schilling of yelling at him. Eventually, Harvey stopped returning Schilling's phone calls. Compounding these problems was Harvey's difficulty in separating his anger about health care reimbursement reductions and the hospital's rocky relationship with the VPG physicians from his work in the hospital.

Dr. Ray Brandon is also an orthopedic surgeon. Brandon was on the district board during the PHO, where he took a more introverted role.

During a closed-door meeting of the board, however, he did not hide his animosity towards the VPG physicians who formed the PHO with the hospital. He is also frustrated about health care reimbursement. Symptoms of the breakdown in communications with the CEO were also becoming apparent with Brandon. Occasionally, Brandon appeared to disregard state law that applied to tax-district hospitals and their governance. The law requires that two or more board members of a district hospital must discuss hospital issues only in a public meeting. Meetings where proprietary information is discussed are exempt from the state's "open meetings" requirement. At one orthopedic surgery committee meeting, he spoke privately with Harvey, for example. On another occasion, in a board meeting where proprietary matters were being discussed, Brandon wanted to legally challenge physicians who refused to take ER call. He was frustrated about the breakdown in the relationship between physicians and hospital governance. After the open board meeting that followed, Brandon pulled aside the hospital legal counsel and asked him to research taking legal action against the physicians who refused to take ER call. Schilling had advised all board members to approach this issue more diplomatically and not attract media attention. Schilling undertook a more politically acceptable solution by gathering benchmarking data from surrounding hospitals and offering to pay on-call physicians the average of the market. Physician groups were then asked to bid for taking ER call.

Dr. Karl Pearl, a neurologist with privileges at the hospital, is the third district board member who was on the district board during the years of the PHO. He is the board member who was most bitter about how VPG "ruined" the PHO, and he publicly criticized them. Pearl's resentment toward the decrease in health care reimbursement is a topic he often pontificates on at board meetings. Like the other physician board members, his clinical privileges at the hospital have been perceived as a conflict of interest. He has publicly criticized the large size of the management staff. The CEO took this as a personal affront and a blow to morale.

The fourth member of the board is also a clinician. Aaron Travis is an osteopath with privileges at a competing community hospital. He respects Schilling and accepts his advice. Travis boasts of "saving" the hospital during the PHO by asking "a few simple questions" about the hospital's performance that, at the time, nobody could answer. This led to other questions and the eventual financial turnaround of the hospital. Unfortunately, Travis has his own limitations that affect his ability to be an effective district board member. He is openly angry about his experiences during the PHO when his car was vandalized and he received threatening phone calls.

The fifth board member, Stephanie Stewart, is a businesswoman in the community. She has a lot of respect for Schilling and is willing to work with him. Stewart had a difficult time grasping the complexity of the hospital's operations and its finances when she first became a board member. The reality that what the hospital charges for services is not what the hospital is paid was an illogical way to do business in her mind. She wants to be a team member and at times becomes frustrated with the physician members' negativism. She and Travis have often asked the physician board members to "move on from the past."

THE NEW CEO

Three of the five district board seats were up for election. Before the November elections, the board asked Schilling to become the new CEO. Schilling was the former CEO of a not-for-profit hospital and had spent his entire 45-year professional career as a hospital administrator. Schilling has a history of back problems. When he arrived on the job, however, he appeared to be in good health. He was originally hired by the district board to help the hospital dissolve its relationship with the physician group in the PHO. He successfully returned the hospital to district control. He eliminated the hospital's $2 million per month deficit. The number of FTEs had been decreased to very low levels during the affiliation with the PHO. Although this kept expenses for salaries and benefits to a low percentage of hospital revenue, Schilling wanted to increase morale by hiring more staff, reinstating salary increases, and providing better benefits to the employees. He also began to put resources back into the hospital by making desperately needed upgrades to the facility. These changes greatly increased employee trust and respect for Schilling and his warmth and caring attitude toward his employees helped him gain their loyalty.

LEADERSHIP STYLE

The board members, physicians, and employees gave Schilling accolades for returning the hospital to profitability. Schilling's leadership style, however, was quickly criticized when later financial projections showed a $24 million loss for the next year. The physicians described his leadership style as patriarchal and paternalistic. The physicians, nurses, and managers were accustomed to a culture of teamwork that had been supported and fostered by the former CEO. Schilling became frustrated when his authority was questioned, not only by the medical staff and nurses but also his own executive team. Schilling actually felt his team was sophomoric. Most were good at taking direction from him and his COO, but they felt that the absence of a strategic plan impeded their ability to focus on a common goal. Schilling delegated the authority to run all executive team meetings to his COO, Daniel Porter. Porter was not well respected by the team because of his authoritarian leadership style and his lack of listening skills. The dynamic in the executive meetings would either break down into arguing or nobody would contribute ideas. A lack of leadership was becoming apparent throughout the organization.

LOSING SUPPORT

By increasing morale, renovating the facility, and bringing in some of his own executive team, Schilling was able to stabilize BMH. A strategic plan had been developed and presented to the hospital board. Schilling's approach to keeping the strategic plan confidential until it was ready to be launched, however, made many of the management, physicians, and hospital staff uneasy. Unfortunately, because of the politics involved when physicians felt that their turf was threatened, it was impossible to increase market-driven, revenue generating services. Orthopedic and open-heart surgery were two such services. When pressed to expand the orthopedic surgery service by recruiting new surgeons, the physicians threatened to go to neighboring hospitals. The orthopedic surgeons had been there for many years and were comfortable with the department's current status. Added to the equation was the physician board members' reluctance to make enemies. The PHO experience had left a bitter taste in the board members' mouths; they appeared to be paralyzed by past events. Schilling began to lose support.

The board criticized even highly successful decisions made by the CEO. The last major decision the board made at his recommendation was to get out of risk pool agreements with the insurance companies. Schilling presented two options to the district board: increase revenue or decrease expenses. The board had agreed to decrease expenses by renegotiating the hospital's insurance contracts, but later claimed Schilling waited too long to present this information to the board. In fact, Schilling had been trying to persuade the board to get out of risk pool agreements for more than 2 years.

A TROUBLED PHYSICIAN

The vice chief of staff, Clara Mavory, M.D., was a practicing anesthesiologist during this time. She was praised for her commitment to BMH's survival as a freestanding facility. Mavory had helped lure Schilling from a neighboring hospital to help bring the hospital back to district ownership. Mavory had a troubled history with VPG; she was asked to leave the VPG after being disciplined for disruptive behavior 7 years prior to establishing her own medical practice. A year after Schilling became CEO, Mavory began to demand confidential files, including legal records and peer review files. Mavory disagreed with many sections of the medical staff bylaws and recommended revisions. This caused a slowdown in preparation for The Joint Commission on Accreditation of Healthcare Organizations (Joint Commission) survey because the quality department had to refocus its energy on legal counsel's approval of the revisions. The Joint Commission requires all bylaws changes to be in place a year before a survey. When Mavory did not receive all the confidential files she demanded, she criticized Schilling publicly and began to persuade other physicians to distrust his administration. She had done the same thing to the prior administration.

The board members began to feel bullied by Mavory. The three physician board members with hospital privileges disagreed with Mavory's demands, but found it easier to acquiesce. A peer review file on Mavory's clinical performance prepared by the quality department showed several instances of questionable clinical judgment. Also in this file were complaints about Mavory's inappropriate behavior toward patients and hospital staff. Schilling had felt protective as a friend and obligated to Mavory for his position as CEO at BMH. Although her peer review file had gone to a peer review committee, no disciplinary action had been taken against her. Schilling kept her file locked away in a file in the clinical quality department's office. According to the hospital's attorneys, the only way to remove a physician's privileges is to substantiate evidence of poor-quality medical practice in accordance with the medical staff bylaws.

Schilling later realized how critical the information in her peer review file could have been in stopping Mavory from causing a rift between the medical staff and the administration. The file still existed and could be acted upon. Because his relationship with Mavory had become adversarial, however, reporting Mavory might have appeared vindictive considering the time lapse from when the events originally occurred. Schilling's only recourse had been to persuade the board to support him in blocking her demands for confidential information. Over the last year, however, Schilling received no support from the board in disciplining Mavory on her behavior towards the hospital staff. Schilling's numerous attempts to telephone Harvey had been futile. Harvey would not return his calls.

Schilling also wrote memoranda to all the board members when Mavory demanded information. These memoranda often included responses to Mavory and explanations to the board as to why certain information was confidential or not appropriate for Mavory to see. Schilling's weekly memoranda went unanswered by all of the board members. Verbal communications had become infrequent and were limited to the board meetings. Harvey, along with the other board members, felt Schilling was not healthy enough to continue in his role as CEO. Their attitude toward his health clouded their ability to trust Schilling's decision making. They also preferred to ignore Mavory instead of dealing with her. As fellow clinicians, the four physicians on the board felt obliged not to criticize Mavory.

REORGANIZING THE BOARD

Schilling trusted his intuition and 45 years of experience as he tried to make better use of two board members who still supported his ideas and remained loyal to his leadership. He developed a plan to organize the board into subcommittees to better use the support of these two board members to sell ideas to the other three members. The subcommittees included strategic planning, finance, emergency room on-call coverage (which was a short-term commitment), and governance. The membership on each subcommittee consisted of two board members, the CEO, and other designated administrative staff. The proposal for the new subcommittees was presented at an evening public board meeting and passed unanimously by the board. This restructuring was the first step towards solving the communication problems and increasing the level of trust the other three board members had in him.

SUCCESSION PLANNING

Schilling's contract was to end next fall. Should he retire or should he seek to renew his contract? As much as he did not want to admit it, his health was deteriorating and maintaining relationships that were in turmoil was becoming too demanding. Major surgery relieved a back condition but his general health improved only minimally. Schilling had succeeded in what he had been hired to do—getting the hospital back into district control and stabilizing the organization. Continued success depended on regaining support from his board and the trust of the medical staff. After adding staff and upgrading the facility, however, the hospital's expenses now exceeded revenues. Financial projections showed that the hospital would soon repeat history by losing $2 million a month. Patient volumes were very low in most services. Nursing ratios were high, but the culture of the organization demanded lower patient ratios in return for not increasing salaries, a compromise that a strong in-house nursing union supported.

Unfortunately, almost all of the board members were less interested in following the CEO's advice to improve the numbers because they no longer believed that he knew what he was doing. As the date for his contract renewal loomed closer, employees, too, began to question Schilling's continuation as their leader. Morale declined further as employees began to fear the instability of a possible change in leadership at the hospital. Employees feared that a for-profit hospital system would buy the hospital. This would completely change the culture of the BMH, and possibly cause lay-offs. During the PHO period, employees had been laid off, salaries frozen, and benefits cut. The employees did not want that to happen again. The local branch of a statewide union brought in their leadership to organize the nonnursing employees after receiving a phone call from a BMH employee. The nurses and facility engineers were already unionized. Schilling did not have the motivation to stop the infiltration of the union, which could ultimately unionize all hospital employees.

CHIEF OF STAFF

Mavory was elected vice chief of staff after successfully running against several opponents. The medical staff bylaws provided that the vice chief of staff would automatically become chief of staff if the election was uncontested. Mavory had stated that she would refuse to take the salary usually paid to the chief of staff because she considered it a conflict of interest. As the election drew near, her only opponent withdrew after she confronted him by telling him that his candidacy was causing a rift in the medical staff. His withdrawal made an election unnecessary and Mavory became chief of the medical staff.

In response to Mavory's criticism of Schilling's power over the board, Schilling recommended that the hospital change its bylaws to make the CEO a nonvoting member. As Schilling's presence waned due to health problems, Mavory requested that the hospital board make her a voting member because she was chief of staff. This action would require a change in the hospital and medical staff bylaws. The board members did not act on her request.

TERMINATION FROM VPG

Seven years ago Mavory had been forced out of VPG because of disruptive behavior. This appeared to be the only possible motivation Schilling could think of for Mavory to make enemies of the VPG physicians by publicly attacking them in the medical staff's newsletter and at the medical staff executive meetings. This group was 50% of the hospital's physicians and they were essential to its continued financial health. Schilling thought her disruptive behavior would wane if she were not confronted. He hoped that by ignoring her behavior Mavory would lose her audience. Unfortunately, this did not prove to be the case. On a weekly—and sometimes daily—basis, she would demand access to computer files, legal correspondence between the medical staff office employees and the hospital attorney, and files on malpractice cases. Mavory demanded the right to attend confidential department meetings and verbally abused physicians who disagreed with her. She constantly tried to pit the medical staff against administration. She appeared to want the physicians to become a unionized bargaining unit.

OBSTRUCTING PREPARATION
FOR JOINT COMMISSION

In one meeting that focused on Joint Commission preparation, Mavory demanded a change in an organizational diagram that showed the flow in communications throughout the hospital. During the last Joint Commission visit the surveyors had actually praised the hospital on this excellent tool for representation of how all hospitals should expedite communications through the layers of bureaucracy. Mavory felt that the chart appeared to show the medical staff reporting to the CEO.

As soon as she became chief of staff, Mavory tried to dissolve the medical executive committee and change most of the membership of the physician committees. She wanted most representatives of administration removed even if they served as support staff to the committees. These would be violations of the medical staff bylaws and could compromise The Joint Commission accreditation survey only six months away. The only Type 1 violation the hospital had received in the previous survey was the medical staff's failure to comply with its own bylaws. Mavory wanted the vice president of quality, Harold Fredrick, removed from all meetings and eventually fired. Mavory said she did not like Fredrick because they had a personality conflict. Mavory thwarted changes to many policies and procedures that also were reviewed and approved by the medical executive committee. She added and removed appointments to joint medical staff and administrative committees and stalled bylaws revisions for months and even as long as a year. According to the VP of quality, this jeopardized Joint Commission accreditation because all approvals by the Medical Staff Chiefs' Committee (MSCC) that must also be approved by the board should be in place for at least a year before a Joint Commission survey (see Exhibit 3). The manager of the medical staff office quit, citing high levels of stress over the last year.

Mavory made it clear to all hospital employees and physicians that she was everyone's boss. When the copy room informed her that she could no

---

REMOVAL OF COMMITTEE MEMBERS

. . . A committee member appointed by the chief of staff may be removed by a two-thirds vote of the Medical Staff Chiefs' Committee. A committee member appointed by the department chief may be removed by a two-thirds vote of the department medical staff membership or the Medical Staff Chiefs' Committee . . .

Exhibit 3. Proposed medical staff bylaws provision thwarted by Dr. Mavory.

longer make personal copies at the hospital's expense, she told one of the mail room supervisors, "Do you know who I am? I am the most powerful physician in the hospital. I am your boss. You will do as I say!"

COMPENSATION FOR ER ON-CALL PANEL

It appeared that Mavory searched for issues or problems to pit physicians against administration. Knowing that physicians were demanding pay for being ER on-call, she coached one plastic surgeon to take this issue to the MSCC to be discussed. When some members of the MSCC asked the plastic surgeon for benchmarking data on what other hospitals are paying for ER on-call physicians, the physician claimed he was "too busy" to conduct research on this issue. The plastic surgery group became the most frustrated with not being paid for being on-call in the ER. They gave the administration a deadline to begin on-call payments that the hospital could not meet. None of the physicians would agree to do research or benchmark how much other hospitals were paying physicians for on-call service. Some board members wanted to report some of the physicians to the state authorities for writing an ultimatum to administration saying they would refuse to take call. Patients not seen in the ER because there were too few physicians would have to be transported to other hospitals. Some board members were concerned that this could be a violation of the Emergency Medical Treatment and Active Labor Act, which could become very expensive in fines for the hospital and bad public relations. Administration thought this was unlikely, however. The two board members on the on-call subcommittee came to the MSCC meeting to show their willingness to resolve the issue and to get feedback from the physicians as to what they believed the solution to be. They were well received by the physicians attending this meeting after the board members encouraged the physicians to help find solutions to the problem. Ultimately, the CEO proposed a solution that was accepted by the physicians. Physicians would be paid $300.00 for carrying an ER pager; physicians called in to the ER would be paid $1,000.00 per 8-hour shift.

NO STRATEGIC PLAN IMPLEMENTED

The board would not sell or close the money-losing cancer unit because the physicians providing that service might take their other patients to a competing hospital. They also were worried that these VPG doctors would become wealthy because of the financial arrangement. Schilling believed that the board was uneasy about a change in the hospital's services. After the PHO, they seemed reluctant to cut services that could possibly make even one hospital physician angry or add services that could make one of them "wealthy."

Dr. Mavory's replacement as vice chief of staff was the secretary/treasurer of the medical staff, Dr. Barry Landon. He was the only open-heart surgeon at BMH. This violated state law requiring hospitals performing open-heart procedures to have a two-surgeon team. When the director of strategic planning, Kelly Nelson, approached Landon about recruiting another cardiovascular surgeon, Landon wanted to have her fired. Landon felt threatened by Nelson's recommendation. He wanted full control over the open-heart surgery. Mavory supported Landon in efforts to remove Nelson, calling her "no good."

SCHILLING'S RESIGNATION

Schilling decided to resign. He did not want to be blamed for the demise of the hospital and felt responsible for solving its financial problems. His attempts to rebuild his relationship with his board and the chief of staff, however, seemed futile. He did not have the energy because of his poor physical health to strengthen his relationship with employees, managers, and physicians. Schilling agreed to stay until the district board hired a consultant as the interim CEO.

CONSULTANT HIRED

Jena Carson agreed to take the interim CEO position. Carson's 20 years of experience as a "turnaround" expert made her an obvious choice. She had many decisions to make in her new role. How would she approach improving the financial position of the hospital? How would she approach increasing patient volumes? Could she use the old strategic plan or would she need to develop a new one? Would the board support her decisions? Could she stop other hospital employees from unionizing? How could she control the chief of staff's divisiveness? Could she focus the organization on completing its preparation for The Joint Commission? How would she manage her board members and executive team into becoming effective leaders to assist her in turning the hospital around and perhaps making the hospital a market leader? Most important, what priority should be assigned to these problems?

PART IV

Resource Utilization and Control

18

Regional Health System

The Satellite Health Park Strategy

Jonathon S. Rakich
Indiana University Southeast, New Albany, Indiana

Michael F. Rolph
First Health of the Carolinas, Pinehurst, North Carolina

As he prepared for the December 1993 board meeting, Michael Reynolds, Senior Vice President and Chief Financial Officer of Regional Health System (RHS) felt exhilarated by the bold strategic initiatives that were implemented by RHS in July. The change to the organization had been breathtaking and the manner in which RHS delivered health services was fundamentally different from that of just a year ago. Reynolds was, however, still worried about the increasingly turbulent and threatening health services delivery environment. He knew that if "you rest you rust." He was still somewhat apprehensive about RHS's future and survival. The always-present prospect of marginal financial performance, or worse, the specter of acquisition by an aggressive for-profit hospital system remained in the deep reaches of his mind.

As the "money man" of the $140 million a year organization, Reynolds felt confident that the satellite health park strategy to be presented for consideration by the board at its December 1993 meeting was financially viable. Still, he had a sinking feeling that other considerations and external forces could affect the potential success of the strategy.

Reynolds, age 49, has always been comfortable with numbers. His MBA and CPA background, 5 years' teaching experience as a professor of accounting at a major university, and 20 years' experience in various financial positions at two nonprofit hospitals and a managed care insurance company provided him with an in-depth understanding of the financial dimensions of health services delivery. He had witnessed the industry evolve from rather simple reimbursement systems two decades ago to the exceedingly complex systems of today. He thought to himself:

> Can we keep up with the fast-paced changes? It seems that today's market place pressures, especially from government, managed care organizations, large third-party payers, and competitors, including physicians, have turned traditional health services delivery upside down. I know what the numbers tell me. Robert Meek [President and CEO] and I should strongly recommend to the board that the satellite health park strategy be seriously considered for implementation. Yet, the numbers don't tell all. There are other considerations, some beyond control, that might affect them or cause them to unravel.

BACKGROUND

Prior to July of 1993, RHS was a stand alone 342-bed not-for-profit acute care hospital that served a predominantly elderly community in Florida. The hospital had been operationally profitable during the 1980s even after the implementation of the Medicare prospective payment reimbursement system (PPS) in 1983. Under PPS, the federal government reimbursed hospitals for Medicare acute care inpatient services based on diagnosis-related groups (DRGs). Each DRG represents an associated fixed reimbursement amount by case/discharge regardless of the hospital's cost in delivering the service. In the early 1990s, however, the hospital had begun to see its operating margin suffer as the federal government's efforts to reduce its deficit translated into reduced Medicare reimbursement.

Approximately 45% of the population of the hospital's primary and secondary markets are age 65+ compared to a national average of 13%. Due to the greater than proportionate utilization of health services by the elderly, the hospital's Medicare payer mix was and still is greater than that of 99% of hospitals nationally. The hospital's operating and capital costs of providing inpatient care per case/discharge for Medicare patients had been increasing at a rate in excess of 7% each year since 1983, while the Medicare program has provided less than a 3% reimbursement rate increase each year through the same period. Given the situation of declining margins, in July of 1992 Meek appointed Reynolds as chair of the strategic planning committee with the responsibility of exploring alternatives that would enhance revenues and the financial viability of the hospital. Meek said,

> Mike, we must respond to this deteriorating financial situation. We have to do something to increase revenues since inpatient dollars for Medicare patients will continue to be limited by the Feds. Remember, missions are nice, but no bottom line residual money means no long-term mission accomplishment. Put your pen to work, crunch the numbers, and give me the committee's recommendations by December.

With extensive analysis and review, Reynolds and the strategic planning committee conceived and evaluated numerous strategic alternatives that could meet Meek's charge of enhancing hospital revenues. All were framed within the planning premise of specifically choosing not to expand Medicare inpatient care but to expand other services to the senior and other market segments that would be eligible for alternate forms of reimbursement. The committee's report was submitted to Meek in December of 1992.

Reynolds's pen did indeed work wonders. Based on the committee report and with Reynolds at his side, Meek recommended to the board the following strategies that would transform the hospital into a vertically integrated health system. They were:

1. *Convert 36 general acute care medical/surgical beds to a Medicare certified hospital-based skilled nursing unit.* Meek told the board that "this unit would provide an alternative setting within which patients and others would receive rehabilitation, transfusion, and other skilled care. With treatment in such a unit, revenue would be enhanced beyond the Medicare inpatient acute care DRG fixed amount and would be based upon the actual cost of providing the services."

2. *Acquire a Medicare certified hospital-based home health agency.* Meek explained to the board that a home health agency "presents an opportunity to provide health services traditionally performed in a hospital acute care setting in a less costly setting, thereby increasing reimbursement and reducing costs while maintaining quality. We have a unique opportunity to acquire an existing agency which is the dominant home health provider in our service area."

3. *Acquire a 120-bed free-standing nursing home.* Meek was particularly
   excited as he presented this strategy to the board. He indicated that at
   this time there was not a critical shortage of nursing home beds in the
   service area. Based on future growth projections, however, "we can
   seize a rare opportunity to acquire an upscale nursing home from private investors who want to sell." He added that state certificate-of-
   need regulations prohibit the building of more nursing home beds in
   our area. "If we do not purchase this facility now there is little likeli-
   hood that another opportunity would present itself for many years.
   There will be barriers to entry."

Since all three strategies met the criteria of being financially viable
and enhancing revenues, the board approved them at its January 1993
meeting. The three strategies were implemented by July 1993.
Furthermore, to facilitate implementation, the board approved a restructuring of the hospital and changed its name (effective July 1993) to RHS
in order to reflect the fact that it had now become an integrated health
system offering a range of services beyond just that of acute inpatient
care.

REGIONAL HEALTH SYSTEM 1993

Throughout his 23-year career as a hospital manager, Meek has always
been an idea and big picture person. Having earned his MHA degree from
a leading university in 1970, he gained substantial experience at three different hospitals before joining what is now RHS as President and Chief
Executive Officer (CEO) in 1990. His success was largely due to his
aggressiveness. One of the most telling events in his career was the fact
that the 400-bed not-for-profit hospital where he was previously the Chief
Operating Officer (COO) was sold to a for-profit hospital chain. When
informed that his services were no longer needed he vowed to himself that
he would never let the for-profits "zap" him again. Meek's proclivity to initiate programs and strategies without clearly assessing all factors and environmental forces beyond the financials or how they could affect the financials was known to Reynolds. In their meetings Meek would often say to
Reynolds, "Just show me the numbers."

In late August of 1993 Reynolds returned from a well-earned vacation. The task of implementing the skilled nursing unit, home health
agency, and nursing home acquisition strategies by July 1993 had been delegated to him by Meek. Drained, he looked forward to a few months of
peace and calm. This was not to be. During the monthly meeting of senior
managers, Meek told those assembled that he thought that RHS should

embark on another strategy that he called the Satellite Health Park. Turning to Reynolds, Meek said, "Reconvene and chair the strategic planning committee, run the numbers, and make a recommendation to me by November. I want to make a presentation to the board at its December meeting and, if the health park strategy is approved, implementation would begin in 1994."

THE SATELLITE HEALTH PARK STRATEGY— BACKGROUND DATA

Meek visualized the satellite health park strategy as a means to expand RHS's outpatient services to a nonhospital site. The satellite health park would include the following: (a) an ophthalmology surgery center, (b) a diagnostic facility, and (c) a rehabilitation facility, in addition to the building and sale of physician office condominiums. Meek told Reynolds,

> Progressive advances in technology have significantly increased the ability of health care providers to deliver traditionally inpatient care in settings such as the health park. The setting offers the opportunity of enhanced reimbursement while also providing economies that result in reduced overhead and other costs. Also, because of the need for a critical mass, I believed that all components of the health park must be included. It is an all or nothing proposition.

In terms of resources, Reynolds knew that RHS had approximately $6,000,000 of proceeds remaining from a recent bond issue that had an effective interest cost of 7%. An additional $10,000,000 of capital was available from a board-designated fund for plant replacement and expansion. That fund has been professionally managed in recent years and was expected to continue yielding 9% per annum. Accordingly, incremental cost of capital is a weighted average of 8.25%. The health park strategy would require approval from the State Agency for Health Administration in the form of a certificate of need (CON). It was anticipated that such approval would be forthcoming.

At the committee's request, the Planning Department conducted a demographic study of the RHS market and provided Reynolds and the committee with information and several exhibits that were of assistance in evaluating the financial viability and long range strategic value of the health park. The population age distribution, for example, indicated the significant contrast in age of this community from the national average. Nearly 45% of the RHS service area is age 65+ as compared to the national average of only 13%.

Exhibit 1 (Service Area Population and Market Share Capture) provides 1990 census data for the primary and secondary service area as well as estimates of annual growth rate, projected 1995 census and RHS's market share of outpatient services to be offered at the health park before and after the health park would open. Exhibit 2 (Payer Mix) is the Planning

Service Area	Census 1990	Growth Rate 1991–2000	Projected Census 1995
Primary:			
North	15,099	3.2%	17,674
South	9,262	4.5%	11,542
Center	12,219	2.1%	13,557
East	26,484	5.5%	34,614
Total	63,064	4.1%	77,387
Secondary:			
North	3,695	3.5%	4,389
East	16,353	7.1%	23,043
South	32,407	6.1%	43,573
Total	52,455	6.2%	71,005
Total Service Area	115,519	5.1%	148,392

Outpatient Market Share Capture

Before Addition of Health Park			After Addition of Health Park		
Surgical	Diagnostic	Rehab	Surgical	Diagnostic	Rehab
25.000%	40.000%	50.000%	34.000%	60.000%	64.000%
18.103%	14.921%	19.906%	54.051%	47.204%	69.281%
21.700%	28.000%	35.600%	43.594%	53.877%	66.527%

Exhibit 1.   Service area population and market share capture.

Payer	Health Park	
	Surgery (%)	Other (%)
Medicare	90	65
Medicaid	2	3
Commercial/Other	6	28
Bad Debt/Charity	2	4
Total	100	100

Exhibit 2. Payer mix.

Department's best estimate of the payer mix to be experienced for each of the initiatives contemplated. Again the dominant payer is the Medicare program.

Planning developed estimates of service area use rates per thousand population as a means of computing total market demand for the services contemplated. A summary is provided in Exhibit 3 (Service Area Use Rates). As may be inferred from the exhibit, advent of the Medicare prospective payment system, managed care, and technology advances in surgery and medicine, all contributed to a national and regional shift from inpatient to outpatient utilization. Planning analyzed population growth, use rate trends, and other factors in projecting the volume of services for each health park component and they are presented in Exhibit 4 (Projected Service Volume).

Cost data specific to each health park component were compiled by the Fiscal Services Department, Management Engineering, key operating personnel, and others. The Operations Standards presented in Table 1 provide a summary of their effort to identify relevant variable and fixed operating costs. The cost/volume relationships may be assumed to be valid in later years. All costs with the exception of initial outlay and depreciation are assumed to inflate at an average rate of 4% per annum. Depreciation of building and equipment is based upon the useful life of the assets.

	Year	
Healthcare Encounters	1990	1995
Inpatient Discharges	211.1	172.0
Outpatient:		
Surgeries	36.1	37.1
Diagnostic Tests	1,922.40	1,999.30
Rehab. Therapy Visits	289.7	298.4

Exhibit 3. Service area use rates.

Description	Service		
	Surgery	Diagnostic	Rehab
A. Use Rate per 1,000 (Exhibit 3)	37.1	1,999.30	298.4
B. Projected Population (1,000's) (Exhibit 1)	148.392	148.392	148.392
C. Projected Total Market (A x B) (Rounded)*	5,505	296,680	44,280
D. Market Share (%) After Addition of Health Park (Exhibit 1)	43.594%	53.877%	66.527%
E. Market Share After Addition of Health Park (Rounded)	2,400	159,843	29,458
F. Market Share (%) Before Addition of Health Park (Exhibit 1)	21.700%	28.000%	35.600%
G. Market Share Before Addition of Health Park (Rounded)	1,195	83,071	15,764
H. Market Share Increase (E–G)	1,205	76,772	13,694
I. Percent of Hospital Volume to Shift to the Health Park	100.000%	40.000%	40.000%
J. Hospital Volume Shift to Health Park (G x I)	1,195	33,228	6,306
K. Total 1995 Volume at Health Park (H + J)	2,400	110,000	20,000
L. Total 1994 Volume at Health Park (K x 50%)	1,200	55,000	10,000

*Projected market is assumed to remain constant through 1998 to simplify the case. A more exact solution would require total market to change with projected use rate and population each year.

Exhibit 4. Projected service volume.

THE HEALTH PARK STRATEGY— FINANCIAL ANALYSIS

As Exhibit 1 illustrates, RHS's service area growth rate (1991–2000) was projected to be the greatest in the secondary market, particularly in the east and south. Growth, as well as the industry trend toward greater outpatient utilization per capita, appears to assure an adequate demand for services proposed for the health park.

The Planning Department's estimates of the cumulative shift in market from competitors and from the RHS Hospital itself to the health park are provided in Exhibit 1 (Market Share Capture). The capture rate in conjunction with use rates and service area population provide the basis upon which the projected service volumes given in Exhibit 4 (Projected Service Volume) were developed.

In order to obtain additional information on the economic viability of the health park strategy, Reynolds and his committee engaged a project management firm to evaluate the proposed site to determine construction cost, adequate access, environmental impact, and other development issues. The site has two parcels with 39 combined acres. The acquisition cost is $110,000

Table 1. Operations standards

Description of Cost	Surgery	Diagnostics	Rehab
Variable cost/unit	$500	$40	$50
Fixed Expenses:			
Staff and supplies	$175,000	$150,000	$180,000
Allocated overhead	0	0	0
Depreciation	$80,000	$250,000	$110,000

per acre. Site development cost will approximate $2,450,000. The project management firm recommended that the infrastructure be developed for the total acreage even though only 25 acres will be required to accommodate the health park. A number of *bona fide* buyers were known to exist for the remaining 14 acres. After site development, the per acre market value would increase to $250,000. For purposes of this analysis it is assumed that 6 acres will be sold in 1994 with the remaining 8 acres sold in 1995. Table 2 shows the capital investment costs that will be required for each health park service.

The physician offices that will be built will be divided into office condominiums and sold during 1994 at a total net sales price of $2,330,000. Title to the land will remain with RHS and a land lease executed with each physician purchasing an office. The lease payments will aggregate $145,000 per year and will run a term of 99 years. At the completion of the term, all leasehold improvements will revert to RHS. Working capital requirements will approximate $1,100,000.

Medicare reimbursement for free-standing ophthalmology surgery and diagnostic services is based upon a fee schedule. The surgical procedures will be primarily cataract, which will be reimbursed at $795 per procedure in 1994. Diagnostics are expected to have a Medicare reimbursement rate of $85 per procedure in 1994. The Medicare reimbursement rate is expected to increase 3% per annum.

Medicare reimburses certified outpatient rehabilitation facilities (CORF) based on actual cost. Cost is computed as the direct cost of oper-

Table 2. Capital investment costs for surgery, diagnostics, rehabilitation, and physician offices

	Building	Equipment
Ophthalmic Surgery	$1,050,000	$270,000
Diagnostics	1,680,000	850,000
Rehabilitation	2,090,000	195,000
Physician Offices	2,025,000	0
Total	$6,845,000	$1,315,000

ating the facility (operating expenses and depreciation) plus allocated overhead from support departments such as RHS administration using a complex cost finding process. For purpose of this case it is assumed that the reimbursement rate will be $80 per therapy in 1994 and increase at 4% per annum.

Medicaid reimburses free-standing centers for surgery, diagnostic, and rehabilitation services in a manner similar to Medicare. Thus, the Medicare and Medicaid payer mix may be combined in analyzing total reimbursement received from those programs.

Patient charges per procedure in 1994 will be $1,200 for cataract surgery, $120 for diagnostic tests, and $100 per rehabilitation visit. Rate increases are projected to approximate 7% per annum. Commercial/other payers receive a 10% discount from charges during the entire forecast period.

Procedures captured from the RHS Hospital will reduce contribution margin there. The revenue and variable expense relationships at the RHS Hospital are similar to those projected for the health park. Thus, it may be assumed that the contribution margin lost at the RHS Hospital due to the shift in services to the health park will equal the contribution margin per unit generated at the health park multiplied times the health park volume captured from the RHS Hospital. All of the ophthalmology but only 40% of the diagnostic and rehabilitation volume will shift to the health park.

Determining the Cost–Benefit of the Health Park Strategy

Knowing that Meek and the board required a complete financial analysis of the health park strategy, Reynolds worked on a cost–benefit analysis for the 5 year period, 1994–1998. His analysis of cash flow from operations covering the years 1994–1998 for the (a) surgery, (b) diagnostic, and (c) rehabilitation services is provided in Exhibits 5–7. Exhibit 8 provides the contribution margin lost by the hospital for each service. Exhibit 9 presents the cost–benefit analysis for the years 1994–1998 for all three services, as well as the sale of physician offices.

Reynolds provided this information to you, his assistant. His instructions to you were to use the Operations Standards information, the information provided in Exhibits 5–8, and an interest rate of 8.25% to do the following:

1. Calculate the payback in years (the number of years for the net cash flow to equal the initial investment outlay).

2. Calculate the net present value (present value of benefits less initial outlay).

3. Calculate the profitability index (present value of benefits divided by initial outlay).

4. Based on your analysis, make a recommendation to me whether the health park strategy should be recommended to Meek and the board.

	1994	1995	1996	1997	1998
Patient Volume by Payer:					
Medicare/Medicaid (95%)	1,140	2,280	2,280	2,280	2,280
Commercial/Other (3%)	36	72	72	72	72
Bad Debt/Charity (2%)	24	48	48	48	48
Total Patient Volume (100%)	1,200	2,400	2,400	2,400	2,400
Reimbursement Rate Per Case ($):					
Medicare/Medicaid	795.0000	818.8500	843.4155	868.7180	894.7765
Commercial/Other	1,080.0000	1,155.6000	1,236.4920	1,323.0464	1,415.6597
Bad Debt/Charity	0.0000	0.0000	0.0000	0.0000	0.0000
Operating Revenue ($):					
Medicare/Medicaid	906,300	1,866,978	1,922,987	1,980,677	2,040,097
Commercial/Other	38,880	83,203	89,027	95,259	101,927
Bad Debt/Charity	0	0	0	0	0
Total Operating Revenue ($)	945,180	1,950,181	2,012,014	2,075,936	2,142,024
Variable Expenses ($)	660,000	1,372,800	1,427,712	1,484,820	1,544,213
Contribution Margin ($)	285,180	577,381	584,302	591,116	597,811
Fixed Expenses ($):					
Staff and Supplies	175,000	182,000	189,280	196,851	204,725
Depreciation	80,000	80,000	80,000	80,000	80,000
Total Fixed Expenses ($)	255,000	262,000	269,280	276,851	284,725
Income (Loss) from Operations ($)	30,180	315,381	315,023	314,265	313,086
Expenses Not Requiring Cash ($):					
Depreciation	80,000	80,000	80,000	80,000	80,000
Cash Flow from Operations ($)	110,180	395,381	395,023	394,265	393,086

Exhibit 5. Cash flow from surgery.

	1994	1995	1996	1997	1998
Patient Volume by Payer:					
Medicare/Medicaid (74%)	40,700	81,400	81,400	81,400	81,400
Commercial/Other (21%)	11,500	23,100	23,100	23,100	23,100
Bad Debt/Charity (5%)	2,750	5,500	5,500	5,500	5,500
Total Patient Volume (100%)	54,950	110,000	110,000	110,000	110,000
Reimbursement Rate Per Case ($):					
Medicare/Medicaid	85.0000	87.5500	90.1765	92.8818	95.6682
Commercial/Other	108.0000	115.5600	123.6492	132.3046	141.5660
Bad Debt/Charity	0.0000	0.0000	0.0000	0.0000	0.0000
Operating Revenue ($):					
Medicare/Medicaid	3,459,500	7,126,570	7,340,367	7,560,578	7,787,395
Commercial/Other	1,247,400	2,669,436	2,856,297	3,056,237	3,270,174
Bad Debt/Charity	0	0	0	0	0
Total Operating Revenue ($)	4,706,900	9,796,006	10,196,664	10,616,815	11,057,569
Variable Expenses ($)	2,200,000	4,576,000	4,759,040	4,949,402	5,147,378
Contribution Margin ($)	2,506,900	5,220,006	5,437,624	5,667,413	5,910,191
Fixed Expenses ($):					
Staff and Supplies	150,000	156,000	162,240	168,730	175,479
Depreciation	250,000	250,000	250,000	250,000	250,000
Total Fixed Expenses ($)	400,000	406,000	412,240	418,730	425,479
Income (Loss) from Oper. ($)	2,106,900	4,814,006	5,025,384	5,248,684	5,484,713
Expenses Not Requiring Cash ($):					
Depreciation	250,000	250,000	250,000	250,000	250,000
Cash Flow from Operations ($)	2,356,900	5,064,006	5,275,384	5,498,684	5,734,713

Exhibit 6. Cash flow from diagnostic.

	1994	1995	1996	1997	1998
Patient Volume by Payer:					
Medicare/Medicaid (74%)	7,400	14,800	14,800	14,800	14,800
Commercial/Other (21%)	2,100	4,200	4,200	4,200	4,200
Bad Debt/Charity (5%)	500	1,000	1,000	1,000	1,000
Total Patient Volume (100%)	10,000	20,000	20,000	20,000	20,000
Reimbursement Rate Per Case ($):					
Medicare/Medicaid	80.0000	83.2000	86.5280	89.9891	93.5887
Commercial/Other	90.0000	96.3000	103.0410	110.2539	117.9716
Bad Debt/Charity	0.0000	0.0000	0.0000	0.0000	0.0000
Operating Revenue ($):					
Medicare/Medicaid	592,000	1,231,360	1,280,614	1,331,839	1,385,113
Commercial/Other	189,000	404,460	432,772	463,066	495,481
Bad Debt/Charity	0	0	0	0	0
Total Operating Revenue ($)	781,000	1,635,820	1,713,386	1,794,905	1,880,594
Variable Expenses ($)	500,000	1,040,000	1,081,000	1,124,864	1,169,000
Contribution Margin ($)	281,000	595,820	632,386	670,041	711,594
Fixed Expenses ($):					
Staff and Supplies	180,000	187,000	194,688	202,476	210,575
Depreciation	110,000	110,000	110,000	110,000	110,000
Total Fixed Expenses ($)	290,000	297,000	304,688	312,476	320,575
Income (Loss) from Operations ($)	(9,000)	298,820	327,698	357,565	391,019
Expenses Not Requiring Cash ($):					
Depreciation	110,000	110,000	110,000	110,000	110,000
Cash Flow from Operations ($)	101,000	408,820	437,698	467,565	501,019

Exhibit 7. Cash flow from rehabilitation.

	1994	1995	1996	1997	1998
Surgery:					
Health Park Contribution Margin ($)	285,180	577,381	584,303	591,116	597,811
Health Park Volume	1,200	2,400	2,400	2,400	2,400
Contribution Margin per Unit Volume ($)	237.6500	240.5754	243.4596	246.2983	249.0880
Volume Shift from Hospital to Health Park	1,195	1,195	1,195	1,195	1,195
Contribution Margin Lost by Hospital ($)	283,992	287,488	290,934	294,327	297,660
Diagnostic:					
Health Park Contribution Margin ($)	2,506,900	5,220,006	5,437,624	5,667,414	5,910,192
Health Park Volume	55,000	110,000	110,000	110,000	110,000
Contribution Margin per Unit Volume ($)	45.5800	47.4546	49.4330	51.5220	53.7290
Volume Shift from Hospital to Health Park	33,228	33,228	33,228	33,228	33,228
Contribution Margin Lost by Hospital ($)	1,514,532	1,576,821	1,642,560	1,711,973	1,785,307
Rehabilitation:					
Health Park Contribution Margin ($)	281,000	595,820	631,787	670,041	710,735
Health Park Volume	10,000	20,000	20,000	20,000	20,000
Contribution Margin per Unit Volume ($)	28.1000	29.7910	31.5894	33.5021	35.5368
Volume Shift from Hospital to Health Park	6,306	6,306	6,306	6,306	6,306
Contribution Margin Lost by Hospital ($)	177,199	187,862	199,203	211,264	224,095

*The change in the contribution margin per unit each year is based upon the net effect of a combination of reimbursement rate changes by payer and unit variable expense increases.

Exhibit 8.   The contribution margin lost by the hospital to the health park for surgery, diagnostic, and rehabilitation.

	Outlay	1994	1995	1996	1997	1998
Cost ($):						
Land	4,290,000					
Site Development	2,450,000					
Construction	6,845,000					
Equipment	1,315,000					
Working Capital	1,100,000					
Contribution Margin Lost by Hospital						
Surgery		283,992	287,488	290,934	294,327	297,660
Diagnostics		1,514,532	1,576,821	1,642,560	1,711,973	1,785,307
Rehabilitation		177,199	187,862	199,203	211,264	224,095
Total Cost ($)	16,000,000	1,975,723	2,052,171	2,132,697	2,217,564	2,307,062
Benefit ($):						
Cash Flow from Operations						
Surgery		110,180	395,381	395,023	394,265	393,086
Diagnostics		2,356,900	5,064,006	5,275,384	5,498,684	5,734,713
Rehabilitation		101,000	408,620	437,099	467,566	500,160
Land Sales		1,500,000	2,000,000			
Physician Office Sales		2,330,000				
Land Lease		145,000	145,000	145,000	145,000	145,000
Total Benefit ($)		6,543,080	8,013,007	6,252,506	6,505,515	6,772,959
Net Cost/Benefit ($)	(16,000,000)	4,567,357	5,960,836	4,119,809	4,287,951	4,465,897

Additional Financial Analysis:

Payback Period (years)	
Present Value of Net Benefits ($)	
Outlay ($)	(16,000,000)
Net Present Value ($)	
Profitability Index	

Exhibit 9. The cost–benefit analysis for the years 1994–1998 for surgery, diagnostic, and rehabilitation.

19

The ER that Became the Emergency

Managing the Double Bind

Earl Simendinger

Mary Anne Watson

Mike Jasperson

Bryan Boliard
University of Tampa, Florida

FRIDAY SENIOR STAFF MEETING

"I finally have some good news concerning our marketing activities," Bill Coffman said with a smile at the weekly senior staff meeting. "Our radio advertising and other marketing efforts over the past 5 months seem to be paying off. In the last $2\frac{1}{2}$ months, we've seen a dramatic increase in our emergency room visits, and I feel quite positive about the increase in demand." It was easy to see that Bill, the Chief Financial Officer of Community Memorial Hospital (CMH) was quite pleased about his monthly report.

From Simendinger, E., Watson, M. A., Jasperson, M., and Boliard, B. (1998). "The ER that became the emergency: Managing the double bind." *Business Case Journal*, 6(2). Used by permission.

Ralph Peterson, Chief Executive Officer of the hospital, returned Bill's grin and responded, "That's great, Bill, especially since 30% of all of our admissions come through our emergency room."

Bill went on to note that admission increases were directly related to the growth in the amount of emergency room visits. He estimated that ER visits were expected to rise 15%–20% next month.

"Do we have enough staff, or should we start looking at hiring more physicians and nurses?" Ralph asked.

Bill promised he would look into the staffing matter before next week's meeting. As Bill continued with his report, Ralph's attention kept drifting back to the new ER figures on the income statement and balance sheet. For some unexplained reason, an uneasy feeling settled in his gut. He couldn't help but think something didn't fit—it seemed too good, too quick, and too lucky that the increase in admissions had occurred almost solely through CMH's marketing efforts. He wondered if the 15%–20% increase in ER visits in such a short time was realistic. The advertising seemed a bit too effective. One of his friend's favorite sayings popped into his head: "If it seems too good to be true, it probably is!"

In an attempt to gain more information from Bill about the emergency room activity, Ralph interrupted Bill's report and asked whether he had analyzed the ER visit numbers, tracking what types of new patients are using the emergency room. He also wanted to know when and from where they had come and what the payer mix was. "I don't have that information right here," Bill answered, "but we assumed that the payer mix was the same as it had been for the past 2 or 3 years. Why would it be any different?" (Payer mix is a term in health care that refers to the fact that different insurers, such as Medicare, Medicaid, HMOs, and PPOs, reimburse the hospital at different rates for the same service to patients.)

"Let's get the numbers. I have an uneasy feeling about this one," Ralph replied with an irritated shake of his head.

After a few minutes, the burn intensified, and Bill, visibly frustrated, replied, "Do you realize how much time that analysis would take, and I'm up to my ears right now just trying to get the financials, capital, and operating budgets out on schedule!"

Ralph sat there thinking for a moment, wondering if there was something he was missing. As the senior staff at the meeting paused, Ralph finally answered. "Bill, do the analysis please."

As the Friday senior staff meeting concluded and everybody got ready to go home for the weekend, Ralph caught up with Bill on the way out. "Could you get me that ER information as soon as possible?" he asked.

BACKGROUND

CMH, a 400-bed medical/surgical hospital, is located in Middleville, Ohio, a mid-sized city of about 650,000 residents. It is a private, not-for-profit facility that has been located in the downtown area for 75 years. There has always been strong community support for the hospital. Its medical staff consists of 350 physicians and the hospital employs 1,700 people. The payer mix is typical of many hospitals with 25% private pay, 50% Medicare, 10% Medicaid, and the rest composed of HMO, medically indigent, and self-pay patients. The Medicaid program provides medical aid by the federal government although administered at the state level to provide benefits according to established criteria for the poor, aged, blind, disabled, and dependent children. The hospital's clinical reputation has been positive but community members, the board, and the medical staff have raised some concerns regarding its declining financial situation over the past 5 years.

City Hospital, a very well respected, 600-bed health care facility, is located about a quarter mile from CMH. City Hospital has two primary missions: (1) It is a teaching hospital and trains large numbers of residents in conjunction with the local medical school; (2) given its location in the poorest part of the city and its distinction as the city's only publicly funded hospital, it takes care of the city's Medicaid patients as well as other categories of medically indigent patients. A medically indigent patient is one who has insufficient income or savings to pay for medical care without having to sacrifice other essentials for living (i.e., food, clothing, shelter). Treating high numbers of these patients, coupled with the physician training programs, is extremely costly and produces very high operating costs for the City Hospital facility. The Emergency Medical Treatment and Active Labor Act (EMTALA) requires that hospitals receiving federal reimbursement treat, stabilize, and admit (as needed) all patients (regardless of payment) who present at their emergency departments. Patients whose conditions require capability that the hospital lacks may be sent elsewhere after the hospital stabilizes them. City tax funds make up any loss sustained each year by City Hospital for the cost of taking care of this population. The funds transferred to City Hospital have increased to $10 million over the past few months. Jim Harding, who has been the administrator at the City Hospital for the last five years, has worked with the mayor and other city commissioners to try to reduce City Hospital's high operating expenses. Despite several cost-cutting initiatives and two rounds of layoffs, City Hospital still is predicted to have a loss of $12 million for the coming year. The city can't cover this loss with its tax funding, and Mr. Harding is feeling a lot of pressure to, as the mayor says, "find a way."

In addition, there are five other hospitals throughout the city that provide medical care to the residents of the area. St. Marks, a 350-bed, religious-based hospital, is located on the north side of town, approximately 12 miles from CMH. OhioCare, a for-profit, 300-bed, medical/surgical hospital, is situated on the south side of the city about eight miles away from CMH. A third facility, Health Associates, is a specialty hospital, concentrating on serving cancer victims. The Ohio Women's Center Hospital, which is located on the east side of town, is a 200-bed facility that provides services primarily to women and children. Finally, Doctor's Hospital, another medical/surgical facility that has been in town for 20 years, is located on the west side of the town and is an osteopathic hospital.

CMH has competed aggressively with the other hospitals in the city through an expensive, active marketing campaign to get its occupancy rate up from 56%. With the recent increase in emergency room visits, CMH's efforts seemed to be paying off. Then, Bill Coffman did the analysis and found some alarming data on the new ER patients.

FOLLOW-UP MEETING (RALPH, I HAVE THE INFORMATION YOU ASKED FOR)

Over the weekend, Bill Coffman went into the office because he couldn't stop thinking about the strained interaction he had had with Ralph, his concerns regarding the ER payer mix, and from where the new patients were coming. Sitting at his computer, feeling like Sherlock Holmes, he pored through the ER data with a fine-toothed comb. "From where are they coming? Let's look at the zip codes. When are they coming? How are they paying (type of insurance coverage)—or are they?" The printer was buzzing, pumping out the information. Sipping on his cold coffee and munching a sandwich from the vending machine, Bill began to analyze the stack of computer printouts on his desk. After looking at several sets of data, Bill began to shake his head in amazement and tried to avoid the sinking feeling in the pit of his stomach. "I'm seeing, but I don't believe it!" he said to himself. There was a clear pattern emerging as he looked at the information. Not only were the majority of new ER patients medically indigent patients, but also the zip code analysis showed that they were coming primarily from a high demand area not seen before. They were primarily coming in on the weekends during the busiest times for ERs and the most likely time to draw medically indigent patients. Bill sat back in his chair and thought, "Ralph isn't gonna believe this!" Looking more closely at the figures, he was shocked to learn that the medically indigent patient increases were going to be responsible for CMH losing $70,000 to $80,000 this coming month. He groaned and reached for the phone to call Ralph but changed his mind when he looked at his watch and saw it was 1:30 A.M. He realized that waking Ralph in the middle of the night, combined with delivering the bad news, would be an unwise move, especially considering the interaction they had had in the staff meeting.

The following morning, Ralph received a message from Bill Coffman asking if they could get together to discuss the findings that he had come up with concerning the jump in patient activity. At 10 A.M., Ralph popped his head into Bill's office. "So what did you find out, Sherlock?"

"I don't think you're gonna like it—you're not going to believe what's happening and it makes no sense to me. I can't figure it out," Bill said, grimacing. "That jump in emergency room activity was all made up of medically indigent patients coming from one zip code area, and it'll cause a huge ER loss this month."

Ralph sat back in his seat abruptly, and said, "I knew it," and asked for the zip code map. "They're from 00010," Bill stated abruptly. "Get a zip code map, Bill," Ralph commanded.

As soon as Ralph's eyes hit the location on the map, he knew. "These patients are coming from City Hospital's area!" Ralph asked Bill, "What times were the peaks occurring?"

"Peak ER times—the weekends," was the glum reply.

"I think it's time to have a little chat with Jim Harding at City Hospital," Ralph said emphatically. "I'll set up a meeting with him and get to the bottom of this."

TUESDAY MEETING WITH MR. HARDING

Jim Harding, City Hospital's CEO, appeared as scheduled at Ralph's office at 10 A.M. sharp on Tuesday and remarked, "I knew it was just a matter of time before we would be sitting down and discussing this particular issue." He went on to discuss the problems that City Hospital was having with the lack of staffing in its emergency room. Even with the additional government funding, it was unable to afford the number of physicians, residents, and nurses needed to meet the demands of patients coming through its facility. City Hospital's concern for patients' quality of care and lack of staffing, Jim explained to Ralph, was the reason that City Hospital's diversion process had commenced. Diversion is the tactic used by hospital ER administrators to reroute patients to other facilities' emergency rooms when they have reached their capacities. Sometimes this tactic can be used deceptively: A hospital ER may go on diversion to avoid the high costs associated with taking certain types of ER patients, specifically those who provide low reimbursement to the hospital. Jim also admitted that

CMH would be the logical choice for patients diverted from City Hospital based on proximity and patient safety/liability issues. Ralph broke in and said, "I understand your circumstances and why you're going on diversion, but is there any way we can form some kind of financial relationship when you send us your patients? When you go on diversion, can we at least have some kind of a cost-based reimbursement arrangement for the medically indigent patients we take from you?" As the meeting came to a close, Jim agreed that a relationship between the two hospitals would be a good idea and that he would put together a cost-based reimbursement proposal in the next few days for Ralph to consider.

A week later, Ralph received a proposal on his desk from Jim and quickly sent it to Bill Coffman to analyze. Bill quickly ran the numbers and stopped into Ralph's office with the report. After giving Ralph a minute for an initial glance he summed it up, "So . . . the reimbursement of $100 per visit to CMH that City Hospital is offering us to reduce the expenses isn't even close to covering the losses from the influx of its medically indigent patients. At best they would only reduce our average losses by 20%. In 6 months we will be in serious financial trouble."

Ralph thanked Bill for the fast turnaround on the information as he left the office. Frustrated, he thought to himself, "Okay, I've got an ER that's bleeding us to death. What's my next move?"

Ralph immediately called Jim and told him the proposal was unacceptable based on CMH's financial situation. Jim responded by saying, "I'm not surprised, but that's the best I can do." In the conversation that followed, Jim inadvertently shared the fact that City Hospital received $550 a visit for medically indigent patients from city funds. Ralph immediately challenged him, "OK, Jim, let me get this straight. If a medically indigent patient in our city walks through your ER doors, the city gives you a visit rate of $550 as an all-inclusive amount, but if the same patient comes through my doors we will only receive $100 a visit? How is that fair?!" Jim reiterated, "Like I said, that's the best I can do given our financial situation. Sorry."

A WEEK LATER (MEETING WITH COMMISSIONERS)

Finding no acceptable alternatives in his conversation with Jim, Ralph decided his next step was to call a couple of the city commissioners he knew and ask their advice on the situation. Inasmuch as it had to do with city funds, they suggested that Ralph needed to speak with the mayor. After getting off the phone with the last city commissioner, feeling somewhat like a basketball being tossed around in warm-ups, Ralph finally realized he needed to go to the top. He phoned the mayor's office and was able to get an appointment for the following Friday morning.

FRIDAY MEETING WITH THE MAYOR

Ralph made his way promptly to his first ever meeting with the mayor. To his surprise, the mayor, Bill Cane, walked in on time despite his very busy schedule and escorted Ralph into his office. Feeling very impressed and a little intimidated by being in the mayor's office, Ralph brought the mayor up to date on the situation. He proposed that the city increase funding to City Hospital to deal with its financial situation. He also suggested that CMH would be willing to help with the diversion problem but it would need reasonable funding from the city for the care of the city's medically indigent patients.

The mayor expressed understanding: "I see your predicament, but right now the city is battling its own health care financial crisis. We're significantly lacking in funding for health care. You may not know that currently the tax funds can only be spent on medically indigent patients that receive care in a city facility. Any changes will take some time to get passed. We could try to change the city code that was passed with the health tax referendum but, as you are well aware, it is a very long, complex process. As you know, it typically takes 3 years to complete all the procedural and legal steps, even before it could be put to the voters."

With the meeting coming to an end, it was clear to Ralph that the city's financial problems and the politics behind trying to get something done were digging a financial grave for CMH.

As Ralph drove back to CMH, he started realizing the lack of options and began to contemplate the extent of the double bind he was facing. First, he thought the hospital would reach a serious financial problem within 6 months if the problem weren't resolved quickly. On the other hand, if the hospital took a stance of refusing to accept the city patients coming through the ER doors, CMH could experience severe bad press that would bring a negative image on the facility and him. All Ralph could picture was the front page of the city's newspaper with a cartoon picture of himself holding the ER doors closed, preventing a bleeding, medically indigent patient, on his knees, from getting needed medical care. Ralph trembled to think of the board reaction to that picture.

Observing the traffic jam growing in front of him, Ralph turned to take an alternate route home. As he drove past Doctor's Hospital, it suddenly occurred to him that this issue went beyond CMH. Other hospitals might feel threatened as well, even though they were not currently affected by an influx of medically indigent patients. He thought a brainstorming session with other hospital administrators might be in order. As Ralph passed by City Hospital en route to his facility, he felt a slow burn across his back thinking about the fact that City Hospital could divert patients with no flack but he shuddered to think what would happen if CMH diverted just one patient. Over time, diversion of medically indigent patients had become an accepted practice from City Hospital. Although infrequent, City Hospital's ER was sometimes understaffed and unable to deal with the incoming patient volume. As a result, the facility went on diversion without notice or criticism. In the past, however, the duration of the diversion was typically short and involved only a few patients. Never had so many patients been diverted for so long!

SUGGESTED MEETING WITH OTHER CEOs

As soon as Ralph returned to the office, he made phone calls to each of the local hospital CEOs asking them to attend a meeting to discuss the situation. He was sure that he would be able to convince the other hospitals' administrators, his friends, to take their fair share of medically indigent patients for the city.

As a week passed, Ralph was very frustrated at the lack of response from any of the other hospitals' administrators concerning the proposed meeting. In an attempt to get answers, Ralph called his good friend, Dick Rusk, CEO of Health Associates, to find out why he hadn't heard from him. Dick remarked, "I know what you're going through over at CMH and understand why you called the meeting, but we at Health Associates wouldn't want to change a system that would increase our costs." Dick also added he, as most of the other hospital CEOs, felt that they were already taking their fair share of medically indigent patients! Dick concluded by saying, "City Hospital has the funding support through the local referendum to take responsibility for a larger percentage of the area's medically indigent patients. Let them deal with the problem." As Ralph got off the phone, he realized that if he were one of the other CEOs he would probably do the same thing.

MEETING WITH HIMSELF

Later that afternoon, Ralph sat staring through his window at work. The image of getting doors slammed in his face—first Jim Harding's, the mayor's, the city commissioners', then all those hospital CEOs' who were his supposed friends—kept running through his head. Although Ralph realized the problem was complex and had financial, political, and public relations implications, he was humbled by the fact that he had no clear idea what to do next. As he sat perplexed at his desk, the wail of an ambulance siren grew louder, and then passed directly below his window. "Oh, great," he thought, "there goes another 550 bucks out the window!"

20

Attica Memorial Hospital

The Ingelson Burn Center

Bonnie Eng-Suess
Central Health MSO, Inc., Covina, California

Robert C. Myrtle
University of Southern California, Los Angeles,
California

INTRODUCTION

In late 2001, Attica Memorial Hospital purchased and absorbed its nearest competitor, Delphi Hospital, in what was termed an alliance. Attica Memorial's plans were to consolidate duplicate services and to realign all remaining units. Services unique to the acquired hospital were thoroughly evaluated in order to determine if they would survive the alliance. Services that were not essential to the community or added minimum value to Attica Memorial would not be supported. The Ingelson Burn Center was one of those unique lines of service that Attica Memorial thoroughly evaluated in order to determine its fate.

BACKGROUND

Attica Memorial and Delphi Hospitals competed for more than 40 years for patients, physicians, and favorable insurance reimbursement rates. The two hospitals were nonprofit, acute care facilities located in Norton County, less than a half mile from each other, and both offered similar types of services, creating a fiercely competitive environment. Many Attica Memorial physicians also had privileges at Delphi Hospital and could refer patients to either hospital. Physicians took their patients to the hospital that offered greater pay and benefits. In addition, both hospitals competed for limited resources such as staff, health plans, and medical group contracts. Before Attica Memorial acquired Delphi Hospital, health plans and medical groups pitted the hospitals against each other in order to obtain favorable reimbursement rates. Attica Memorial CEO Richard Ponti was left with the dim view that "Any contract rate is a good rate," even if the health plan reimbursed the hospital $4,000.00 for an open-heart procedure. When Delphi's parent organization placed the hospital for sale, Attica Memorial saw a strategic opportunity to purchase its long-time competitor and strengthen its position in the marketplace.

The initial plan of the alliance was to have both hospitals as recognizable "Center of Excellence" facilities by completely realigning the services between the two structures. Attica Memorial transitioned into an acute care inpatient facility while Delphi Hospital became an ambulatory care outpatient pavilion. The original Attica Memorial facility became Attica Memorial East Campus (AMH East Campus) and Delphi Hospital was renamed Attica Memorial West Campus (AMH West Campus). By combining resources with Delphi Hospital, the new Attica Memorial became a stronger and more vital community presence. The hospital would be able to expand its spectrum of patient care by offering new services, more outreach, improved access to care, and an increased focus on quality. Achieving the efficiencies promised by the consolidation of redundant services, however, required careful evaluation of each department and service line, transfers of personnel, and, inevitably, layoffs.

MACRO ENVIRONMENT

Before the 1980s, hospitals did not worry much about charges since they were reimbursed at fee-for-service rates (i.e., their charges were paid at full-price rates). The 1980s, however, brought dramatic changes to the health care environment. The trend was toward continual increases in the cost of health care due to increased costs of pharmaceuticals, aging of the general population, advancements in medical technology, shortage of nurses, and increases in the number of higher-acuity patients. Managed care organizations (MCOs) started to monitor hospital services closely in order to control health care costs. Health maintenance organizations (HMOs) began dictating the length of stay and reimbursement rates for hospitals, making competition for market share extremely difficult in Norton County, which contained a dense concentration of hospitals. In response, the demand for health care services shifted dramatically from the inpatient to the outpatient setting, leaving too many hospital beds for the shrinking number of inpatients. At the same time, the federal government attempted to contain and reduce costs by reimbursing hospitals' Medicare patients on diagnosis-related group (DRG) rates. Reimbursement for services from health plans and Medicare declined substantially. Hospitals started to see their revenue streams shrink on lower reimbursement and discounted fee-for-service rates, making it very difficult to cover costs.

COMPETITIVE ENVIRONMENT

Not only was Attica Memorial affected by trends in the macro environment brought on by the evolution of managed care, but also pressures were even greater in the competitive environment. In Norton County, competition was fierce for market share because there were too many hospitals within a small geographic area. Within a 5-mile radius, Attica Memorial was surrounded by seven other hospitals, all competing for patients, physicians, and health plan contracts. Within a 10-mile radius, Attica Memorial's competition increased to more than 16 hospitals. The managed care penetration in Norton County was approximately 46%—almost double the national average of 24.3%—thereby creating concerns for managed risk and contract liability.

Excess capacity in hospitals was an increasingly steady trend; in 2000, the hospital room occupancy rate in the state was 45.6%, while Norton County's hospital room occupancy rate was slightly lower at 42.6%. A further external threat pressuring hospitals was California State Bill 1953 (SB 1953). This legislation mandated retrofitting of existing hospitals to current building seismic safety codes by the year 2008 and required significant capital expenditures and interruption of services of many hospitals. In addition, the health care market was experiencing a nursing shortage, thereby increasing costs and competition for quality staff.

ANALYSIS OF THE INGELSON BURN CENTER

Nature of Burn Injuries

Burn injuries are unique occurrences. Burn is a service line unlike obstetrics, in which OB physicians can estimate how many deliveries they will perform within a given time based upon patient base. Burns can be the result of fire, the sun, chemicals, heated objects, heated fluids, and electricity. The injury resulting from burn can be diagnosed as minor burn, needing non-emergent care, or major burn, needing life saving emergent care. The degree of burn is determined by the damage to the tissue of the body.

Burn Statistics

In the United States, approximately 2.4 million burn injuries are reported per year. Medical professionals treat approximately 650,000 of the injuries; 75,000 are hospitalized. Of those hospitalized, 20,000 have major burns involving at least 25% of their total body surface. Between 8,000 and 12,000 patients with burns die, and approximately 1 million sustain substantial or permanent disabilities resulting from their burn injury.

The Bureau of Labor Statistics published the following burn statistics for 1992:

- 41,000 heat burns resulted in an average of 4 lost days of work each. Breakdowns of industrial burns were as follows: 16,500 retail trade; 9,500 manufacturing; 8,600 service industry (e.g., restaurants).

- 15,700 chemical burns resulted in an average of 2 lost days of work each. Breakdowns were: 5,800 manufacturing (e.g., chemical manufacturers); 3,200 service industry; 2,600 retail industry.

Children age newborn to 2 years old are the most frequently admitted patients for emergency burn treatment. The kitchen is the most common area in the home where burn injuries occur for children of these ages. The next most frequent area is in the bathroom, where scalding hot water burns children. Scalds are the leading cause of accidental death in the home for children from birth to age 4 and are 40% of the burn injuries for children up to age 14.

Burn Center Background

In 1993, Dr. Craig Ingelson felt that there was a need to provide his unique standard and continuum of care to burn victims in three large counties by establishing a burn center in Norton County. The center would serve as a regional Center of Excellence by utilizing the same coordinated approach to the acute, surgical, and rehabilitative continuum of burn services for which he first established Ingelson Burn Center, 50 miles from Delphi Hospital. In 1997, Dr. Ingelson helped Delphi Hospital establish the Ingelson Burn Center as a state-of-the-art, six-licensed inpatient bed facility coupled with a dedicated outpatient burn center adjacent to the hospital, with himself as the Medical Director. The Ingelson Burn Center of Norton County had earned a reputation for excellent care delivery and superior outcomes by a highly motivated and trained team. The burn center received referrals from other hospitals, employers, insurance companies, and fire departments for both acute inpatient care and continuing outpatient reconstructive and therapy treatments.

Patient Care

Once a patient arrived at the emergency department, the team, consisting of emergency medical physicians, nurses, and emergency medical technicians, all of whom were fully trained in specialized burn care, conducted a preliminary assessment and performed emergency treatment of the patient's injuries based upon the category of burn. The emergency team was in contact with the team of burn surgeons, headed by Dr. Ingelson, relaying all information regarding the status of the patient's injuries. The patient was admitted to the inpatient burn unit where the progress of the patient's injuries was monitored for 48–72 hours postinjury. Burn care specialists coordinated patient care.

Staff

The staff of a burn team was comprised of a variety of members. It consisted of plastic surgeons; neurologists; psychologists; infectious disease physicians; neonatologists; pulmonologists; ophthalmologists; nurses; occupational, physical, recreational, respiratory, and speech therapists; and case managers.

All staff were trained in the most current treatment protocols for burn care, receiving continuous education throughout the year. In addition, all staff was ACLS (advanced cardiac life support) certified and ABLS (advanced burn life support) trained.

Nurse staffing in the inpatient burn center was based on the ratio recommended for any critical/intensive care patient. All specialists utilized were trained in the emergent, acute, immediate, and progressive treatment of burn injuries and were called upon on an as-needed basis after a full evaluation was made of the patient's needs. The burn center had four full-time scheduled personnel, one part-time, and one *per diem* nurse. Normally, the burn center patient–staff ratio was 1:1, 2:1, and 3:1, respectively, which was based on patient classification and patient care needs.

Staffing needs were continuously assessed and adjusted based on patient census and condition fluctuations, the staff's experience and training, technological equipment used, and degree of supervision needed. Policy required not less than two nursing personnel physically present in the unit when a patient was present, with at least one of the nursing personnel an RN.

On average, approximately 20% of the Ingelson Burn Center's patients were children. To serve this special population, the burn center provided a bilingual licensed clinical social worker on staff who was paneled by State Children's Services. The social worker provided recreational therapy and worked with the children and their families to address concerns and fears in dealing with their burn injury.

Communication among the burn team and a patient's employer, insurer, and medical management representative was critical to delivering quality patient care. In order to maintain continuous flow of communication among all members of the team, the burn center coordinated weekly patient care conferences moderated by the case manager. The purpose of the conferences was to discuss and evaluate all inpatient and outpatient burn cases in order to ensure a complete continuum of patient care.

Quality/Image

Dr. Ingelson was a nationally recognized plastic surgeon, a graduate of Emory University and The University of Tennessee Medical School. He was board certified in general surgery as well as plastic surgery. Dr. Ingelson had a unique method of treating burns, characterized by his high utilization of surgery when he debrided and grafted burn patients, which was less painful than the traditional method of debridement and grafting. He was able to combine an extensive burn and reconstruction surgical practice with an aesthetic surgical practice.

The Ingelson Burn Center of Norton County had earned a reputation in the community for excellent care delivery and superior outcomes by a highly skilled and patient-focused team. Patients of the burn center were referred from local and regional hospitals, employers, insurance companies, and fire departments for both acute patient care and continuing outpatient reconstructive and therapy treatments.

License Requirements

In order to have a burn unit, the hospital had to comply with the California State Code of Regulations for both state operations codes and state building codes.

State Operations Codes   According to the Department of Licensing, regulations dictate that a burn center must be a dedicated, closed unit.

In order to treat severe burns, the burn center beds must be licensed for the treatment of burn patients only. In addition, due to the lowered immune response of the burn patient, the unit must be isolated from traffic.

- A burn unit is defined as an intensive care unit (ICU) with services and staff specializing in burn treatment, used solely to treat burns or similar/related conditions.

- A burn unit must be located to prevent through traffic.

- A burn unit must have a minimum of four beds and no more than twelve.

- A burn unit must treat at least 50 burn patients per year.

State Building Codes According to the architecture firm contracted by Attica Memorial, a burn center, as defined in the state building codes, described a unit that must meet requirements for the operation of an intensive care unit, a rehabilitation space, and a respiratory care service space.

The code did not state or imply that any of these referenced areas may be shared, but only that the design guidelines for a burn center needed to comply with requirements needed for an intensive care unit, rehab unit, and a respiratory care service space. Given the unique nature of the treatment and potential for airborne contamination in a burn center, the architects believed it was the intention of the code to designate this department to function as a stand-alone department or unit. In the past, the Office of State Health and Licensing had categorized the Ingelson Burn Center as a separate unit used for the treatment of burn patients.

Burn center regulations closely paralleled the state building codes for the operation of an intensive care unit. The following summarize the key requirements:

- At least one negative pressure isolation room shall be provided for patients with an airborne communicable disease (state building code)

- Nursing station with control desk, charting space, lockable medicine cabinet, refrigerator, and hand wash fixture (state building code)

- At least 132 square feet of floor space per bed with no dimension of less than 11 feet, at least 4 feet of clearance around the bed, and at least 8 feet between beds (state building code)

- 24-hour coordination and physical space requirements for Respiratory and Rehabilitation (state building code)

Physician and Nursing Supervision

There were very specific California state operation codes regulations related to supervision of a burn center. Based on these requirements, Attica Memorial would be required to provide medical and nursing staff with significant burn care experience and training as follows.

- Two accredited physicians experienced in burn therapy shall be responsible for supervision and performance of burn care (state operation code).

- Continuous in-house physician coverage is required (state operation code).

- A registered nurse with at least 6 months of experience in treating burn patients and with evidence of burn care continuing education shall be responsible for nursing care and management in the burn center (state operation code).

- A registered nurse with at least 3 months' experience in treating burn patients shall be on duty each shift (state operation code).

Members of the medical and nursing staff at Attica Memorial and Delphi Hospitals were interviewed to determine the level of experience and interest in the treatment of burn patients. Based on those interviews, it was determined that many of the RNs who had already trained in burn care had resigned from Delphi Hospital. It was the opinion of the Attica Memorial intensive care unit (ICU) and critical care unit (CCU) leadership that the staff of Attica Memorial did not have the necessary competencies in burn treatment to continue the required level of care.

STATE CHILDREN SERVICES (SCS) IMPACT

California State Children Services (SCS) is the body that regulates the treatment of Medicaid children aged birth to 21 years who experience disabilities resulting from congenital anomalies or severe debilitating injury. SCS certification was vital to the operation of the burn center. According to the director of business development for the Ingelson Burn Center, SCS patients represented 74% of the pediatric inpatient burn volume and 26% of all pediatric outpatient visits in 2000. For the first and second quarters of calendar year 2001, 59% of inpatients and 31% of outpatients were SCS.

SCS Certification Requirements

State Children Services (SCS) guidelines provided for specialized care of pediatric patients and for adults with delayed mental development in an acute care environment. These guidelines consisted largely of policies and procedures designed to support the psycho-social and emotional well-being of the pediatric patients. Meeting SCS certification requirements had very little impact on the normal operations of a burn unit. The following applied to SCS requirements:

- Pediatric playroom and age-appropriate toys

- Increased security provisions for pediatric patients

- Specialized pediatric burn intake and admission nursing protocols

- Cribs and crib nets functional 24 hours

- Pediatric Crash carts, thermometers, scales, BP cuffs, and so forth

- Pediatric PT available 24 hours

- Child life therapist available 24 hours

SCS Current State

The Ingelson Burn Center applied for SCS certification 3 years ago but was granted only provisional status because the burn center had not fulfilled all the requirements dictated by the Department of Health Services. The provisional status was to expire on October 31, 2001. If this status were allowed to expire without immediate written notification to SCS regarding the future of the center, the burn center would no longer be reimbursed for treating the largest percentage of its pediatric burn patients. Recertification was unlikely if provisional status was allowed to lapse.

Even if the provisional status was renewed after October 31, 2001, SCS could not be applied to the burn center at Attica Memorial East Campus since SCS status was not transferable from one facility to another. Applying for SCS accreditation was an extensive process that could take more than two years. Without SCS, the burn center would not be able to treat pediatric patients and would have to transfer them to University Hospital, 5 miles to the south. University Hospital was able to treat pediatric burn patients under its SCS medical center umbrella policy; however, the medical center was applying for SCS specifically to treat pediatric burn patients, which would be a threat to Attica Memorial's ability to capture this important burn population.

FACILITY CONSTRAINTS

Based on the findings regarding the licensing and regulatory requirements of operating a burn center, the burn unit was required to be located near critical/intensive care because of the severity of burn injuries and the complications that could arise. Because infection was so threatening to a burn victim, both positive and negative pressure rooms were required to handle the most critical patients. Children typically comprise 50% of all burn patients. In order to treat pediatric burn inpatients, SCS required a playroom within the burn unit. The playroom was for parents to visit with their children, adolescents to visit with their friends, and for staff or social workers to perform play and recreational therapy with children. According to the business director for the burn center, the existing playroom was too small (190 square feet) and needed to be expanded by 5%.

A hydrotherapy room was a critical element in the treatment of a severe burn. Hydrotherapy cleaned the burn area, allowed the removal of dressings, and performed gentle skin debridement.

Hyperbaric oxygen therapy (HBO) was the second critical element in treating burn. HBO was the process of placing a patient in an environment that allowed them to breathe and be surrounded by oxygen at two to three times atmospheric pressure. HBO had proven to be significant in promoting rapid healing.

Equally important was the third element of the Ingelson Burn Center, the Outpatient Burn Center, located close to Delphi Hospital. At the Outpatient Burn Center, the patient's progress was continually monitored and modified when appropriate, not only by the physicians, psychologist, and nurses, but also by the therapists and the burn case manager.

CAPACITY ANALYSIS

Based on the findings regarding the licensing and regulatory requirements of operating a burn center, a capacity analysis was conducted to locate space for the integration of a dedicated burn unit into the existing Attica Memorial East Campus physical plant. The current East Campus ICU/CCU space was identified as a potential location for the burn center. Two capital build-out scenarios were considered: (1) integration of a burn unit into current ICU/CCU configuration, and (2) expansion of inpatient space through a full unit build-out. Based on ICU/CCU post–campus integration capacity constraints and the state operation code and state building code regulations, it was determined that it was not feasible to integrate the burn unit into the existing ICU/CCU unit. Therefore, a new unit would have to be built to accommodate the program. The architecture firm determined the cost for a full build-out of a dedicated six-bed burn unit would be approximately $1,604,958; a dedicated four-bed burn unit full build-out would cost approximately $1,505,525. There would, however, be potential cost savings if the burn unit moved to the Attica Memorial rehabilitation space. Moving the burn unit to the rehabilitation space would cost approximately $820,147 for a six-bed burn unit, or approximately $735,618 for a four-bed burn unit (see Exhibit 1, p. 312).

PHYSICIAN RELATIONS

Dr. Ingelson was the medical director of the Ingelson Burn Center. He was not, however, an on-site physician at Delphi Hospital. Dr. Ingelson and his team of burn surgeons were only on site for difficult and acute burn patients; otherwise, Dr. Fred Peace was the local burn physician who managed all the burn cases that came through the Ingelson Burn Center. Dr. Peace then reviewed all the burn cases with Dr. Ingelson for a confirmed patient treatment plan. All phases of inpatient care were coordinated on the same unit and were supervised by Dr. Ingelson and his team of specially trained burn physicians. Nurses, therapists, and other allied health professionals had all been trained to treat and deal with burn injuries and issues associated with burn. The continuity of care continued to the Outpatient Burn Center with familiar physicians and staff working with the patients and their families on a daily basis toward full physical and emotional recovery.

Edward Totino, former CEO of Delphi Hospital, stated that Dr. Ingelson was an extraordinary physician and commanded special treatment from clinical and administrative staff. Whenever Dr. Ingelson was needed at Delphi, the hospital provided limousine service for his trip to the burn center. Totino gave a firm warning that if Attica Memorial did not treat Dr. Ingelson correctly, Dr. Ingelson would leave and set up his burn service elsewhere. A burn center without Dr. Ingelson would no longer be regarded as a Center of Excellence in Norton County. Therefore, burn patients would have to use other burn centers that might not be well known for their burn treatment. In addition, the hospital would lose a vital source of revenue generated from the Ingelson Burn Center.

PHYSICIAN POLITICS

When Attica Memorial CEO Rick Ponti surveyed the physicians with practicing privileges at both Attica Memorial East and West Campuses and who knew of Dr. Ingelson and his burn practice, all the physicians had negative comments about Dr. Ingelson. The physicians categorized Dr. Ingelson as a "Diva Physician." They did not like the fact that the administration gave special treatment to Dr. Ingelson and did not treat all physician staff the same. Attica Memorial East Campus physicians had mixed feelings about the Ingelson Burn Center joining their facility. Some of the physicians were indifferent to the burn program; however, there was a lack of support from all of the general surgeons and plastic surgeons interviewed. The surgeons did not like Dr. Ingelson's customary practice of reserving large blocks of OR time each week since that blocked OR time was typically underutilized (see Exhibit 3, p. 314).

When Dr. Ingelson met with Ponti and his executive team for a tour of the East Campus, it was noted that Dr. Ingelson's requested location of the burn unit would be extremely expensive. If the hospital determined to transition the Ingelson Burn Center to East Campus, a dedicated unit just for burn would have to be built out, requiring tearing down existing structures and shifting around services. Dr. Ingelson's request to convert the RN's rest area into the burn pediatrics playroom was not well received by Debra Walker, the VP of Patient Care. Converting the physician work-out room into the HBO facility was also not well received by the physicians.

COMMUNITY IMPACT

Through Dr. Ingelson's dedication to superior patient care, continuing education, and community outreach, the burn center had earned the respect and support of local fire departments. In interviews regarding the Ingelson Burn Center, all local firefighters contacted supported the burn center. One interviewee had been treated at the Ingelson Burn Center and was extremely satisfied with his outcome. According to a local fire department spokesperson, they preferred the Ingelson Burn Center treatment to the University Hospital burn treatment. The firefighters stated in their memorandum of understanding (MOU) that if they were ever victims of burn, they preferred to be treated at the Ingelson Burn Center over other burn centers.

The Progressive Group health care consultants claimed that burn units should admit 100 patients annually for 3 consecutive years in order to maintain the appropriate level of proficiency with burn care. Based on Norton County statistics, University Hospital admitted approximately 384 burn patients from 1998 to 2000 and its burn center was meeting NCOS standards. The Ingelson Burn Center had approximately 279 admissions for the same period. In addition, 85% of the burns treated in Norton County were 0%–20% burns, not considered "severe" burn. Lower severity burns could be treated in nondedicated inpatient units and through the emergency department. These statistics indicated that there might not have been a need for two burn centers serving Norton County.

Dr. Matthew Suess, Medical Director of Norton County, stated that a preliminary study of burn treatment in Norton County indicated that University Hospital provided more than adequate coverage for the county. Dr. Suess did not support the continuation of the Ingelson Burn Center and did not support Dr. Ingelson's methodology of treating burn with extensive plastic surgery that was not within the norm of burn treatment. Dr. Suess felt that there was no need for two programs in Norton County based on the low volume of critical burn cases and he claimed Norton County would not be affected by having the University Hospital as the sole provider for burn treatment.

OPPORTUNITY FOR MARKET GROWTH

With the Ingelson Burn Center as a Center of Excellence, there was potential for branding Attica Memorial and driving up volume with Dr. Ingelson's treatment for burn care. As part of the center's continuum of service, the Ingelson Burn Center provided outreach and educational services to pre-hospital personnel, emergency department personnel, schools, employers, and insurance carriers. The center hosted educational seminars, participated in community and employer health fairs, and provided in-service training, utilizing materials on burn safety, first aid for burn injuries, and breakthrough treatments of burn injuries and other pertinent information. In addition to hosting burn educational seminars, the Ingelson Burn Center held an annual Burn Survivors Reunion for all former and current patients, their families, and friends. Attica Memorial could establish relationships with local medical centers and community physicians in order to secure transfers post-stabilization and pre-admission.

Opportunities for market growth could be dimmed, however, by significant competition with University Hospital's burn center nearby. This leading burn center reported greater volume due to a Level 1 trauma emergency department, and had 123 inpatient cases reported in 1999. Without Level 1 trauma, the Ingelson Burn Center was limited to receiving only burn patients and was not able to treat patients with combinations of burn and other non-burn emergency injuries. According to Norton County's Emergency Medical Services, in the past 3 years, burn volume had been trending down from 23% to 15% of all emergencies.

Obtaining workers' compensation, patients could be limited because patients must either predesignate a program or wait 30 days postadmission to transfer to a different burn center. In an interview, Dr. David Carpenter, owner of a large medical group contracted with Attica Memorial, stated that his medical group would not use the Ingelson Burn Center for his occupational patients because of Dr. Ingelson's high cost of treating burn patients. Although Dr. Ingelson's plastic surgery approach to treating burn had impressive outcomes, his treatment costs were more than the norm. Dr. Carpenter referred all of his occupational patients to University Hospital because it was known to have positive outcomes and the burn treatment costs were within the norm.

PROFITABILITY

Based on the financial data provided by Delphi Hospital's decision support system and factoring in the impact on inpatient surgery, the Ingelson Burn Center's net margin in FY 2000 was $309,939, while FY 2001 decreased to $232,745 (see Exhibit 1).

If the Ingelson Burn Center were moved to Attica Memorial East Campus, the capital expense for a full build-out expansion of six beds was $1,604,958, based on either FY 2000 or FY 2001 financials. The payback of this capital investment was 5.18 years based on FY 2000 patient volume and revenue, or 6.9 years based on FY 2001.

If the burn program were moved into the present rehabilitation space at Attica Memorial East Campus, the capital expense could be lowered to $820,147 for six beds, with payback of the full build-out expansion in 2.65 years based on FY 2000, or 3.52 years based on FY 2001 (see Exhibit 1).

	FY 2000	FY 2001	FY 2000	FY 2001
Contribution Margin				
Net Revenues	$1,901,953	$1,904,538	$1,901,953	$1,904,538
Variable Expenses	967,066	1,047,561	967,066	1,047,561
Fixed Expenses	433,068	432,352	433,068	432,352
	$501,819	$424,625	$501,819	$424,625
Impact to Inpatient Surgery	191,880	191,880	191,880	191,880
Burn Center Net Margin	$309,939	$232,745	$309,939	$232,745

	Moved to present rehabilitation space at Attica Memorial East		Moved to Attica Memorial East (full build-out expansion)	
Capital Expense—6 Beds	$820,147	$820,147	$1,604,958	$1,604,958
Capital Expense—4 Beds	$735,618	$735,618	$1,505,525	$1,505,525
Analysis				
Payback (in years)—6 Beds	2.65	3.52	5.18	6.90
Payback (in years)—4 Beds	2.37	3.16	4.86	6.51

Exhibit 1. Ingelson Burn Center summary (without loss of SCS).

Moving Ingelson Burn Center to the East Campus, whether into a new building or into the existing rehabilitation space, however, meant that the loss of SCS certification had to be considered. Because SCS status would not transfer to the AMH East Campus, the financial health of the program quickly worsened. According to the financial analysis for FY 2001, lost SCS contribution margin was $114,885. The lost savings for surgery call coverage was ($70,080), and the lost cost savings for a blood bank technician was ($32,120); therefore, the total net margin was $12,685. Without SCS certification, the payback of the capital investment in the burn program for a full build-out expansion for six beds was 126.52 years; if the program moved to the AMH East Campus rehabilitation space, the payback for six beds was 64.65 years. The dramatic financial impact of the loss of SCS status could make it financially untenable for the hospital to support such a unique program (see Exhibit 2).

The practice of reserving large blocks of OR time by the Ingelson Burn Center Physician Medical Group would dramatically affect the Attica Memorial Surgical Services if the burn center moved to AMH East Campus. The burn physician group currently scheduled two $4\frac{1}{2}$-hour OR time blocks per week at the West Campus in anticipation of as-needed surgical services. According to Attica Memorial's Surgical Services Coordinator, it was standard practice at East Campus to release OR time 72 hours in advance. The burn physician group, however, released blocked OR time for rescheduling only 14 hours in advance, at 5:00 P.M. on the day prior to blocked time that had no scheduled sur-

	FY 2001	FY 2001
Loss of State Children Services		
Lost Contribution Margin	$114,885	$114,885
Lost Savings	102,200	102,200
Burn Center Net Margin	$12,685	$12,685
	Present rehab space at AME	Moved to AME (full build-out)
Capital Expense—6 Beds	$820,147	$1,604,958
Capital Expense—4 Beds	$735,618	$1,505,525
Analysis		
Payback (in years)—6 Beds	64.65	126.52
Payback (in years)—4 Beds	57.99	118.69

Exhibit 2. Ingelson Burn Center summary (with loss of SCS).

geries. The surgical services coordinator claimed that the late cancellation practice of Dr. Ingelson would result in idle OR time and affect scheduling and hospital revenues.

Attica Memorial East Campus OR suites were operating at or near capacity and constraints on OR scheduling were anticipated when services from the West Campus were integrated. In addition, interviews with Attica Memorial West Campus Surgical Services personnel revealed that the Ingelson Burn Center Physician Medical Group was currently under-utilizing its block schedule by 3 hours each week, which impacted inpatient surgery at the Attica Memorial East Campus facility. The practice of reserving large blocks of OR time might affect Attica Memorial East Campus Surgical Services by $191,880 (see Exhibit 3). When the capital expenditure for a new, six-bed, dedicated burn unit at the East Campus of $820,147, when using rehab space, or $1,604,958 for the full build-out, was coupled with a decrease in the overall inpatient surgery contribution margins, the burn program would have a negative impact on the financial health of AMH East Campus.

EASE TO IMPLEMENT

Intentions to close the Ingelson Burn Center were met with great resentment by the former Delphi Hospital's staff and administration. Delphi's

Total Inpatient Cases	1,420
Avg. Gross Revenue Per Inpatient Case	$35,920
Avg. Deduction Inpatient Case	24,406
Net Revenue Per Inpatient Case	$11,514
Avg. Variable Costs Per Inpatient Case	6,773
Avg. Direct Fixed Costs Per Inpatient Case	1,051
Avg. Contribution Margin Per Inpatient Case	$3,690
Number of Inpatient Procedures Impacted Each Week by Underutilization of Blocked Operation Room Time	1
Impact Per Week	$3,690
Number of Weeks Per Year	52
Impact Per Year	$191,880

Note:
According to Jamie Patel in the Surgical Services Department at AMH West Campus, Dr. Ingelson on average underutilizes his Operating Room time by 3 hours each week. Assuming that average inpatient surgery takes 3 hours and Operating Room time is near or at capacity, the underutilization of OR time will impact 1 surgery per week.

Exhibit 3.   Impact on inpatient surgery contribution margins.

former CEO believed that Dr. Ingelson's reputation for his burn treatment and outcomes were far superior to nearby competitors that had medical residents treating burn patients. In addition, with provisional SCS status, Attica Memorial West Campus would be able to drive up volume and surpass University Hospital, its nearest competitor. Following the alliance's plan for an East Campus acute/inpatient care facility and a West Campus ambulatory care facility would, however, require moving the program to the East Campus and building a new critical/intensive burn unit and hyperbaric facilities.

Implementing the burn center at the East Campus would require investment to train all emergency clinical and critical/intensive care staff in emergency burn care. In addition, during the interim transition, essential burn staff would be required to train the East Campus clinical staff that will be administering burn treatment. In addition, some of the current burn nurses had expressed discontentment working with Dr. Ingelson and with burn patients, and had stated they want to transition out of the burn unit. The burn center had a trend of high nursing staff turnover because, as one burn nurse stated, working with Dr. Ingelson could be challenging, and hiring and training burn nurses was costly.

THE INGELSON BURN CENTER DECISION

After Ponti reviewed the burn center analysis, he knew that a decision had to be made on the fate of the program. In order to clearly delineate the implications and ramifications of whichever course was to be taken with the burn center, there were a number of issues that Ponti need take into consideration. In deciding, Ponti knew that the community impacts and emotional issues could not be overlooked, but that the financials were vital to the decision about whether to continue the burn center. Three alternatives emerged from the analysis: (1) Status Quo—The Ingelson Burn Center remains at Attica Memorial West Campus, the former Delphi Hospital; (2) Relocation—The Ingelson Burn Center transitions to Attica Memorial East Campus; (3) Termination—Attica Memorial closes the Ingelson Burn Center.

21

West Florida Regional Medical Center (A)

Curtis P. McLaughlin
University of North Carolina at Chapel Hill

Now that West Florida Regional Medical Center (WFRMC) had success-fully completed the Joint Commission on Accreditation of Healthcare Organizations (JCAHO) survey, John Kausch, its administrator/CEO, felt that he and his management team should start 1992 by focusing on their continuous quality improvement (CQI) process. There were a number of issues that he and the quality improvement council could address, includ-ing (1) performance reviews under CQI, (2) speeding up the work of the task forces, (3) focusing the process more on key competitive issues, and (4) deciding how much money to spend on it.

WEST FLORIDA REGIONAL MEDICAL CENTER

The WFRMC is a Hospital Corporation of America (HCA) owned and operated, for-profit hospital complex on the north side of Pensacola, Florida. Licensed for 547 beds, West Florida Regional operated approxi-mately 325 beds in December 1991, plus the 89-bed psychiatric pavilion, and the 58-bed Rehabilitation Institute of West Florida. The 11-story office building of the Medical Center Clinic, P.A., is attached to the hos-pital facility, and a new cancer center is under construction.

The 130 doctors practicing at the Medical Center Clinic and its satellite clinics admitted mostly to WFRMC, whereas most of the other doctors in this city of 150,000 practiced at both Sacred Heart and Baptist hospitals downtown. Competition for patients was intense, and in 1992 as much as 90%–95% of patients in the hospital were admitted subject to discounted prices, mostly Medicare for the elderly, CHAMPUS for military dependents, and Blue Cross/Blue Shield of Florida for the employed and their dependents.

The CQI program had had some real successes during the past 4 years, especially in the areas where package prices for services were required. All of the management team had been trained in quality improvement techniques according to HCA's Deming-based approach and some 25 task forces were operating. The experiment with departmental self-assessments, using the Baldridge award criteria and an instrument developed by HCA headquarters, had spurred department heads to become further involved and begin to apply quality improvement techniques within their own work units. Yet Kausch and his senior leadership sensed some loss of interest among some managers, while others who had not bought into the idea at first were now enthusiasts.

THE HCA CQI PROCESS

Kausch had been in the first group of HCA CEOs trained in CQI techniques in 1987 by Paul Batalden, M.D., corporate Vice-President for Medical Care. Kausch had become a member of the steering committee for HCA's overall quality effort. The HCA approach is dependent on the active and continued participation of top local management and on the Plan-Do-Check-Act (PDCA) cycle of Deming. Exhibit 1 shows that process as presented to company employees. Dr. Batalden does not work with a hospital administrator until he is convinced that that individual is fully committed to the concept and is ready to lead the process at his own institution, which includes being the one to teach the Quality 101 course on site to his own managers. Kausch also took members of his management team to visit other quality exemplars, such as Florida Power and Light and local plants of Westinghouse and Monsanto.

In 1991, Kausch became actively involved in the total quality council of the Pensacola Area Chamber of Commerce (PATQC), when a group of Pensacola area leaders in business, government, military, education, and health care began meeting informally to share ideas in productivity and quality improvement. Celanese Corporation (a Monsanto division), the largest nongovernmental employer in the area, also supported PATQC.

FOCUS-PDCA

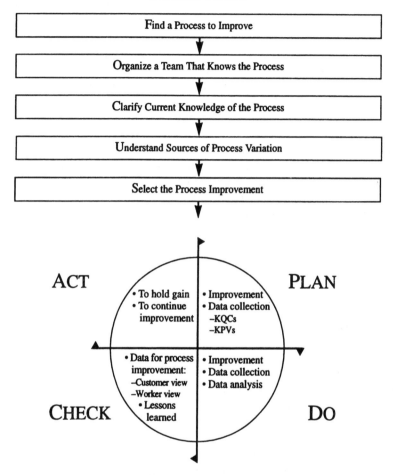

Exhibit 1.   The FOCUS-PDCA problem-solving approach.

From this informal group emerged the PATQC under the sponsorship of the chamber. The vision of PATQC was "helping the Pensacola area develop into a total quality community by promoting productivity and quality in all area organizations, public and private, and by promoting economic development through aiding existing business and attracting new business development." The primary employer in Pensacola, the U.S. Navy, was using TQM (total quality management) extensively and was quite satisfied with the results and supported the chamber program. In fact, the first 1992

1-day, community-wide seminar presented by Mr. George F. Butts, consultant and retired Chrysler Vice President for Quality and Productivity, was to be held at the Naval Air Station's Mustin Beach Officers' Club.

The CQI staffing at WFRMC was quite small, in keeping with HCA practice. The only program employee was Ms. Bette Gulsby, M.Ed., Director of Quality Improvement Resources, who serves as staff and "coach" to Kausch and as a member of the quality improvement council. Exhibits 2 and 3 show the organization of the council and the staffing for quality improvement program support. The "mentor" was provided by headquarters staff, and in the case of WFRMC was Dr. Batalden himself. The planning process had been careful and detailed. Appendix A shows excerpts from the planning processes used in the early years of the program.

WFRMC has been one of several HCA hospitals to work with a self-assessment tool for department heads. Exhibit 4 shows the cover letter sent to all department heads. Exhibit 5 shows the scoring matrix for self-assessment. Exhibit 6 shows the scoring guidelines, and Exhibit 7 displays the five assessment categories used.

FOUR EXAMPLES OF TEAMS

Intravenous Documentation

The nursing department originated the IV documentation team in September 1990 after receiving documentation from the pharmacy department that, over a 58-day period, there had been $16,800 in lost charges related to the administration of intravenous (IV) solutions. The pharmacy attributed the loss to the nursing staff's record keeping. This was the first

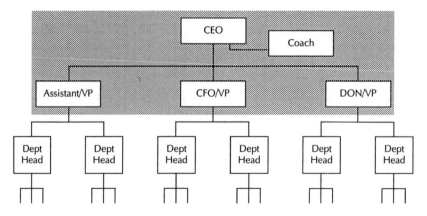

Exhibit 2. Organization chart with quality improvement council (shaded box).

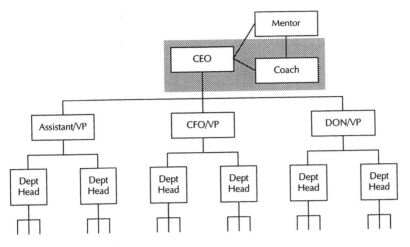

Exhibit 3. Organization chart with CEO QIP support (shaded box).

time that the nursing department was aware of a problem or that the pharmacy department had been tracking this variable. There were other lost charges not yet quantified, resulting from recording errors in the oral administration of pharmaceuticals as well.

> In an effort to continue to monitor and implement elements of improvement and innovation within our organization, it will become more and more necessary to find methods that will describe our level of QI implementation.
>
> The assessment or review of a quality initiative is only as good as the thought processes that have been triggered during the actual assessment. Last year (1990), the quality improvement council prepared for and participated in a quality review. This exercise was extremely beneficial to the overall understanding of what was being done and the results that have been accomplished utilizing various quality techniques and tools.
>
> The departmental implementation of QI has been somewhat varied throughout the organization and, although the variation is certainly within the range of acceptability, it is the intent of the QIC to understand better each department's implementation road map and, furthermore, to provide advice/coaching on the next steps for each department.
>
> Attached please find a scoring matrix for self-assessment. This matrix is followed by five category ratings (to be completed by each department head). The use of this type of tool reinforces the self-evaluation that is consistent with continuous improvement and meeting the vision of West Florida Regional Medical Center.
>
> Please read and review the attachment describing the scoring instructions and then score your department category standings relative to the approach, deployment, and effects. This information will be forwarded to Bette Gulsby by April 19, 1991, and, following a preliminary assessment by the QIC, an appointment will be scheduled for your departmental review.
>
> The review will be conducted by John Kausch and Bette Gulsby, along with your administrative director. Please take the time to review the attachments and begin your self-assessment scoring. You will be notified of the date and time of your review.
>
> This information will be utilized for preparing for the next department head retreat, scheduled for May 29 and 30, 1991, at the Perdido Beach Hilton.

Exhibit 4. QI assessment cover letter sent to department heads.

APPROACH	DEPLOYMENT	EFFECTS (Results)
* HQIP design includes all eight dimensions[a] * Integration across dimensions of HQIP & areas of operation	(Implementation) * Breadth of implementation (areas or functions) * Depth of implementation (awareness, knowledge, undertsanding and application)	* Quality of measurable results

100% ───

* World-class approach: sound; systematic; effective; HQIP based; continuously evaluated, refined, and improved * Total integration across all functions * Repeated cycles of innovation/improvement	* Fully in all areas and functions * Ingrained in the culture	* Exceptional, world-class, superior to all competition; in all areas * Sustained (3–5 years), clearly caused by the approach

80% ───

* Well-developed and tested, HQIP based * Excellent integration	* In almost all areas and functions * Evident in the culture of all groups	* Excellent, sustained in all areas with improving competitive advantage * Much evidence that they are caused by the approach

60% ───

* Well-planned, documented, sound, systematic, HQIP based: all aspects addressed * Good integration	* In most areas and functions * Evident in the culture of most groups	* Solid, with positive trends in most areas * Some evidence that they are caused by the approach

40% ───

* Beginning of sound, systematic, HQIP based; not all aspects addressed * Fair integration	* Begun in many areas and functions * Evident in the culture of some groups	* Some success in major areas * Not much evidence that they are caused by the approach

20% ───

* Beginning of HQIP awareness * No integration across functions	* Beginning in some areas and functions * Not part of the culture	* Few or no results * Little or no evidence that any results are caused by the approach

0% ───

[a] The eight dimensions of HQIP are: leadership constancy, employee-mindedness, customer-mindedness, process focused, statistical thinking, PCDA-driven, innovativeness, and regulatory proactiveness.

Exhibit 5.   QI scoring matrix for self-assessment.

The team formed to look at this problem found that there were some 15 possible reasons why the errors occurred, but that the primary one was that documentation of the administration of the IV solution was not entered into the medication administration record (MAR). The MAR was

In order to determine your department's score in each of the five categories, please review the scoring matrix for self-assessment. The operational definitions for Approach, Deployment, and Effects are listed in the small boxes on the top of the scoring matrix. Each criterion is divided into percent of progress/implementation (i.e., 0%-100%). For example, you may determine that your departmental score on category 3.0 (QI Practice) is:

APPROACH	DEPLOYMENT	EFFECTS
20%	20%	20%

This means that your departmental approach has fair integration of QIP practice, your departmental deployment is evident in the culture of some of your groups, and it is not actually evident that your departmental effects are caused by the approach.

Please remember that this is a *self-assessment* and only *you* know your departmental progress. This assessment is not a tool to generate documentation. However, if you would like to bring any particular document(s) to your review, please do so. This is only meant to provide a forum for you to showcase your progress and receive recognition and feedback on such.

Remember, review each of the self-assessment criteria of approach, deployment, and effects and become familiar with the levels or percentages described. You have three scores for each Departmental QI Assessment Category (categories 1.0–5.0).

Exhibit 6.   The QI scoring guidelines used.

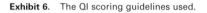

kept at the patient's bedside and, each time that a medication was administered, the nurse was to enter documentation into this record.

The team had to come to understand some terms as they went along. The way that the pharmacy kept its books, anything that was sent to the floors but not billed within 48–72 hours was considered a "lost charge." If an inquiry was sent to the floor about the material and what happened and a correction is made, the entry was classified as "revenue recovered." Thus the core issue was not so much one of lost revenue as one of unnecessary rework in the pharmacy and on the nursing floors.

The team developed Pareto charts showing the reasons for the documentation errors. The most common ones were procedural (e.g., patient moved to the operating room, patient already discharged). Following the HCA model, these procedural problems were dealt with one at a time to correct the accounting for the unused materials. The next step in the usual procedures was to get a run chart developed to show what was happening over time to the lost charges on IVs. Here the team determined that the best quality indicator would be the ratio of "lost" charges to total charges issued. The pharmacy management realized, at this point, that it lacked the denominator figure and that its lack of computerization led to the lack of that information. Therefore, the task force had been inactive for 3 months, while the pharmacy implemented a computer system that could provide the denominator.

Ms. Debbie Koenig, Assistant Director of Nursing, responsible for the team, said the next step would be to look at situations where the MAR was not at the patient bedside, but perhaps up at the nursing station, so that a nurse could not make the entry at the appropriate time. This was an especially bothersome rework problem, because of nurses working various shifts or occasionally an agency nurse who had been on duty and was not available to consult when the pharmacy asked why documentation was not present for an IV dose of medication.

1.0 DEPARTMENTAL QI FRAMEWORK DEVELOPMENT

The QI Framework Development category examines how the departmental quality values have been developed, how they are projected in a consistent manner, and how adoption of the values throughout the department is assessed and reinforced.

Examples of areas to address:

- Department mission
- Departmental quality definition
- Departmental employee performance feedback review
- Department QI plan
- QI methods

APPROACH	DEPLOYMENT	EFFECTS
_____ %	_____ %	_____ %

2.0 CUSTOMER KNOWLEDGE DEVELOPMENT

The Customer Knowledge Development category examines how the departmental leadership has involved and utilized various facets of customer-mindedness to guide the quality effort.

Examples of areas to address:

- HQT family of measures (patient, employee, etc.)
- Departmental customer identification
- Identification of customer needs and expectations
- Customer feedback/data review

APPROACH	DEPLOYMENT	EFFECTS
_____ %	_____ %	_____ %

3.0 QUALITY IMPROVEMENT PRACTICE

The Quality Improvement Practice category examines the effectiveness of the department's efforts to develop and realize the full potential of the work force, including management, and the methods to maintain an environment conducive to full participation, quality leadership, and personal and organizational growth.

Examples of areas to address:

- Process improvement practice
- Meeting skills
- QI storyboards
- QI in daily work life (individual use of QI tools, i.e., flowchart, run chart, Pareto chart)
- Practice quality management guidelines
- Departmental data review
- Plans to incorporate QI in daily clinical operations
- Identification of key physician leaders

APPROACH	DEPLOYMENT	EFFECTS
_____ %	_____ %	_____ %

Exhibit 7.   The five QI assessment categories used.

4.0 QUALITY AWARENESS BUILDING

The Quality Awareness Building category examines how the department decides what quality education and training is needed by employees and how it utilizes the knowledge and skills acquired. It also examines what has been done to communicate QI to the department and how QI is addressed in departmental staff meetings.

Examples of areas to address:

- JIT training
- Employee orientation
- Creating employee awareness
- Communication of QI results

APPROACH	DEPLOYMENT	EFFECTS
____ %	____ %	____ %

5.0 QA/QI LINKAGE

The QA/QI Linkage category examines how the department has connected QA data and information to the QI process improvement strategy. Also examined is the utilization of QI data-gathering and decision-making tools to document and analyze data (how the department relates the ongoing QA activities to QI process improvement activities).

Examples of areas to address:

- QA process identification
- FOCUS-PDCA process improvement
- Regulatory/accreditation connection (JCAHO)

APPROACH	DEPLOYMENT	EFFECTS
____ %	____ %	____ %

Universal Charting

There was evidence that a number of ancillary services results, or "loose reports," were not getting into the patients' medical records in a timely fashion. This was irritating to physicians and could result in delays in the patient's discharge, which under diagnosis-related groups (DRGs), essentially fixed payment per case, meant higher costs without higher reimbursement. One employee filed a suggestion that a single system be developed to avoid running over other people on the floor doing the "charting." A CQI team under Ms. Debbie Wroten, Medical Records Director, was authorized. The 12-member team included supervisors and directors from the laboratory, the pulmonary lab, the EKG lab, medical records, radiology, and nursing. They developed the following "opportunity statement":

> At present, six departments are utilizing nine full-time equivalents 92 hours per week for charting separate ancillary reports. Rework is created in the form of re-pulling in-house patient records, creating an ever-increasing demand for chart accessibility. All parties affected by this process are frustrated because the current process increases the opportunity for lost documentation, chart unavailability, increased traffic on units creating congestion, and prolonged charting times, and provides for

untimely availability of clinical reports for patient care. Therefore, an opportunity exists to improve the current charting practice for all departments involved to allow for the efficiency, timeliness, and accuracy of charting loose reports.

The team met, assessed, and flow charted the current charting processes of the five departments involved. Key variables were defined as follows:

Charting timeliness—number of charting times per day, consistency of charting, and reports not charted per charting round

Report availability—indicated by the number of telephone calls per department asking for reports not yet charted

Chart availability—chart is accessible at the nurses' station for charting without interruption

Resource utilization—staff hours and number of hours per day of charting

Each department was asked to use a common "charting log" for several weeks to track the number of records charted, who did the charting, when it was done, the preparation time, the number of reports charted, the number of reports not charted (missed), and the personnel hours consumed in charting. The results are shown in Exhibit 8. These data gave the team considerable insight into the nature of the problem. Not every department was picking up the materials every day. Two people could cover the whole hospital in .75 hour each or one person in 1.5 hours. The clinical chemistry laboratory, medical records, and radiology were making two trips per day, while other departments were only able to chart every other day and failed to chart over the weekends.

The processes used by all the groups were similar. The printed or typed response had to be sorted by floors and room numbers added if missing, then taken to the floors and inserted into patient charts. If the chart was not available, they had to be held until the next round. A further problem was identified in that, when the clerical person assigned to these rounds was not available, a technical person who was paid considerably more and was often in short supply had to be sent to do the job.

A smaller team of supervisors who actually knew and owned the charting efforts in the larger departments (medical records, radiology, and clinical chemistry) was set up to design and assess the pilot experiment. The overall team meetings were only used to brief the department heads to gain their feedback and support. A pilot experiment was run in which these three departments took turns doing the runs for each other. The results were favorable. The pilot increased timeliness and chart availability by charting four times per day on weekdays and three on weekends. Report availability was improved and there were fewer phone calls. Nursing staff, physicians, and participating departments specifically asked

Department	Mean records per day	range	Mean hours per day	range	Comments
Medical Records	77.3	20–140	1.6	0.6–2.5	Daily
Pulmonary Lab	50.3	37–55	1.0	0.7–1.5	MWF
Clinical Lab	244.7	163–305	3.2	1.9–5.4	Daily
EKG Lab	40.2	35–48	0.8	0.1–1.0	Weekdays
Microbiology	106.9	3–197	1.4	0.1–2.2	Daily
Radiology	87.1	6–163	1.5	0.1–2.9	Daily

Exhibit 8. Results of each department tracking the number of records charted, who did the charting, when it was done, the preparation time, the number of reports charted, the number of reports not charted (missed), and the personnel hours consumed in charting.

for the process to be continued. The hours of labor dropped from 92 weekly to less than 45, using less highly paid labor.

The team decided, therefore, that the issues were important enough that they should consider setting up a separate universal charting team (UCT) to meet the needs of the entire hospital. "However, an unanticipated hospital census decline made impractical the possibility of requesting additional staffing. Consequently, the group reevaluated the possibility of continuing the arrangement developed for the pilot using the charting hours of the smaller departments on a volume basis. It was discovered that this had the effect of freeing the professional staff of the smaller departments from charting activities and a very minimal allocation of hours floated to the larger departments. It also increased the availability of charters in the larger departments for other activities." The payroll department was then asked to develop a system for allocating the hours that floated from one department to another. That proved cumbersome, so the group decided to allocate charting hours on the basis of each department's volume. "In the event that one or more departments experience a significant increase/decrease in charting needs, the group will reconvene and the hourly allocation will be adjusted."

The resulting schedule had the lab making rounds at 6 A.M. and 9 A.M. and radiology at 4 P.M. and 9:30 P.M. Monday–Friday, while medical records did it at 6 A.M., 1 P.M., and 8 P.M. on Saturdays and Sundays. Continuing statistics were kept on the process, which is shown in Appendix B. The system continues to work effectively.

Labor, Delivery, Recovery, Postpartum (LDRP) Nursing

Competition for young families needing maternity services had become quite intense in Pensacola. WFRMC obstetrical (OB) services offered very traditional services in 1989 in three separate units—labor and delivery, nursery, and postpartum—and operated considerably below capacity.

A consultant was hired to evaluate the potential growth of obstetrical services, the value of current services offered by WFRMC, customers' desires, competitors' services, and opportunities for improvement. Focus group interviews with young couples (past and potential customers) indicated that they wanted safe medical care in a warm, homelike setting with the lowest possible number of rules. More mothers were in their thirties, planning small families with the possibility of only one child. Fathers wanted to be "actively involved" in the birth process. The consultant challenged the staff to come up with their own vision for the department based on the focus group responses, customer feedback, and national trends.

It became clear that there was a demand for a system in which a family-centered birth experience could occur. The system needed to revolve around the customers, rather than the customers following a rigid traditional routine. Customers wanted all aspects of a normal delivery to happen in the same room. The new service would allow the mother, father, and baby to remain together throughout the hospital stay, now as short as 24 hours. Friends and families would be allowed and encouraged to visit and participate as much as the new parents desired. The main goals were to be responsive to the customers' needs and provide safe, quality medical care.

The hospital administration and the six obstetricians practicing there were eager to see obstetrical services grow. They were open to trying and supporting the new concept. The pediatricians accepted the changes, but without great enthusiasm. The anesthesiologists were opposed to the change. The OB supervisor and two of the three head nurses were dead set against it. They wanted to continue operations in the traditional manner.

When the hospital decided to adopt the new LDRP concept, it was clear that patients and families liked it, but the nursing staff, especially nursing management, did not. The OB nursing supervisor retired; one head nurse resigned, one was terminated, and the third opted to move from her management position to a staff nurse role. Ms. Cynthia Ayres, R.N., Administrative Director, responsible for the psychiatric and cardiovascular services, was assigned to implement the LDRP transition until nursing management could be replaced.

One of the issues involved in the transition was clarification of the charge structure. Previously each unit charged separately for services and supplies. Now that the care was provided in a single central area, the old charge structure was unnecessarily complex. Duplication of charges was occurring and some charges were being missed because no one was assuming responsibility.

Ayres decided to use the CQI process to develop a new charge process and to evaluate the costs and resource consumption of the service. Ayres had not been a strong supporter of the CQI process when it was first introduced into the organization. She had felt that the process was too slow and rigid, and that data collection was difficult and cumbersome. Several teams were organized and assigned to look at specific areas of the LDRP process.

To reach a simplified charge process, as well as a competitive price, all aspects of the process had to be analyzed. Meetings were held with the nursing and medical staff. Management of the OB patient and physician preferences in terms of supplies and practices were analyzed. A number of consensus conferences were held to discuss observed variations. Each of the six obstetricians, for example, specified a different analgesic for pain control. Each drug appeared effective for pain control, but their cost per dose ranged from $10 to $75. The physicians agreed that the $10 product was acceptable, because the outcome was the same.

Another standard practice was sending placentas to the pathology laboratory for analysis after every normal delivery. This involved labor time, lab charges, and a pathologist's fee for review. The total procedure cost $196. When questioned about the practice, the current medical staff did not feel it was necessary medically nor the current practice nationally, but that they were just following the rules. Upon investigation, the team found that an incident involving a placenta had occurred 15 years ago that led the service chief (since retired) to order all placentas sent to the lab. The obstetricians developed criteria for when it was medically necessary for the lab review of a placenta. This new rule decreased the number of reviews by 95%, resulting in cost savings to the hospital and to patients.

The charges team reviewed all OB charges for a 1-year period. They found that in 80% of normal deliveries, 14 items were consistently used. The other items were due to variations in physician preferences. The teams and the physicians met and agreed which items were the basic requirements for a normal delivery. These items became the basic charges for package pricing.

The charges team met weekly for at least 1 hour for over a year. Some meetings went as long as 5 hours. Initially, there was a great deal of resistance and defensiveness. Everyone wanted to focus on issues that did not affect themselves. The physicians objected that they were being forced to practice "cookbook medicine" and that the real problem was "the hospital's big markup." Hospital staff continued to provide data on actual hospital charges, resource consumption, and practice patterns. The hospital personnel continued to emphasize repeatedly that the physicians were responsible for determining care. The hospital's concern was to be consistent and decrease variation.

Another CQI team, the documentation team, was responsible for reviewing forms utilized previously by the three separate units. The total number of forms used had been 30. The nursing staff were documenting vital signs an average of five times each time care was provided. Through review of policies, standards, documentation, and care standards, the number of forms was reduced to 20. Nurses were now required to enter each care item only once. The amount of time spent by nurses on documentation was reduced 50%, as was the cost of forms. Data entry errors were also reduced.

The excess costs that were removed were not all physician-related. Many had to do with administrative and nursing policies. Many were due to old, comfortable, traditional ways of doing things. When asked why a practice was followed, the typical response was, "I don't know; that's just the way we've always done it." The OB staff are now comfortable with the use of CQI. They recognize that although it requires time and effort, it does produce measurable results. The OB staff are continuing to review their practices and operations to identify opportunities to streamline services and decrease variation.

Pharmacy and Therapeutics Team

In late 1987, a CQI team was formed jointly between the hospital's pharmacy and therapeutics (P&T) committee and the pharmacy leadership. Their first topic of concern was the rapidly rising costs of inpatient drugs, especially antibiotics, which were costing the hospital about $1.3 million per year. They decided to study the process by which antibiotics were selected and began by asking physicians how they selected antibiotics for treatment. They reported that most of the time they order a culture of the organism causing the infection from the microbiology lab. A microbiology lab report would come back identifying the organism and the antibiotics to which it is sensitive and those to which it is resistant. Some physicians reported that they would look down the list until they came to an antibiotic to which the organism is sensitive and order that. That list was in alphabetical order. A study of antibiotic utilization showed a high correlation between use and alphabetical position, confirming the anecdotal reports. Therefore, the team recommended to the P&T committee that the form be changed to list the antibiotics in order of increasing cost per average daily dose. The doses used would be based on current local prescribing patterns rather than recommended dosages. The P&T committee, which included attending physicians, approved the change and reported it in their annual report to the medical staff. Exhibit 9 shows what happened to the utilization of "expensive" antibiotics (more than $10 per dose) from 1988 to 1991. These costs were not adjusted at all for inflation in drug prices during this period. The estimated annual saving was $200,000.

Given this success, the team went on in 1989 to deal with the problem of the length of treatment with antibiotics. Inpatients did not get a prescription for a 10-day supply. Their IM and IV antibiotics were continued until the physician stopped the order. If a physician went away for the weekend and the patient improved, colleagues were very reluctant to alter the medication until he or she returned. The team wrestled with how to encourage the appropriate ending of the course of treatment without hassling the physicians or risking undue legal liability. They settled on a sticker that went into the chart at the end of 3 days stating the treatment had gone on for 3 days and that an ending date should be specified, if possible. The hospital newsletter and the P&T committee annual report noted that the physician could avoid this notice by specifying a termination date at the time of prescribing. This program seemed to be effective. Antibiotic costs again dropped, and there were no apparent quality problems introduced as measured by length of stay or by adverse events associated with these system changes.

In 1990, the team began an aggressive drug usage evaluation (DUE) program, hiring an Assistant Director, Pharmacy Clinical Services, to administer it. The position had to be rigorously cost justified. DUE involved a review of cases to determine whether the selection and scheduling of powerful drugs matched the clinical picture presented. If the physician prescribed one of three types of antibiotics known to represent a risk of kidney damage in 3%–5% of cases, for example, the DUE administrator ordered lab tests to study serum creatinine levels and warn the

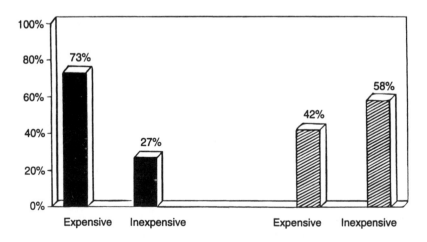

Exhibit 9.   Utilization of "expensive" antibiotics (more than $10 per dose) from 1988 to 1991.

physician if they rose, indicating kidney involvement. There was a sharp decline in the adverse effects caused by the use of these drugs. This program was expanded further to looking at other critical lab values and relating them to pharmacy activities beyond antibiotics, the use of IV solutions and potassium levels, for example. By 1991, the unadjusted antibiotic costs for roughly the same number of admissions had dropped to less than $900,000.

LOOKING AHEAD

One of the things that had concerned Kausch during 1991 had been the fact that implementation had varied from department to department. Although he had written in his annual CQI report that the variation had certainly been within the range of acceptability, he was still concerned about how much variation in implementation was appropriate. If maintaining enthusiasm was a concern, forcing people to conform too tightly might become a demotivator for some staff. This issue and the four mentioned in the introductory paragraph should all be addressed in the coming year.

APPENDIX A: PLANNING CHRONOLOGY FOR CQI

Initiation Plan: 3–6 Months, Starting May 25

May 25:	Develop initial working definition of quality for WFRMC.
May 25:	Define the purpose of the quality improvement council and set schedule for 2 P.M.–4 P.M. every Tuesday and Thursday.
May 25:	Integrate HQT into continuous improvement cycle and hold initial review.
June 2:	Start several multifunctional teams with their core from those completing the leadership workshop, with topics selected by the quality improvement council using surveys, experience, and group techniques.
June 2:	Department heads complete "CEO assessment" to identify customers and expectations, determine training needs, and identify department opportunities. To be discussed with assistant administrators on June 15.
June 16:	Present to QIC the task force report on elements and recommendations on organizational elements to guide and monitor QIP.
June 20:	Division meetings to gain consensus on department plans and set priorities. QIC reviews and consolidates on June 21. Final assignments to department heads on June 22.
June 27:	Draft initial statement of purpose for WFRMC and present to QIC.
June 29–July 1:	Conduct first facilitators' training workshop for 16.
July 1:	Task force reports on additional QIP education and training requirements for:
	Team training and team-members handbook
	Head nurses
	Employee orientation (new and current)
	Integration of community resources (colleges and industry)
	Use of HCA network resources for medical staff and board of trustees
July 19:	Task force report on communications program to support awareness, education, and feedback from employees, vendors, medical staff, local business, colleges and universities, and HCA.

August 1:   Complete the organization of the Quality Improvement Council.

Implementation Plan: 9 Months

Fall: Pilot and evaluate "patient comment card system."

Oct. 21:   QIC input to draft policies/guidelines regarding: forming teams, quality responsibility, and guidelines for multifunctional teams. Brainstorm at October 27 meeting, have revisions for November 10 meeting, and distribute to employees by November 15.

Oct. 27:   Review proposals for communicating QIP to employees to heighten awareness and understanding, communicate on HCA and WFRMC commitments; key definitions, policies, guidelines; HQT; QIP; teams and improvements to date; responsibility and opportunities for individual employees; initiate ASAP.

Nov. 15:   Prepare statements on "On further consideration of HCA's quality guidelines"; discuss with department heads, hospital staff; employee orientation; use to identify barriers to QI and opportunities for QI. Develop specific action plan and discuss with QIC.

Dec. 1:   Identify and evaluate community sources for QI assistance—statistical and operational—including colleges, companies, and the Navy. Make recommendations.

Early Dec.:   Conduct Quality 102 course for remaining department heads. Conduct Quality 101 course for head nurses and several new department heads.

Jan. 1, 1989:   Develop and implement a suggestion program consistent with our HCA quality guidelines, providing quick and easy way to become involved in making suggestions/identifying situations needing improvement; providing quick feedback and recognition; and interfacing with identifying opportunities for QIP.

Implementation Plan: Next 9 Months

Aug. 1:   Survey department heads to identify priorities for additional education and training.

Sept. 14–15:   Conduct a management workshop to sharpen and practice QI methods; to include practice methods;

	to increase management/staff confidence, comfort; to develop a model for departmental implementation; to develop process assessment/QIP implementation tool; to start quality team review.
September:	Develop a standardized team orientation program to cover QI tools and group process rules.
Fall:	Expand use of HQTs and integrate into HQIP—improve communication of results and integration of quality improvement action plans. Psychiatric pavilion to evaluate and implement HQT recommendations from "patient comment card system"—evaluate and pilot.
October:	Incorporate QIP implementation into existing management/communication structure. Establish division "steering committee functions" to guide and facilitate departmental implementation. Identify QI project for each department head/assistant administrator. Establish regular quality reviews in department manager meetings.
December:	Evaluate effectiveness of existing policies, guidelines, and practices for sanctioning, supporting, and guiding QI teams. Include opportunity form/cross functional team sanctioning; team leader and facilitator responsibilities; team progress monitoring/guiding; standardized team presentation format (storyboard). Demonstrate measurable improvement through Baxter QI team.
Monthly:	Monitor and improve the suggestion program.
January:	Pilot the clinical process improvement methodology.
All Year:	In all communications, written and verbal, maintain constant message regarding WFRMC commitment to HQIP; report successes of teams and suggestions; and continue to educate about principles and practices of HQIP strategy.
January:	Successfully demonstrate measurable improvement from focused QIP in one department (medical records).
Spring:	Expand use of HQTs and integrate into HQIP. Pilot HQT in rehab center. Evaluate and implement physicians' HQT. Pilot ambulatory care HQT.
Summer:	Expand use of HQTs and integrate into HQIP. Human resources—Pilot HQT Payers—Pilot HQT

APPENDIX B

Universal Charting Team FOCUS-PDCA Outline

F   Opportunity statement:

At present, six departments are utilizing nine full-time equivalents 92 hours per week for charting separate ancillary reports. Rework is created in the form of re-pulling in-house patient records, creating an ever-increasing demand for chart accessibility. All parties affected by this process are frustrated because the current process increases the opportunity for lost documentation, chart unavailability, increased traffic on units creating congestion, and prolonged charting times, and provides for untimely availability of clinical reports for patient care. Therefore, an opportunity exists to improve the current charting practice for all departments involved to allow for the efficiency, timeliness, and accuracy of charting loose reports.

O   Team members include:

Debbie Wroten, Medical Records Director—Leader
Bernie Grappe, Marketing Director—Facilitator
Joan Simmons, Laboratory Director
Mary Gunter, Laboratory Patient Services Coordinator
Al Clarke, Pulmonary Services Director
Carol Riley, Pulmonary Services Assistant Director
Marlene Rodrigues, EKG Supervisor
Patti Travis, EKG
Debra Wright, Medical Records Transcription Supervisor
Mike West, Radiology Director
Lori Mikesell, Radiology Transcription Supervisor
Debbie Fernandez, Head Nurse

C   Assessed and flow-charted current charting practices of departments.

Clarified and defined key quality characteristics of the charting process:

Charting timeliness—number of charting times per day, consistency of charting, and reports not charted per charting round.
Report availability—indicated by the number of telephone calls per department asking for reports not yet charted.
Chart availability—chart is accessible at the nurses' station for charter without interruption.
Resource utilization—staff hours and number of hours per day of charting.

U   Gathered data on departments' charting volumes and time spent charting.

S   Data gained through the pilot indicated that significant gains were available through the effort to justify proceeding with the development of a universal charting team.

P   The team developed a flow chart of the charting process using a universal charting team rather than previous arrangement. In order to pilot the improvement, the group decided to set up a UCT using current charters from the three major charting departments—medical records, laboratory, and radiology. The team also developed written instructions for both the charters and participating departments. A subgroup of the team actually conducted a 1-day pilot before beginning extensive education to ensure that the UCT would work as planned and to be sure that the charters from each of the large departments were well versed on possible situations that might occur during the pilot.

D   Piloted proposed universal charting team using current charting personnel from radiology, laboratory, and medical records to chart for all departments.

C   Pilot results were positive and indicated the UCT concept offered significant advantages over the previous charting arrangements.

Results were:
   Timeliness/chart availability—Pilot reduced daily charting to four scheduled charting times daily for all departments. Smaller departments did not chart daily prior to pilot. The charting team also reduced the number of occasions that charters from different departments were on the nursing unit needing the same chart.
   Report availability—Telephone calls were reduced and nursing staff, physicians, and participating departments specifically asked for UCT following the pilot.
   Resource utilization—Number of staff hours spent charting and preparing to chart was reduced from 92 hours weekly to less than 45 hours. The improvement also allowed the use of less expensive staff for charting.

A   The group reached consensus that the easiest configuration for the UCT would be to set up a separate UCT that would serve the needs of the entire hospital.
   This was to be proposed to administration by the team as the conclusion of their efforts. However, an unanticipated hospital

census decline made impractical the possibility of requesting additional staffing, and so forth. Consequently, the group reevaluated the possibility of continuing the arrangement developed for the pilot using the charting hours to the smaller departments on a volume basis. It was discovered that this had the effect of freeing the professional staff in the smaller departments from charting responsibilities for a very minimal allocation of hours floated to the larger departments, and it increased the availability of charters in the larger departments for other activities. The payroll department was then involved in order to develop the proper mechanism and procedure for floating hours.

This modification of the previous pilot was piloted for a month with continued good results. Streamlining of the hours floating process may be necessary to place less burden on the payroll department.

Because no major changes were required following the pilot, the group has elected to adopt the piloted LJTC format. Allocation of charting hours is based on a monthly review of charting volumes for each department. In the event that one or more departments experience a significant increase/decrease in charting needs, the group will reconvene and the hourly allocation will be adjusted.

Lessons Learned

Because of the size and the makeup of the team, which included a number of department heads, it was found helpful to set up a smaller team of three supervisors who actually knew and owned the charting efforts in the major departments. This group designed and assessed the initial pilot and actually piloted the pilot before bringing departmental charters into the process. As a result, overall team meetings were primarily used to brief department heads and gain their feedback and consensus.

22

Brunswick Community Hospital Cash Flow Crisis

Michael Wiltfong

Gary R. Wells

William E. Stratton
Idaho State University, Pocatello, Idaho

Peter Butler recently assumed the position of chief financial officer (CFO) at Brunswick Community Hospital (BCH), which was organized under state law as a county institution. As such it is not subject to income, sales, or property taxes. The hospital is managed under contract by a large national hospital management corporation that hires and pays the hospital administrator and provides management oversight. With the exception of the hospital administrator, all individuals working for the hospital are county employees.

Prior to assuming his duties, Peter discussed the situation faced by the hospital with the regional financial vice president and the chief executive officer (CEO) of the hospital services firm. The financial vice president told him, "There is a lot of work to do at Brunswick. Internal reporting is inadequate and no one seems to know about the computer. Most of the problems can be addressed long term, but there won't be a long term unless we can get the cash situation under control."

The CEO was concerned about the cash situation, too, but he had additional concerns for BCH as well. "We can't get anywhere if we don't build revenue," he stated. "To build revenue we must attract new physicians. If we can't free up money for equipment, these doctors won't come. I have just recruited a urologist, and he will need equipment. I know that we are short of cash, but we must buy what these doctors need. We need money for capital expenditure and we need it quickly."

Peter had accepted the job offer at BCH partly because of the challenge it afforded him. After spending a week becoming familiar with the hospital and meeting the other key employees, Peter thought further about the situation. With the words of the regional financial vice president and the CEO still ringing in his mind, Peter wondered what options were available to the hospital, in both the long and short term, to resolve the cash problem. He felt considerable pressure as the CFO to come up with a viable solution and to come up with it soon.

BACKGROUND

Brunswick Community Hospital is a 54-bed acute care hospital with an attached 58-bed long-term nursing care and 16-bed residential care facility providing health care services to residents of its county. The hospital service area covers approximately 35,000 people. Three larger hospitals are within 25 miles of Brunswick. Two are located in a city of 60,000 people and one is in another city of approximately 50,000. One smaller hospital also operates within the county. Brunswick often refers its more specialized cases to the other three larger hospitals. The area hospitals have been discussing the collective purchasing of mobile equipment such as a machine for MRI, CT scanners, and a mammography unit as a way to provide additional services at reasonable cost.

Subsequent to changes in the Medicare program, BCH experienced trends common among hospitals throughout the healthcare industry in the United States. The Medicare program funds a majority of health care costs for patients covered by Social Security. Historically, the payments provided by the Medicare program were changed from a cost-based system to a fixed payment system. In place of billing for the actual costs of treating a patient, under the fixed payment system hospitals received a set fee for a given diagnosis, regardless of the expense incurred in treating any specific patient. In conjunction with this change, Medicare, as well as other insurance payers, began to challenge the appropriateness of care provided to their covered beneficiaries. The processes implemented to control alleged inappropriate delivery of care resulted in an initial decline in activity at

BCH. Recently, extended care and residential care suffered additional declines (see Table 1).

During the same time, the percent of patient days devoted to Medicare/Medicaid increased from 43.0% to 49.7% (see bottom of Table 1). These changes led to significant decreases in cash inflows, which were covered by bank loans during the past two years.

An additional possible impact on the hospital cash flows was the conversion of the hospital computer system in October of Year 4 (see the Appendix for a description of the computerized charging system). The conversion was blamed by some for all the problems the hospital was currently experiencing. The business office manager represented the opinion of many of the employees involved in the collection of the patient accounts when he stated, "We never had these problems in the past. We were always current in paying our bills until we decided to change that blasted computer."

The conversion included all data processing systems. In November of Year 4, shortly after the conversion, receivables climbed to an average of 140 days outstanding. Industry averages were approximately 80 days. The effect was to decrease the hospital's operating cash by $36,000 over a period of just 30 days. This result led to the forecast of a critical cash crisis for Year 5 (see Table 2). The cash flows from operations are expected to accrue evenly throughout the year. The capital expenditures are sched-

Table 1. Brunswick Community Hospital patient days and occupancy rates (for the year ended June 30)

	Patient Days			
	Year 1	Year 2	Year 3	Year 4
Hospital				
Adults & Children	5,649	5,525	5,148	5,576
Newborn	861	834	800	804
Extended Care	19,922	19,839	20,602	19,907
Residential Care	5,905	6,391	5,871	5,329

	Occupancy Rate			
	Year 1	Year 2	Year 3	Year 4
Hospital				
Adults & Children	28.7%	28.0%	26.1%	28.3%
Newborn	19.7%	19.0%	18.3%	18.4%
Extended Care	97.5%	96.8%	97.0%	94.0%
Residential Care	77.0%	83.2%	96.6%	91.3%
Medicaid/Medicare Inpatient Utilization of Hospital (Inpatient Days)	43.0%	46.9%	44.0%	49.7%

Table 2. Brunswick Community Hospital cash forecast
(for the year ending June 30)

	Year 5
Cash Flow from Operations	$450,000
Capital Expenditures	(200,000)
Deposits designated for capital improvements	(100,000)
Increase of funds on hand	(100,000)
Decrease in A/P held in excess of term	(150,000)
Increase in Due to Third-party Payers	75,000
Decrease in Unsecured Debt	(100,000)
Cash Deficit	−$125,000

uled for the first 6 months of the year. Peter's immediate challenge is to develop a plan to meet the predicted cash deficit.

ALTERNATIVE APPROACHES TO A SOLUTION

Long-Term Financing Options

Hospital policy regarding long-term financing limited the courses of action open to Peter. The board of trustees, as a matter of principle, wanted to avoid all unsecured debt and to liquidate all debt currently outstanding.

Revenue Bonds   Long-term financing, such as a revenue bond, was a possibility. Two weeks after arriving at BCH, Peter met for the first time with the finance committee of the board of trustees, whose membership included county commissioners and other community leaders. Peter presented an overview of the cash situation at BCH to the committee and recommended they consider increasing long-term borrowing by issuing revenue bonds for the hospital. His proposal received little support and one committee member, the treasurer of the board of trustees, stated, "If the hospital tries to borrow money, people in this community will string us up." Such financing would require a vote of the citizens of the county, with a positive outcome in no way assured. The school district had recently made several attempts to obtain voter approval for long-term debt, and all of them were unsuccessful. Peter's meeting with the finance committee ended with no progress made toward resolving the cash crisis of the hospital. The finance committee, and by extension the board of trustees, was reluctant to consider long-term borrowing to provide the needed infusion of cash, although it had not been ruled out categorically.

Deferred Compensation Plan Funds   Other possible sources of financing are two alternative off-balance-sheet sources of financing available to the hospital. The first involves the deferred compensation plan sponsored by the hospital, which is structured and operated under the provisions of the Internal Revenue Code Section 457 (457 Plan). Under this plan, salary is withheld tax-free from an employee's current pay and deposited with a third-party administrator. The funds are invested in fixed interest contracts with a highly rated insurance company.

Brunswick Community Hospital operates as a governmental entity under the Internal Revenue Code, which is more liberal for governmental entities than for nongovernmental entities. In governmental units, the 457 Plan funds are legally general assets of the entity. Under other types of deferred compensation plans, the funds are assets of the individual participant. Governmental entities are allowed to use deferred compensation funds to meet current obligations. In a bankruptcy proceeding, the participants in the deferred compensation plan would be treated as general creditors of BCH instead of preferential creditors. Withdrawal of funds from the plan is available at any time to governmental entities without paying a penalty assessed under other types of deferred compensation plans. In addition, pension plans for nongovernmental entities require minimum funding by the entity based on an actuarial evaluation. A governmental entity is not required to fund its plan.

For a 457 Plan of this type, generally accepted accounting principles require that the deferred compensation be shown as an asset and a liability on the hospital's balance sheet. The amount of the hospital's 457 Plan funds held by the third party administrator on June 30 of Year 4 was $967,763.

Pension Plan Funds   Another source for increasing the availability of cash funds is the hospital sponsored pension plan. The hospital maintains a defined benefit plan. As a governmental pension plan, contributions can be delayed until pay-outs are made to the beneficiaries. In fact, the hospital had historically deferred funding of the plan during previous cash crises. The available pension assets as a percentage of the present value of projected pension benefits were close to 95% in Year 4. Discontinuing scheduled contributions to the pension plan would increase available cash by $120,000.

Working Capital Options

Another alternative available to Peter is to generate cash through managing components of working capital. The following is a discussion of the components of working capital on June 30 of Year 4.

Cash   The primary cash account is the operating account held in a local bank. Deposits are made to this account daily, and general expenses of the hospital are paid out of it daily as well. The hospital tries to keep just enough money in this account to cover the expenses being paid, with excess funds being invested in short-term, interest-bearing accounts.

Accounts Receivable   Patient receivables/third-party payer receivables represent more than 80% of current assets. The length of time in days that receivables have been outstanding (unpaid) on June 30 of Year 4 is shown in Table 3. Of a total of $2,600,297 owed the hospital, $1,212,786 has been owed for more than 120 days.

The patient receivables by type of payer are shown in Table 4. Accounts are classified by payer based on which source will pay the majority of the bill. Private pay accounts, for example, will be paid by the patient, and insurance accounts will be paid by an insurance company such as Blue Cross or Blue Shield. This table indicates that the largest group of accounts is the private pay category accounting for 38.4% of receivables. This account is followed by the insurance accounts at 27.5%.

Contracts that the primary payers (insurance companies, Medicare, and Medicaid) have with the hospital dictate the terms of payment. These payers dictate the timing and the amount of payment for a given diagno-

Table 3.   Brunswick Community Hospital aging of patient receivables (at June 30)

	Year 4
Days Outstanding	Amount of Receivables
0–30	$768,660
31–60	240,448
61–90	231,592
91–120	146,811
121–360	746,032
Over 360	466,754
	$2,600,297

Table 4. Brunswick Community Hospital patient receivables by type of payer

Type of Account	Year 4
Private Pay	38.40%
Insurance	27.50%
Medicaid	17.30%
Medicare	16.80%
	100.00%

sis or procedure. Potentially more flexibility exists for balances due from private payers. These are amounts due from the patient after payment has been made by the primary payer and include coinsurance and deductible payments and amounts due from patients without primary coverage. Two factors, however, restrict this flexibility. The hospital's largest commercial insurance carrier, accounting for approximately 20% of total revenues, had a favored nation clause in its contracts with all health care providers. The crux of this clause was to guarantee the commercial insurance carrier the best pricing available. The original intent of such a clause was to promote competitiveness in health care pricing. This state's insurance commissioners, however, have concluded that this type of clause has the opposite effect. But as long as the clause exists, offering discounts to private payers to accelerate payment of their bills may result in the commercial insurance carriers requesting the same discount.

The historical terms-of-sale offered to private pay patients also constituted a complicating factor in attempting to lower the level of patient receivables. As a matter of policy, the hospital provided care regardless of the ability of the patient to pay. The hospital had no formal charity policy. Therefore, all write-offs were treated as bad debt. To maximize the cash received from patients, the hospital allowed them to make payments over time without interest. Formal records of the commitments patients had made to the hospital to pay their bills did not exist. Over the years, the number of these accounts had grown to the point that more than 1,200 accounts owing a total of $300,000 fell into this category.

Collection Efforts Along with the favorable terms-of-sale provided to private pay patients, other factors hampered collection efforts. One factor was the previous hospital write-off policy, which dictated an account be charged directly to expense at the time of write-off. To control this expense, write-offs were limited to a maximum of $10,000 per month. This amount included any defaults due to bankruptcy. To avoid exceeding the $10,000 limit, some accounts that the hospital did not consider collectible were maintained in the system as accounts receivable. The lack of formal records of commitments made by private payers combined with personnel turnover resulted in collection efforts on old patient accounts coming to a standstill. One accounts receivable collector summed up her frustration by saying, "I am afraid to come in to work on Monday. I don't know which account will blow up this week. Which account should I make a collection effort on? Which account needs to be billed after six months? There is just no way of knowing." Personnel could no longer determine whether to bill, dun, or write off an account with no activity. In addition, the hospital's billing system complicated the collection of this type of account.

The hospital billing system was designed to facilitate the collection of an account within 120 days of the service date. Three to five days after a patient is discharged, for example, a final bill is generated by hospital staff. This bill is submitted to the patient's insurance carrier or the applicable governmental agency. The employee in accounts receivable then flags the account for follow up at a future date. The follow-up date may be different for each account and requires some judgment on the part of the billing clerk. Typically, 30–60 days later the clerk reviews the account to determine if action has been taken by the insurance carrier or governmental agency. If the appropriate action has been taken, then the clerk bills the patient for the residual amount due on the account. At this same time, the account is flagged again for subsequent follow up. If appropriate action has not been taken by that later time, the clerk ascertains the problem with the account and takes appropriate action and again flags the account for subsequent collection. Due to this billing process, at any one time the billing clerk is only working a small number of the total number of accounts for which he or she is responsible. This process does not readily accommodate accounts making irregular payments for up to 12 years after the patient's discharge. Consequently, the monitoring of this type of account was haphazard.

Supplies Inventory   Inventories consist of two categories—supplies related directly to patient care and those related to general services (see Table 5 for the components of the supplies inventory). Medical, intravenous, pharmacy, central supply, lab, and surgery constitute the inventory of items required for the care of patients. The need for any particular item may be very sporadic. Not having an item in stock when needed, however, may be potentially life threatening. The operating room supervisor stated her opinion concerning inventory management as follows: "I'm not going to jeopardize my patient because of some wild thing called carrying cost." Control is vested with patient caregivers for

Table 5. Brunswick Community Hospital supplies inventory (at June 30)

	Year 4	
Medical Supplies	$29,016	19%
Office Supplies	22,559	15%
Housekeeping Supplies	1,190	1%
Intravenous	4,251	3%
Linens	9,587	6%
Maintenance	187	0%
Pharmacy Drugs	31,149	20%
Central Supply	14,011	9%
Lab Supplies	21,507	14%
Surgery	20,905	14%
Total	$154,362	100%

these inventories. Their primary motivation is to stock inventory at such a level as to provide generous safety stock. General service departments maintain the remaining inventories. The use of these items is more predictable and out-of-stock situations less critical. Physical inventory counts are scheduled once a year. Base safety levels are used to maintain medical supplies inventories. Central supply was in the process of establishing these base safety levels. There was very little interest or understanding by other managers of the idea of efficient inventory levels. Day-to-day management of inventories was largely each department manager's concern. No formal control system was in place to establish or maintain inventory levels.

Prepaid Expenses/Other Current Assets Prepaid expenses comprise annual organization dues and annual maintenance contracts that provide for discounts of 5%–10% for annual up-front payment. Other current assets consist of the quarterly subsidy paid by the county government. By July 31 of Year 6, this balance will be paid in full. A long-term goal of the hospital board of trustees is for the hospital to be self-supporting.

Current Liabilities The cash forecast (see Table 2) outlines the hospital's goals for levels of unsecured debt, accounts payable, and amounts due to third-party payers. These goals could be changed; this would, however, require the approval of the board of trustees of the hospital.

Accounts payable are amounts owed to physicians who are members of the hospital medical staff and to national medical supply companies. The hospital also owes a small amount to local vendors for supply purchases. The local vendor and physician payments are current. National vendors do not emphasize credit worthiness to the extent common in other industries. Generally, community hospitals are good credit risks and some slowness in payment is not a source of concern to these vendors.

The amount due for accrued expenses is mainly attributable to payroll functions. As a practical matter, extending the payment of these accounts is impossible. Historical balance sheets and income statements are presented in Tables 6 and 7.

PETER BUTLER'S DECISION DILEMMA

Peter Butler realized the officers of the national company overseeing the hospital, the hospital administrator to whom he directly reported, and the members of the board of trustees all expected him to come up with a solution to the cash crisis at BCH. Peter knew he had considerable information about the hospital's operations that should be useful in designing a recommended solution. He felt his first job should be to determine exactly how the cash crisis had developed. He wondered what had changed recently compared to prior years when there had been no such problem. He thought this knowledge might then give him some clues as to where solutions may lie.

In general, Peter knew that there were many possible approaches to resolving a cash crisis in any organization. He realized there were several long-term financing options open to the hospital, including issuing revenue bonds, borrowing from deferred compensation funds, or deferring payments to the pension plan. Another set of possibilities included some kind of management intervention in managing the several different working capital accounts—accounts receivable, supplies inventories, prepaid expenses and other current assets, and current liabilities. Peter wondered what he could recommend that would result in the most effective, timely, and permanent solution to the cash crisis being experienced by the hospital.

Table 6. Brunswick Community Hospital balance sheets (at June 30)

ASSETS	Year 1	Year 2	Year 3	Year 4
Current Assets				
Cash & cash equivalents	$53,354	$110,070	$67,698	$43,125
Patient receivables	2,109,146	2,316,550	2,557,518	2,600,297
Less: uncol. & allowances	−380,000	−420,000	−480,000	−1,228,000
Taxes receivable from county	34,950	34,189	35,000	40,700
Due from 3rd-party payers			91,445	
Supplies & inventory	169,084	182,958	192,802	154,363
Prepaid expenses	13,268	18,208	15,797	26,032
Total Current Assets	$1,999,802	$2,241,975	$2,480,260	$1,636,517
Investment & Other Assets				
Interest-bearing deposits designated by board for capital improvements	185,978	236,238	135,565	30,486
Investment in medical office bldg.	227,039	213,759	200,479	187,199
Deferred financing costs	12,554	8,295	4,036	
Deferred compensation plan			822,424	967,763
	$425,571	$458,292	$1,162,504	$1,185,448
Property & equipment at cost	$8,197,389	$8,293,573	$8,442,491	$8,613,363
Less accum. depreciation	3,094,171	3,464,918	3,858,022	4,269,538
	$5,103,218	$4,828,655	$4,584,469	$4,343,825
Total Assets	$7,528,591	$7,528,922	$8,227,233	$7,165,790
Current Liabilities				
Unsecured notes payable to bank			$85,101	$136,334
Current maturities of long-term debt	$129,524	$160,437	117,165	22,589
Accounts payable	260,700	221,372	266,534	348,013
Due to third-party payers	31,960	15,588		75,000
Accrued expenses	226,895	226,309	258,008	301,394
Total Current Liabilities	$649,079	$623,706	$726,808	$883,330
Long-term debt less current maturities	$267,357	$156,947	$41,909	$6,078
Deferred compensation payable			822,424	967,763
Fund balance	6,612,155	6,748,269	6,636,092	5,308,619
Total Liabilities and Fund Balance	$7,528,591	$7,528,922	$8,227,233	$7,165,790

Table 7.   Brunswick Community Hospital statement of revenues and expenses
and changes in fund balance (year ended June 30)

REVENUE AND EXPENSES	Year 1	Year 2	Year 3	Year 4
Net Patient Service Revenue	$5,879,092	$6,181,456	$6,660,092	$6,033,569
Other Operating Revenue	26,895	31,268	4,000	11,563
Total Operating Revenue	$5,905,987	$6,212,724	$6,664,092	$6,045,132
Operating Expenses				
Professional care of patients	$3,815,929	$3,718,098	$4,291,207	$4,753,848
General services	804,724	764,489	820,010	869,964
Fiscal and admin. services	1,259,970	1,225,901	1,270,212	1,453,754
Depreciation	469,128	484,200	512,503	492,287
Total Operating Expenses	$6,349,751	$6,192,688	$6,893,932	$7,569,853
Income from operations	-$443,764	$20,036	-$229,840	-$1,524,721
Nonoperating Gains (Losses)				
Property taxes	$69,900	$69,189	$70,000	$149,700
Income on interest-bearing deposit for capital improvements	22,227	4,296	13,545	6,591
Operating funds	3,872	5,066	25,569	12,175
Gain (Loss) on disposal of equip.	200	-2,038	-1,081	
Unrestricted gifts and requests	1,638	1,380	14,670	7,508
Other	1,030	-7,322	-7,204	-6,876
Net nonoperating gains	$98,867	$70,571	$115,499	$169,098
Rev. & Gains in excess of exp.	-$344,897	$90,607	-$114,341	-$1,355,623
CHANGES IN FUND BALANCE				
Balance, Beginning	$6,950,052	$6,612,155	$6,748,269	$6,636,092
Rev. & gains in excess of exp.	-344,897	90,337	-114,341	-1,355,623
Funds restricted for equipment purchases	7,000	45,777	2,164	28,150
Balance Ending	$6,612,155	$6,748,269	$6,636,092	$5,308,619

APPENDIX

Billing and Collection Processes

Hospital billing and collection processes are unique to the industry. The objective of the BCH computer conversion was to make these processes more efficient. The following is an overview of the BCH computerized billing and collection system.

Charges

Generally the three origins of hospital charges are rooms, procedures, and supplies. Processing each type of charge varies somewhat from the others. Under the previous computer system all charging had been done on a batch basis rather than a continuous online basis. A batch system is more labor intensive, more prone to error, and results in more delays in the billing and collection process than is the case with an online system. The new computer system was designed to process more charges on an online basis.

Room Charges   The charge for a room covers nursing care, food, utilities, depreciation, housekeeping, and linen. The patient is charged a standard rate for each day spent in the facility, except for the day of discharge. If a patient was admitted at 11:00 P.M. on Friday and discharged at 11:00 P.M. on Sunday, for example, the patient would be charged for 2 days.

Under the previous computer system, the room charges were batched daily and entered into the accounts receivable system through a remote terminal. The remote processing center would then run an update. The update would then be reviewed and corrected if necessary.

This system was streamlined by the new computer system. At midnight, the computer checks the room census database. Every account that exists in this database is charged with a room charge.

Procedure Charges   A procedure charge is for the cost of performing a treatment procedure. Most patients admitted for surgery need a chest X ray, for example. These patients are charged a fee for this procedure.

Procedure charges were charged on a batch basis under the previous system. This system required a charge sheet for each procedure. In addition, each charge was entered through the remote terminal. The remote location processed these entries and the input was balanced.

The charging system with the new computer system is more efficient. When a procedure is ordered, the order is entered into the computer. After the procedure has been performed, the results are entered into the computer. The benefit of this system is that the status of the procedure can be checked by referring to the computer. In addition, charging to the patient's account is done automatically at the end of the day.

Supply Charges Supplies are charged as used. All consumable supplies are affixed with a sticker when received. As a supply item is used, the sticker is removed from the item and affixed to a charge card bearing the patient name and account number. These cards are used to enter the charge into the patient's account. This system remains unchanged under the new computer conversion.

Billing

Before a bill can be submitted, all of the above charges must be charged to the patient's account. Submitting charges to a payer after the initial billing significantly increases the time to receive payments. In some cases, late submissions are not paid. Noncharge information also must be submitted with the bill. This information concerns the patient's medical condition and treatment. This subsystem interfaces with the new computer system.

To start the billing process, which determines cash flow, a number of pieces of information must be available. Initially, not all of the new systems to generate this information functioned during the conversion. Some of the breakdowns were attributable to the computer system. Other break-downs were due to employee misunderstanding of the requirements of the new system.

PART V

Human Resource Management and Organizational Dynamics

23

Santorini Hospital

Can Culture Change Save It?

Ronnie Rodrigo Boongaling
North Valley Dermatology Center, Chico, California

Robert C. Myrtle
University of Southern California, Los Angeles,
California

THE NEW JOB

It is January 5, 2007, Nancy Jankowski's first day on the job as Santorini Hospital's new chief executive officer (CEO). She arrives to a hospital full of turmoil. Her predecessor, Alex Roth, who had before been the hospital's chief operating officer (COO), resigned a few months earlier under intense pressure from the medical staff and the community. The interim CEO, Agnes Williams, halted the hospital's expansion project and laid off over 100 nonclinical staff. Physicians, nurses, and support staff were up in arms. The hospital was in the local headlines almost every day.

THE HOSPITAL TODAY

In 1913, Rene Santorini, M.D., performed the first operation in his new hospital in Athens, California. In 1937, Dr. Santorini moved the hospital

---

This case is based on actual events. The organization, its location, and the names of people have been disguised.

to its current downtown location. Today, Santorini Hospital is the center of the medical community in the city of Athens, a community of over 80,000 residents. It has 585 beds and a level III trauma center. Santorini Hospital is Athens's only hospital. In addition, the hospital's market share extends far beyond the city of Athens. The hospital serves over 500,000 residents in a six-county area.

Athens is projected to have an annual population growth of 2%. The growth of the baby boom population will be higher than any other age group. Santorini Hospital is positioning itself for an increasing demand for services as well as for a changing composition of services. Also, because the current medical staff is aging, the hospital needs to attract new physicians to Athens.

Many view the expansion project as quite important to Santorini Hospital's future. The project will cost $140 million and will add 201,000 square feet of additional hospital space, 150 new beds, 15 new operating rooms, and a new emergency department with 36 treatment bays. The construction has already started, with completion expected within 3 years.

RECENT HISTORY

In 2004, some of the nonclinical employees at Santorini Hospital (housekeeping, dietary, and service workers) voted for union representation in an effort to improve their situation—low wages, unaffordable health insurance, insufficient staffing levels, and no job security. Santorini's administration immediately objected to the election results and alleged that some of the ballots were incorrect. The union, Service Employees International Union (SEIU), in conjunction with a well-known professor from Athens State University, validated the employees' grievances with a study showing how Santorini contributes to the growth of Athens's working poor.

The SEIU study revealed that 1 out of 10 employees earned less than $8.00 per hour and 1 out of 4 employees earned less than $10.00 per hour. The median hourly wage was $11.96 per hour. Compared to similar hospitals near Athens, an entry-level housekeeper earned $12.77 per hour, while that same entry-level position paid $7.50 at Santorini. An entry-level certified nursing assistant would have been paid $13.74 per hour at a nearby hospital compared to $9.66 at Santorini. In addition, full-time employees at Santorini Hospital paid between $1,020 and $2,400 annually for their dependent health insurance, while the nearby hospital paid entirely for dependent coverage. The study pointed out that the hospital's "substandard" wages and inadequate benefits caused serious financial hardship to employees, who often had to do without healthcare because of high cost. Finally, the study concluded that the hospital was contributing to the burden on taxpayers because its service employees were using various government programs to supplement their incomes and healthcare.

Despite the negative publicity, Santorini's administration proceeded with its objection to the formation of the union. In a hearing in Athens, an administrative law judge ruled that the election was valid. The hospital appealed the judge's decision to the National Labor Relations Board (NLRB). The NLRB upheld the judge's ruling and ordered Santorini Hospital to bargain with the union, but the administration still refused and sent a letter to the NLRB giving reasons why it refused to comply. The union wrote to the NLRB about the hospital's refusal. The NLRB declared that its decision for Santorini Hospital to bargain with the union was final. Santorini filed an appeal with an appeals court in Washington, D.C. The hospital's attorney attested that if Santorini was not satisfied with the appeals court's decision, it would continue to file appeals to higher courts. Thus, Santorini Hospital did not bargain with the union.

THE FIRE SPREADS

The discontent with the service employees was a catalyst for more unrest in other parts of the hospital. A housekeeper on his own time decided to take cell phone video of overflowing trash bins and medical waste at the hospital. His intent was to show that there were not enough employees to keep the hospital clean. Upon learning of this video, the hospital suspended the employee and then eventually fired him for tardiness. The union cried foul, asserting that Santorini retaliated against an employee who was concerned about safety. The union formally sent a complaint to the Occupational Safety and Health Administration (OSHA) about the hospital's practice of not properly disposing of its medical wastes by letting the waste overflow from trash containers.

Santorini Hospital's reputation in the community was diminishing. More and more articles were being written documenting the conflict between the hospital and the union. Santorini Hospital was now front and center in the local newspapers. One article characterized it as a bully and implored the hospital to bargain. The voices of the union members were heard publicly when the members held a rally in front of the hospital asking Santorini's administration to bargain. The California Nurses' Association, the Athens Teachers' Association, and the California Faculty Association of Athens State University joined the union members' rally. Santorini still stood by its position of not bargaining. In addition, the hospital claimed that it had the support of a separate group of service employees, the secretaries and business office workers, who refused to join the SEIU.

The union fought back. It took aim at Santorini's expansion project. Members were at every public meeting and filed objections to the environmental impact of the expansion. Objections often led to more meetings and studies, which delayed the completion of the project. Each month's delay cost between $500,000 and $1 million.

Residents near Santorini Hospital also joined the union, citing not only environmental issues, but also quality-of-life impacts from the increased automobile traffic and helicopter noise. The Athens City Council ordered the hospital to conduct a more thorough environmental study, adding more delay and project cost. The union also picketed on other sites, such as the office of the vice chair of the board of trustees.

CLINICAL INVOLVEMENT

What started as a dispute with the service workers spread to the clinical sections of the hospital. Less than 2 years after the service workers voted to form a union, the registered nurses gave the leaders of their union the power to call a strike. The nurses' issues involved health benefits for retired nurses, the ability of union leaders to enter the hospital and communicate with nurses, and the practice of "floating," when nurses are assigned to departments in which they normally do not work. Santorini Hospital now had two labor problems to contend with—the service employees and the RNs. And there was more trouble on the way.

PHYSICIAN INVOLVEMENT

Emergency call has never been a popular subject with hospitals and physicians, and Santorini Hospital and its physicians are no exception. Lasting more than a year, recent contract negotiations with the Athens Anesthesiology Group (AAG) led to an agreement in principle. The contract called for certain governance changes at AAG that the hospital claimed would increase efficiency. In addition, AAG would receive $850,000 for signing an exclusive contract with the hospital. A few weeks thereafter, AAG increased its demand to $1.4 million, and then upped the ante to $1.7 million. Alex Roth, the CEO at the time, claimed that the hospital could not meet the demand, so an alternative solution was sought. Santorini's administration decided to contract with a new anesthesiology group headed by a former member of AAG, Dr. Mercedes Celia.

AAG protested, claiming that the governance changes were designed to prevent its members from criticizing the hospital's administration. Dr. Bruno Cris, AAG's former president, also claimed that the third-party negotiator brought in to broker a deal between Santorini Hospital and

AAG had a conflict of interest. AAG had agreed to have Dr. Ricardo Marist as the negotiator because of his clinical background, but AAG later found that Marist was also consulting for the hospital on other matters. In addition, one of the governance changes involved firing certain physicians from AAG, one of whom was Dr. Cris, and imposing a "gag order" against any criticisms about Santorini's administration. Dr. Cris was known to be difficult with the nurses and staff.

Four physicians at AAG quit and found employment outside Athens. AAG gave the hospital notice that in a few days its remaining members would no longer service Santorini Hospital's patients. This announcement sent a shockwave to the community. Shortly thereafter a retired orthopedic surgeon, Dr. Frederick Thompson, placed a full-page advertisement in the local newspaper calling attention to the loss of the four AAG physicians and questioning the capability of hospital management and the quality of care at the hospital. Thompson's ad called the anesthesiologists the "poor boys" compared to other physicians on call, such as the neurosurgeons. At the same time, Thompson built a Web site for medical personnel to give their vote of confidence to Santorini's administration and to make comments. Athens residents were very concerned that the long-trusted anesthesiology group was no longer part of the community. Again, Santorini Hospital was negatively in the headlines.

THE VOTE

The chief of the medical staff, Dr. Felix Jovi, called a special meeting exclusively for the physicians at Santorini Hospital. The current president of AAG, Dr. Donald Foley, gave his account of the events leading to his group's decision to terminate its relationship with the hospital. In his remarks, Dr. Foley did not mention that AAG asked for double the money even though they already had a contract in principle of $850,000 with Santorini Hospital. One of the board members, a physician, explained to the medical staff that taking call was not only a problem for the anesthesiologists, but also for the entire medical staff. He emphasized that physicians do not want to take call, even though the emergency room desperately needs their services. He also added that Santorini's administration did not have enough time to consult with the medical staff about contracting with another anesthesia group because AAG gave only a few days' notice before it decided to terminate its relationship. At that point, Dr. Jovi interceded. He wanted to focus on the administration's failure to consult with the medical staff before a new group was hired.

Dr. Cris, the physician who purportedly was asked to leave AAG as a condition of the contract, enlivened the discussion further when he produced a secretly recorded conversation supposedly implicating his former colleague, Dr. Celia, of taking sides with Santorini Hospital. Dr. Cris alleged that Dr. Celia was ordered by then-CEO Roth to spy on him by driving by his house to check if there was a pro-union sign on his front yard. Dr. Celia, without hearing the tape, gave consent for it to be played. The audiotape did not reveal any such order from Roth, and the stage had been set to steer the discussions away from AAG to Roth exclusively. Dr. Cris argued vigorously that Roth was the cause of all of the hospital's problems. Most of the discussion in the meeting had to do with Roth being dictatorial and vindictive. Some accused him of using "security" as the reason for placing cameras in the hospital as a cover for spying on the staff. The physicians overwhelmingly gave Roth a vote of no confidence.

A SHAKEUP LOOMS

The vote of no confidence was published in the local newspapers and became *the* topic of conversation in Athens. Roth did not comment on the vote and concentrated on the loss of AAG. The Santorini Hospital started prioritizing its surgery schedule. It hired some anesthesiologists from nearby hospitals and employed locum tenens as well. This gave Dr. Celia time to recruit new physicians to Roth's newly formed group, Valley Anesthesiology Partners.

While Roth tried to manage the anesthesiology crisis at Santorini Hospital, he could not stop the momentum that the service employees had started, culminating in the no-confidence vote by the physicians. After extensive coverage in the media, Roth announced his retirement, his last day being the end of the month. The board of trustees announced an immediate search for his replacement. With Roth's departure, half of the board members, including the chair and the vice chair, also announced their resignations. Santorini Hospital was experiencing a broad changing of the guard.

Interim CEO, Agnes Williams, was brought in while the hospital recruited its next CEO. Williams was known for coming into troubled hospitals. In her short stay at Santorini Hospital, she determined that the facility was in financial trouble, so she announced the layoff of 5% of its workforce. This included the same secretaries and business office employees who had refused to join the SEIU. In addition, she questioned the value of the expansion project and halted actions leading to ground breaking.

The issue of not having enough anesthesiologists was still in full swing. Recent patient deaths at Santorini Hospital were prominently covered in the local newspapers. The sheriff's department got involved in the investigations of three deaths, one of which had a clear connection to anesthesiology. The sheriff's department wanted to determine if the hospital's anesthesiology department posed a danger to the public. Several local physicians alleged that Santorini Hospital was supporting the practice of dangerous medicine by hiring out-of-town and locum tenens anesthesiologists.

Other physicians also left the call schedule. Five months after AAG left, the orthopedic group left the hospital. That same month, a prominent vascular surgeon left the call schedule. The cardiac surgeon that Santorini Hospital relied on for its cardiovascular center of excellence left the hospital and took his entire cardiac surgery team with him. Trauma surgeons, radiation oncologists, a hospitalist, a psychiatrist, an interventional cardiologist, and two radiologists also left the hospital. With the exodus of physicians and nurses, a local newspaper labeled Santorini Hospital a dangerous place.

A NEW SKIPPER AT THE HELM

Santorini Hospital's board of trustees selected Nancy Jankowski as the new CEO in January 2007. She brought 25 years of executive management experience with her. Her tenure at her last hospital, Florence Adventist Hospital in Maryland, was a testament to her leadership abilities. Prior to Jankowski's reign there, Florence's administration also received a vote of no confidence. Unlike Santorini, Florence Adventist Hospital was about to lose its accreditation when Jankowski took over. She guided Florence from the brink of collapse to being an award-winning hospital. In addition, the fact that Jankowski was an RN brought her instant credibility with Santorini's nurses and physicians. Jankowski considers herself an "accidental CEO." She readily admits that she did not have formal training to become an executive, but she always had a passion for patient care.

Healthcare professionals at Santorini Hospital received the news of Jankowski's selection with guarded optimism. Their agenda included letting the new CEO know of their concerns, such as lack of openness and transparency. SEIU wanted, at last, to bargain with the hospital's administration. The physicians wanted the hospital's leaders to repair their damaged relationship. Everyone wanted a change in the style of management. When Jankowski arrived, she announced that her primary focus was to change the hospital culture. She set about this task immediately.

EARLY STEPS IN CHANGING THE CULTURE

Even before her arrival, Jankowski ordered a focused review of the surgery and anesthesiology departments. She was establishing a proactive approach to managing the hospital and sought to identify issues before they became problems. The first action Jankowski took after she arrived was to reinstate the laid-off service employees, who also received back pay for the period of their layoff. She recognized the SEIU union, 3 years after the service employees had voted for it. On May 22, 2007, bargaining talks between SEIU and Santorini's administration commenced. Subsequent weekly talks and the content of those meetings were published on the hospital Web site, a first for Santorini Hospital.

On her first days at Santorini Hospital, Jankowski focused on culture change through increased transparency. Communication with employees and the medical staff improved considerably following her arrival. Together with her management team, Jankowski began sending weekly messages on a general voicemail about what was going on in the hospital. Employees and the medical staff could call this voicemail box anytime and listen to her CEO report. Jankowski wanted to let the employees know that messages she left for them through her voicemails were not just her interpretations; they included feedback from all of the managers. She also wanted to put a voice to her name because she recognized that most of the employees had never met her.

She also invited the physicians to a get-to-know-you meeting during which she jokingly told them that they were only allowed one vote of no confidence in their lifetimes. Jankowski also began communicating significant news about the hospital to the medical staff via fax.

THE REGULATORS:
A NEW COMPLICATION FOR JANKOWSKI

Days before Jankowski's arrival, the State Department of Health Services (DHS) sent a nurse to inspect Santorini Hospital in connection with the death in February of a 44-year-old patient, who had been in the hospital for elective shoulder surgery. The inspector reported her findings to the Centers of Medicare and Medicaid Services, which subsequently asked DHS to do a follow-up inspection. On April 3, 2007, the original DHS inspecting nurse as well as a physician carried out a more extensive 5-day survey of the hospital.

In the past, the staff had resisted such surveys. Jankowski emphasized to them that the surveyors were there to help the hospital identify and fix problems. She also expressed that she wanted to change the culture of ignoring problems and fighting those who pointed out problems, as the surveyors had been asked to do. After their inspection, the surveyors told Jankowski that their experience was more positive than in the past. Jankowski immediately put into place corrective actions. This process, however, was for a time interrupted when Jankowski was injured in an accident during a family trip and could not return to work for a few weeks.

During her absence, a team of 10 DHS inspectors arrived to conduct another top-down inspection of the hospital. The survey was unannounced and the surveyors found deficiencies in seven areas, although they were mostly administrative in nature. The surveyors reported that many of the deficiencies found in the April survey had already been corrected and that no problems jeopardized patient care or safety. True to her commitment of transparency, Jankowski published the results of the follow-up survey.

In October 2007, the California Department of Public Health fined Santorini Hospital $50,000 for inadequately monitoring a drug that eases nausea but has dangerous side effects. Jankowski knew that inspections became more frequent when negative publicity and adverse events occurred; however, she was confident that the organization would be better prepared for the next survey.

JANKOWSKI BEGINS TO CHANGE SANTORINI'S CULTURE

Jankowski remains committed to culture change at Santorini Hospital. In addition to being more transparent, she is encouraging accountability within the organization. She expects the staff to follow policies and procedures and holds her senior management team accountable for their performance. Her CEO report is the same report that is presented to the board of trustees as well as to the staff. She holds her management team accountable for the contents of the report.

Jankowski is transforming the management of Santorini into a "self-learning" model. She began by assessing the talent level of all senior managers. Those who could not lead by engaging the staff were let go. Thus, many of the senior managers have taken on added responsibilities until suitable middle managers are found. The self-learning model begins at the top, with senior managers adopting the new management style first. They then teach it to their middle managers, who will in turn teach it to the supervisors, until all employees and medical staff become accustomed to self-managing.

Jankowski knows that this management style will not work for all departments at the hospital. She knows that there are different talent levels; this style requires a more sophisticated manager. She also understands that this type of leadership will thrive in certain departments, such as the emergency department, but may not work well in others, such as food service. Jankowski has lofty goals, but knows that the self-learning model might turn out to be a hybrid of self-management and regimented management.

GOING FORWARD

Jankowski is strongly committed to changing the former culture of not being accountable, finding blame, and not collaborating at Santorini Hospital. She believes it starts with her. She publicly acknowledges she can do very little as a CEO; the job of culture change is really accomplished through other people, such as the staff, RNs, and physicians. Whenever she is in contact with the staff, she makes sure their experience is always positive.

She is even taking the stalled expansion project further. Construction has begun. Jankowski is putting her touch on the entire project by redesigning it from the inside out. In the future, Santorini Hospital will be patient centered. All services will be designed around the patient. The aesthetics, such as the lighting and decor, will be pleasing. Nurses will structure their work around the patients and their families. Jankowski's vision is to have a hospital that employees would want to bring their own families to. She wants a hospital so good that it will be the hospital of choice for the community.

She is very optimistic, believing that the hospital is well positioned in the market. The problems she inherited are not insurmountable. The regulators are more satisfied because the hospital is cooperating and corrections are being made. Although physician call is still a major problem, there are signs of improvement. The new anesthesia group, Valley Anesthesiology Partners, is almost at full strength. Only two more physicians need to be recruited to meet the hospital's minimum requirement of 14 full-time anesthesiologists. In general, more physicians are applying because of the hospital's turnaround.

The bargaining process with the SEIU is still in progress. Jankowski knows she will need to appease the service employees quickly. Because the RNs filed a grievance and authorized their leaders to call a strike only days before Jankowski's arrival, she knows that she will need to bargain with the RNs as well. The emergency room physician call schedule is still not fully covered. There is also the $140 million expansion project that is supposed to be completed within 3 years.

As part of her plan, Jankowski has reached out to nearby hospitals. She is in discussions with their CEOs to share ideas and resources and not to take each other's business. She wants her hospital to work with the others in serving the community.

Jankowski remains positive in continuing the turnaround. She has to. She made a commitment to Santorini Hospital that this is her last stop. She plans to retire from the hospital when the time comes. Jankowski publicly attests that Athens is a great community that deserves a great hospital. And with her leadership, she believes Santorini Hospital can become the big-time hospital with the small-town feel.

Jankowski thinks Santorini Hospital is well under way to achieving her hopes for it to be a great hospital, but she wonders what else she can do to ensure this outcome.

24

Hospital Software Solutions (A)

Elizabeth M. A. Grasby
Jason Stornelli

Richard Ivey School of Business
The University of Western Ontario

IVEY

"Sometimes we just have to do things we don't want to do. Now come on, Natalie, stop complaining. I'm busy and you should be too! Get back to work!"

With her manager's words still ringing in her ears after a disastrous meeting, Natalie MacLachlan fell into her chair with a sigh. It was August 2005, and MacLachlan was three months into her tenure at Hospital Software Solutions. Things were not going well—how could MacLachlan's superiors seemingly perceive her as the office "slacker"? This was certainly not what she had planned for her first job after graduation, and MacLachlan knew she had to fix the situation fast . . . before she was fired.

Jason Stornelli wrote this case under the supervision of Elizabeth M. A. Grasby solely to provide material for class discussion. The authors do not intend to illustrate either effective or ineffective handling of a managerial situation. The authors may have disguised certain names and other identifying information to protect confidentiality.

NATALIE MACLACHLAN

Being labelled as a poor performer was something new for MacLachlan. Before accepting her position at Hospital Software Solutions, she had always been a conscientious student and a high achiever. Originally from Ottawa, Ontario, MacLachlan was attracted to The University of Western Ontario (Western) by the honors business administration (HBA) program at the Richard Ivey School of Business (Ivey), one of Canada's most respected business schools. Because of her strong academic performance and extensive community involvement throughout high school, MacLachlan was pre-accepted into the HBA program before arriving at Western.[1]

During her four years at Western, MacLachlan excelled. She was the recipient of numerous scholarships and awards, including a victory in the Business 020 case competition in her first year. MacLachlan's colleagues at Ivey described her as a good teammate, which was very important in the HBA program, since group work was an important component of the curriculum. Peers considered MacLachlan down-to-earth, articulate, dependable and even-tempered. It was rare to find someone with whom she did not get along. She was ambitious and wanted to do well, but she was not someone who played games to succeed at the expense of others.

MacLachlan extended this sense of thoughtfulness to her activities outside of school. She was active in many charitable, cultural and community organizations in the London area, and she continued to work on behalf of the community when she moved back to Ottawa to begin working for Hospital Software Solutions.

HOSPITAL SOFTWARE SOLUTIONS

History

Hospital Software Solutions (HSS) was founded in 1999 by 10 University of Ottawa software engineering classmates in response to the challenges Ontario hospitals were experiencing when integrating technology into their operations. Deep provincial government budget cuts were forcing hospitals to develop innovative solutions to provide effective and efficient patient care, while keeping costs as low as possible. Many hospitals in Ontario were still using paper systems for tasks such as nursing histories, patient records and medical literature databases.[2] Technology could help streamline these processes and greatly improve service delivery. HSS's customized software solutions promised hospitals an end to the days of lost charts, illegible handwriting and unused capacity with hospital equipment.

Once hospital administrators and physicians were convinced that the computer systems would be as reliable and as easy to use as paper-based methods, HSS's business started to boom. Indeed, the company had uncovered an excellent business opportunity that was easily scalable beyond Ontario. Hospitals around the world were facing similar challenges, and HSS grew very quickly as it expanded into markets in the United States, the United Kingdom and Europe. Much of the company's growth was accomplished through acquisition as the company bought competitors and integrated their operations into the HSS family. By 2005, HSS's financial results were very strong, and the prospects looked good for its future success.

OFFICE CULTURE

Although HSS had grown significantly, the culture at its Ottawa headquarters had not changed significantly. HSS was still run very much as it had been when the company started—like a small business. Because the original 10 partners knew the business best, all strategic decisions had to be cleared through their offices. They worked very hard, putting in long hours and sacrificing their personal lives to put HSS first. It was not unusual to hear the partners talking about missing an anniversary or a child's birthday, and a few had even come to work on the morning of their wedding day. This devotion to the company was what helped to make HSS a success, and the partners expected everyone on staff to work equally hard to move the company forward. Given the business's success to date, the partners believed they had a winning formula, so they had a strong desire to run the company "as it always had been."

Outside of the partners' offices, the culture at HSS was rather individualistic. Everyone concentrated on their own work, and interaction between employees was infrequent. Most staff communicated through instant messaging programs over the computer, and there were few team meetings. Employees received information on the company's strategic direction through a monthly newsletter, which served as the primary link between the company's partners and its employees.

UNEXPECTED BEGINNINGS

Recruiting season during her final year in the HBA program had been a challenge for MacLachlan. She wanted to work for a company that would give her a position with a significant amount of responsibility and would provide opportunity for advancement within the organization. A few friends of MacLachlan had accepted monotonous jobs, such as data entry, and she knew that she would not be happy unless she was being challenged. MacLachlan had also just married, and a position in Ottawa would allow her and her spouse to be close to both sides of their family.

When MacLachlan saw HSS's posting for a project manager position, she was elated:

> The project manager position had exactly what I wanted. The responsibilities were fantastic, and I could really see myself getting into my work on a daily basis. I've always been interested in computers and technology, and I worked on a large project during HBA that uncovered problems with the installation of a new computer system in a hospital in London, so I was already familiar with the industry. Compensation was more than what I was seeking, which I thought would certainly help with paying back my student loans, and the job was in Ottawa. Not only were our families there, but also, the Ottawa technology community was both tight-knit and growing. I thought the position at HSS would be a great opportunity to make contacts in the industry that would really help me in the future. At the time, I couldn't have asked for anything more.

MacLachlan's interviews with Derek Chow (vice-president, customer care), Marcus Nardi (manager, customer care) and Allan Densmore (vice-president, human resources) went well. All three men expressed numerous times during the interview process how perfect MacLachlan would be for the position. For the most part, the company appeared very laid-back and relaxed, although Chow and Densmore each had to step out of the room a few times to answer phone calls during the interview. MacLachlan left the interview convinced that HSS would be a good fit for her personality.

At the beginning of February 2005, MacLachlan received an offer over the telephone for the project manager position, effective July 1, 2005. Even though the company advised her to take a few weeks to consider, MacLachlan believed the job would be perfect for her, and she insisted on accepting over the telephone. She cancelled her upcoming interviews with other firms the next day.

A few weeks later, Densmore called MacLachlan to tell her that the company was changing its offer: they were now planning to hire her as a Customer Care Team Lead, which was a newly created role. Densmore assured MacLachlan that the team lead position was more prestigious than a project manager job, but he could not provide her with many details on her expected responsibilities because the job was so new. MacLachlan was reluctant to accept the team lead position:

> It was unclear what I would be doing as a team lead, and I really liked the project manager role. I think Densmore could tell I was upset—he kept saying on the phone how the team lead job was much better, but he could not give me a firm reason why. I reluctantly accepted, on the condition that they would provide me with a full written job description within two weeks. I don't like to start things when I don't know what I'm getting into.

When MacLachlan received the customer care team lead job description (see Exhibit 1), she had a few concerns, chiefly that she did not have the

Customer Care—Team Lead

Basic Purpose

This position requires a self-motivated, highly organized and independent individual, responsible for working with Sales and Operations team members to deliver outstanding Customer Service to our Top 150 Public Health Care Accounts. The incumbent will demonstrate productivity, profitability and quality, ensuring excellent customer service is provided to clients at all levels. The incumbent will develop strategies to improve overall Customer Satisfaction Scores. As the "voice of the Customer," the successful person will develop processes to improve internal communication and optimize Help Desk policies and procedures. Key initiatives that derive high value-creating benefit for our customers need to be defined, implemented and measured for their effectiveness. Develop streamlined reporting statistics for Account Management, and work with the Sales Team to articulate the value proposition of maintenance revenues. The successful candidate will have excellent customer service skills and communication skills, coupled with strong technical skills and a positive team player attitude.

Essential Duties and Responsibilities

1. Leadership / Management
   - Streamline processes, increase productivity, gain efficiencies and enhance value.
   - Develop and communicate a clear vision of goals and objectives, philosophies about growth, revenue generation and profitability, in particular the corporate customer care agenda relating to the "Customer is No. 1."
   - Generate, maintain and review with management, annual, quarterly and monthly revenue statistics (leading and lagging indicators) that represent customer satisfaction trends, financial statistics, productivity rates and overall improvement trends.
   - Maintain communications on daily activities, issues and potential challenges.

2. Customer Support / Sales
   - Deliver an effective long-term customer care program for top 150 clients, and implement and maintain client support initiatives.
   - Facilitate in-house training sessions, client training sessions and regional conferences for clients and potential clients.
   - Assist company personnel in the collection and assessment of Customer Care generated client information, and produce documentation relating to program usage, special function, instruction and promotions.
   - Assist in the development and maintenance of competitive intelligence programs and generate industry direction reports to support the development of new features and products.
   - Approve and co-ordinate the administration of customer satisfaction and information gathering surveys and other communication tools.

Exhibit 1. Team lead job description. *Source:* Company files.

(continued)

3. Controlling / Internal
   Review with Management:
   - Annual, quarterly and monthly revenue results/forecasts and costs.
   - Participate in the development of special projects, as well as relationships with various levels of government organizations, other private/ public sector organizations (e.g., FTA, State, local government).
   - Participate in the development of internal department policies and programs to support quality and growth.

Education and Work Experience
Bachelor's degree in business or technical field (engineering or IT).
Typically requires minimum three years of customer applications support experience.

Technical and Functional Skills
Excellent customer service skills, including a patient, courteous manner and a clear voice.
Excellent oral and written communication skills.
Managing project-related activities.
Defining and improving processes.
Demonstrated team leadership.
Ownership of issues through to resolution.
Ownership of customer satisfaction and improving scores.
Excellent knowledge of all HSS products, documentation, add-ons and reports.

Equipment and Applications
Knowledge of Hyperion, MS Office, MS Project, Lotus Notes and Maximizer.
Previous experience with incident reporting/bug reporting/call tracking systems an asset.

Work Environment and Physical Demands
General office environment.
Moderate levels of stress may occur at times.
Irregular hours at times.
No special physical demands required.
Travel may be required.

Exhibit 1. *(continued)*

required three years of support experience with customer service applications; however, she decided not to say anything, fearing Densmore would realize his mistake and rescind the offer.

In early May, MacLachlan and one of her classmates, who had also been hired at HSS, received e-mails from Chow requesting that they start immediately—the office was short-staffed and a client was requesting a complicated software installation. MacLachlan had purposefully booked travel plans before the starting date in her offer, and she really did not want to cancel them. She also wanted to attend her HBA convocation, which was taking place in mid-June. When MacLachlan explained why she would be unable to start work right away, Chow became rather upset. MacLachlan apologized but, at the same time, reminded him that her contract did not begin until July 1. Thankfully, MacLachlan's classmate responded that he was at the end of his vacation and he had a flexible airline ticket, so he could start early. MacLachlan's classmate later told her that Chow had made a point of thanking him for his devotion to the company.

THE FIRST MONTH

No Supervisor

On July 1, MacLachlan arrived at HSS headquarters. Despite the initial issues, MacLachlan was excited to begin the first day of her career; however, her enthusiasm soon waned when she arrived at the reception desk to ask for her manager, Marcus Nardi. She was told he had been fired three weeks earlier. Given her difficulties with Densmore and Chow, Nardi was the only member of the interview team she had not yet disappointed. MacLachlan was told that Chow would be supervising her for the next month until Nardi's replacement, April Worthington, returned from her maternity leave (see Exhibit 2).

MacLachlan proceeded to her desk. Due to a shortage of space, her work area was next to the programming staff area, on the other side of the building from the rest of the customer care team (see Exhibit 3). Chow stopped by soon thereafter; he appeared very rushed and flustered, but he did not mention or appear upset about her refusal to start the job early. Chow told MacLachlan that, unfortunately, he did not have time to train her, since there were too many outstanding projects awaiting completion. In

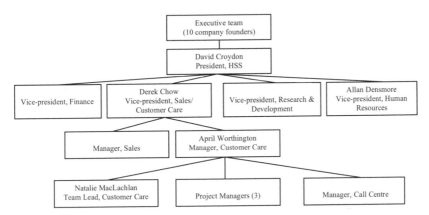

Exhibit 2. Partial Hospital Software Solutions organizational chart. *Source:* Field.

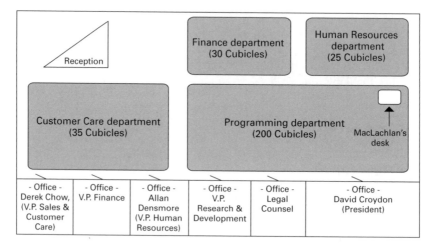

Exhibit 3. Floor plan of Hospital Software Solutions Ottawa headquarters.

the interim, he was not quite sure what to do with her, so she would have to work on data entry and database cleanup tasks for a few weeks. MacLachlan was disappointed. She believed these menial tasks did not fit with the customer care team lead job description Densmore had given her, and she had been looking forward to developing those required skills right away. Nevertheless, Chow seemed like a reasonable person, and MacLachlan did not want to risk further hindering her relationship with him.

Data Entry

Like most people beginning a new position, MacLachlan frequently had questions about her tasks, especially surrounding the HSS computer systems, and she often stopped by Chow's office to ask for clarification. He would usually interrupt his typing or phone call to give her a one-word answer and then go right back to work. MacLachlan thought this was odd, but she deduced that Chow was just busy.

After approximately three weeks, MacLachlan was much more comfortable with her tasks. She devised some time-saving measures to make the data entry more efficient, and she was particularly proud of herself when she was able to clean a significant amount of redundant data off the system. Excited about her progress, MacLachlan sent Chow an e-mail highlighting her efforts to date and asking for his feedback on her performance, but Chow replied with a short response reminding her of the importance of following established procedures (see Exhibit 4).

TO: Derek Chow

FROM: Natalie MacLachlan

SUBJECT: My performance?

Hi Derek,

Just wondering if you could give me some feedback on my performance as of late. I have been working hard on the data entry tasks you gave me, and I think I have come up with a way to tabulate the information without requiring a manual check. This makes the process significantly faster. I have attached the files for your review.

Thanks,

Natalie

Natalie MacLachlan, HBA
Team Lead, Customer Care
Hospital Software Solutions

TO: Natalie MacLachlan

FROM: Derek Chow

SUBJECT: Re: My performance?

Natalie,

Regarding your request for feedback, unfortunately I have not been able to devote much attention to your work lately, as I have been occupied with other matters.

However, I will remind you to follow HSS's data entry procedures as outlined in your employee manual. These procedures are in place for a reason, and deviating from them may cause data anomalies. Please ensure that the work you have done conforms to these specifications before submitting it.

Regards,

Derek Chow

Exhibit 4.   E-mail correspondence between Derek Chow and Natalie MacLachlan. *Source:* Field.

Shortly thereafter, serious problems began to develop with the systems on which MacLachlan was working. She was certain the issues did not relate to her work; nevertheless, she heard from others in the office that Chow was unhappy with her performance. Since she had already asked for feedback in an e-mail and felt that she was bothering Chow, MacLachlan chose not to say anything further.

MacLachlan looked at the pile of data entry sheets sitting on her desk. She believed the established processes Chow had reminded her to follow were redundant, and they were clearly a waste of time. For example, they required a lot of manual checking of figures, when the program had the capability to do that automatically. Chow had asked her to go back and check all her numbers again, which basically meant doing the past three weeks' work over again, even though she knew the numbers were right. "What a waste of my time . . . I don't think I'll bother," she whispered under her breath. This wasn't even what she had signed on for—the customer care team lead position was supposed to help her build skills and give her a significant degree of responsibility, not force her to sit in front of a computer and type in numbers all day.

MacLachlan was very frustrated and, since her work did not require collaboration with others, she decided to start working from home. She assumed this was not a problem, since Chow seemed too busy to spend any time with her and the programming staff (who sat around her) had flexible schedules, often arriving and leaving at odd hours.

THE SECOND MONTH

April Worthington

A few days into MacLachlan's second month at HSS, she met her supervisor, April Worthington, who had returned from her maternity leave.

Worthington had worked at HSS for her entire career (about 10 years), joining the company directly from high school. She held a correspondence diploma in management from a local community college. She had held a number of different positions at the same level within the company over the past three years. As one of the managers of customer care, Worthington was responsible for overseeing many different functions, including sales, technical support and complaint resolution. This responsibility required her to develop skills in a number of different areas and, as a result, she often felt overloaded.

Worthington was a very hard worker, and she appeared very dedicated to the company and its processes. It was not unusual to find her at the office late at night after a 12-hour day. Although she had children and a family, she always put her career first. Every task was urgent in Worthington's mind, and she expected the same urgency from her subordinates. She was very ambitious and had mentioned her keen interest in moving up through the organization.

In their first few weeks of working together, the relationship between MacLachlan and Worthington was cordial. Upon Worthington's return to work, MacLachlan was not clear about who she was now working for—Worthington was supposed to be her immediate supervisor, but she still had outstanding projects from Chow. Because she knew both managers were quite busy, MacLachlan decided not to say anything to either Worthington or Chow, and instead decided to complete all her delegated tasks from home, where there were fewer distractions.

The Phone Call

A few days before the end of her second month at HSS, MacLachlan was working through data entry on her home computer when she received a phone call from Worthington. She seemed particularly agitated that MacLachlan was not in the office, and told her that it would be in her best interest to be at her desk immediately. MacLachlan rushed to the office, only to find Worthington standing at her cubicle, waiting for her:

MacLachlan:

> "Hi April. Was there something you needed to talk to me about? The weather wasn't too great this morning, so I felt like working from home today. I have so much on my plate right now."

Worthington:

> "Why don't you know you're not supposed to be working from home? I expect you to be here when I'm here. I really needed your help yesterday and today on the presentation to the executive board, and I haven't been able to find you. You knew this seminar was very important."

MacLachlan:

> "Well, nobody told me I couldn't log in from home. After all, the programmers do it all the time. I think this is going a bit far. I'm kind of wasting my time at the office doing this data entry stuff anyhow. Do you really want a time sheet from me?"

Worthington:

> "No, I don't think I'm that controlling. However, to be honest with you, maybe I should be. I hear your work on the Ontario hospitals database was very disappointing. I've heard you're not following any of the proper procedures."

MacLachlan:

> "Well, I wasn't trained. Besides, I was just trying to make things more efficient. I came into this job expecting to take a leadership role, and I was trying to do that by improving the processes. Data entry isn't really what I was expecting, given my job description."

Worthington:

> "Your job description is two sentences long. Sometimes we just have to do things we don't want to do. Now come on, Natalie, stop complaining. I'm busy and you should be too. Get back to work!"

As MacLachlan was about to show Worthington the two-page job description from Densmore, Worthington snarled, "If you really want to do something different, do a system format! Have it done by this afternoon." She then stormed off.

Dejected, MacLachlan sat down at her desk. As she turned on her computer, an e-mail from Chow arrived saying that the system problems were getting worse. There appeared to be serious problems with the integrity of the data that needed her immediate attention. In addition to the fact her superiors thought she was a slacker, MacLachlan was now faced with conflicting instructions from two bosses. There was no way she could complete the work for both managers on time.

To add to her troubles, in the course of her data entry, MacLachlan had found problems with the way some of the system processes had been created by the programmers. These processes were unrelated to the data she was entering, but they still affected the computer system as a whole. MacLachlan thought this might be the cause of the problems that had been occurring lately, so she documented her findings. Chow and Worthington probably had no idea there was any problem with the processes, since they had so many other tasks to focus on. Regardless, she was not particularly motivated to share her concerns with either of the two managers, given their recent behavior toward her.

WHAT NEXT?

"Now what?" MacLachlan thought to herself. She knew a town-hall meeting[3] with HSS's president was coming up in a week and that the executive team had specifically asked for feedback on management styles and work processes. This was a meeting for non-management staff only, so Worthington and Chow would not be attending. MacLachlan had met the president a few times in passing, and he seemed like a nice man. She had heard from her colleagues that he was easy to talk to, and he genuinely wanted to do anything that would improve the company. MacLachlan had many ideas about how to improve the workflow at HSS, and she was eager to share them with someone who would listen. She wondered whether she should approach the president at the town hall meeting and raise her concerns. Could this be her chance to make a difference?

"Or maybe I should just talk to Worthington and Chow," thought MacLachlan. After all, a lot of the problems seemed to stem from misunderstandings. After all, Worthington had specifically mentioned that MacLachlan's job description was two sentences long, which was not the case. Had Chow and Worthington thought she was recruited to be doing something different? Maybe a good chat would clear things up. But, what would MacLachlan say? What would be the best way to approach the situation? Should she be threatening? Conciliatory?

MacLachlan knew she could quit, but that would leave her without a job, and she was still paying bills from her wedding and her school debt. It would be very difficult to make ends meet financially. The information technology community in Ottawa was also small, and news of her poor performance and early departure from HSS would surely spread quickly.

MacLachlan knew she had to act quickly. Whatever she decided, she wanted to have a detailed plan of action, with no more mistakes. How could she get herself out of this mess?

ENDNOTES

1. The HBA program was a "2+2" curriculum wherein students undertook two years of university in a field other than business and then entered the HBA program for their third and fourth years of university. Students with exemplary academic and extra-curricular performance could apply at the end of secondary school to have a spot initially reserved for them in the HBA program. Final acceptance into the HBA program was dependent on the maintenance of a high standard of academic and extra-curricular performance in the first two years of university.

2. Canadian Institute for Health Information. *Hospital Report 2002: Acute Care*, pp. 17–18.

3. "Town-hall" meetings are designed to provide a public link between upper management and front-line personnel. They are usually open to all employees and are often used by management to share corporate strategy or receive feedback from employees in a public forum.

25

A New "Brand" for Senior Health Plus

Rosalie Wachsmuth
Aging and Disability Services Administration,
State of Washington

Robert C. Myrtle
University of Southern California, Los Angeles,
California

THE HEART-WARMING COMMERCIAL

It was the end of the day, and Jamie Richards was exhausted by the time she reached home. She turned the television on to catch the end of the evening news but when she saw the commercial for Senior Health Plus (SHP), a not-for-profit Medicare HMO, she let out a big groan. It wasn't that she hated the ad; she definitely thought that it was catchy and appealed to seniors. Nowhere during the 30-second spot was there any mention of managed care or HMOs. Instead, Wilma, an attractive and vibrant member of SHP's Medicare HMO plan, explained to viewers how SHP had changed her life. After Wilma's hip replacement, SHP had provided her with extensive in-home and personal care services that not only sped up her recovery but also helped her to remain independent at home and in control of her life. The commercial ended with heart-warming shots of Wilma riding a bicycle alongside her grandchildren.

Although Jamie had seen the ad many times before, she couldn't help but feel proud. Her company, SHP, had touched that woman's life, and she knew everything that Wilma had said was true. But when Jamie imagined being back at SHP's corporate offices, she grimaced. Thoughts of the inflammatory complaints she received each day, the sarcastic whispers across cubicles, the unhappy faces in the halls, and the demise of employee morale bombarded her all at once. She thought it was ironic that SHP had become so successful at projecting a positive and appealing external image. If the public knew what it was like to work at SHP, they would certainly have a different opinion of the organization. She shook her head as she wondered about what had gone wrong at SHP.

A GOLDEN OPPORTUNITY

Ten months ago, Jamie joined SHP as the Vice President of Human Resources. She had left her long-time position as Director of Human Resources at Mature Health, a rival senior health plan, for many reasons. Her previous job had been a challenge mainly due to the difficulties of boosting employee morale in the fast-paced, ever-changing managed care environment. She had found that most employees were negatively affected by the stigma of working for an HMO. In Jamie's opinion, HMOs had developed a bad reputation and were one of the most universally hated organizations.

At Mature Health, Jamie had learned a lot about managing the culture of an HMO, but she wanted to apply her skill set to a different organizational setting. When the opportunity to work as the VP of Human Resources at SHP appeared, Jamie jumped at the opportunity. She heard that SHP was a different type of Medicare HMO. For the majority of its 20-year history, it had been known as a grassroots organization focused on preserving the independence of seniors. She was impressed by the CEO's track record of pioneering creative approaches to overcome medical and social challenges. He had guided the organization from a small senior services organization to its current state as an impressive health care system for elderly people.

Jamie was enticed by the idea of joining an organization that had a history of pioneering new ways of serving the elderly. She believed that an organization like SHP, with a strong grassroots foundation, had the power to not only change the way that managed care was delivered to seniors but also remove the stigma of HMOs. In addition, she was attracted to SHP because she felt that the employees there would have more passion for their work when compared with employees at other HMOs.

SHP'S EXPONENTIAL GROWTH

Jamie had come on board during an exciting time at SHP. The organization had been experiencing phenomenal growth both in its Medicare HMO membership and employee workforce. Membership over the past several years had skyrocketed from 10,000 to a whopping 20,000. When Jamie joined SHP, membership was soaring near the 35,000 mark and the number of employees had nearly tripled to more than 400. These numbers were small when compared to the size of rival HMOs, but they were still astounding statistics considering SHP's massive growth rate over the past 3 years.

For these reasons SHP's executive management team saw a need for creating the VP of Human Resources position. SHP's culture was undergoing drastic change to accommodate the huge growth in its workforce. In addition, the executive team planned on adding another 80 positions by the end of 1999 to alleviate the heavy workloads.

SHP was also expanding geographically to meet the needs of its customers. Shortly before Jamie's arrival, SHP had relocated its administrative offices and most of its departments from a modest grassroots base located in the heart of Santa Ana to a posh corporate building in Newport Beach.

They had also created three additional area offices within the past year. This brought the total number of area offices scattered across Southern California to seven. The executive team was concerned about maintaining organizational continuity across the sites and wanted the corporate offices in Newport Beach to be the flagship. That is, the corporate offices would set the standards, and the area offices would be expected to follow suit. The executive team thought that a VP of Human Resources was not only necessary to manage the needs of the growing workforce but also to maintain uniformity across the sites.

Jamie was excited about the challenge of molding SHP's workforce. She knew that her actions would have critical effects. She was in the position to change the culture to meet the needs of the growing organization. She was excited to mold a workforce that was embedded in the grassroots beliefs of SHP. Jamie believed that the employees would be eager to develop a new culture that retained the pioneering spirit of SHP.

She was strongly attracted to SHP's vision of maintaining the independence of seniors. The company had developed four core corporate values: passion, integrity, respect, and responsibility. SHP believed that its employees should be driven by the needs of its customers. Thus, they are expected to seek "innovative solutions on issues affecting their health, independence, and lifestyle choices." In addition, the employees' behaviors should be motivated by the desire to "do the right thing." Also, not only does SHP expect employees to protect and enhance the well-being of its customers but also to value and respect each other as fellow workers. Jamie felt these values set SHP apart from other HMOs and it made her even more eager to mold the workforce.

THE BEGINNING AND END OF A HONEYMOON

Jamie had always been told that the first 90 days of a new job were the honeymoon phase. Everything at SHP seemed too good to be true, at first. She was surprised at how quickly she had been welcomed onto the executive team considering her position was so new. The members reassured her that she would be playing a crucial role at SHP and that they respected her track record. Many of the other executives had also worked at rival HMOs. In fact, it seemed like everyone had jumped ship to join SHP.

During the second day of work, she learned that one of SHP's longtime employees had suddenly died. It was the first time in SHP's history that a current employee had passed away. Understandably, the staff was in shock. Jamie knew that her reaction to the situation would be critically evaluated by the entire organization. She quickly interviewed staff members who were close to the employee and distributed a company-wide memo informing SHP's employees of the death. Jamie also arranged for a company-wide memorial service for the employee and declared a special moment of silence in remembrance of her.

Jamie's delicate handling of the situation impressed the executive team, her human resources staff and employees throughout SHP. They commended her, and she gained immediate respect from the Human Resources staff. Jamie felt that she had proven herself to the executive team and her department and validated the need for her position. After the first 2 weeks on the job, however, it seemed like the honeymoon phase had come to an abrupt end. It was then that she realized that there was a lot about SHP that she didn't know and would soon uncover.

THE BRANDING CAMPAIGN

The CEO had suggested that Jamie meet with Rita Lansing, the VP of Marketing, as soon as possible. He raved about Rita's performance and declared that she was single-handedly positioning SHP for the new millennium. Her marketing department was currently immersed in an intense branding campaign. They were conducting focus groups with older adults from the community to find out everything they thought about the colors, shape, and even the symbolism behind the new brand.

The CEO felt very strongly about developing a brand for his company. He wanted to differentiate SHP from other Medicare HMOs by creating a symbol. He explained to Jamie:

> I have always dreamed about creating a brand for SHP. This brand would help consumers identify the unique services that come from our company. A brand name would not only provide an added value to our company, but also give a name for consumers to associate our services with. Seniors tend to be loyal to brand names that symbolize high quality. Just as Windows 2000 is purely Microsoft and Kleenex is the essence of Kimberly-Clark, my vision is to have the public recognize SHP by our logo and know that we deliver high-quality senior services that set us apart from other Medicare HMOs.

Upon hearing this, it clicked in Jamie's head exactly how crucial her role was in this branding process. Creating a brand wasn't just a physical action; it required a change of thought within the company. She would have to encourage the development of a more corporate, professional culture that was consistent with the brand. This branding campaign was an essential part of shaping the organization's culture. It was the basis for many changes.

This task, however, seemed rather overwhelming to Jamie. How could she develop and establish a uniform corporate culture across all eight SHP sites? The atmosphere was drastically different at each separate office. The satellite sites were professional but did not project the same image as the corporate offices. If the culture of the corporate offices represented SHP's new image, then it was crucial for the other sites to replicate it. This was significant because SHP's clients often visited the satellite sites and rarely interfaced with the corporate offices. Thus, it would be important to uphold the SHP image at the satellite sites.

The first thing that Jamie wanted to do was arrange an appointment with Rita. Jamie was eager to meet Rita and find out how she could help carry out the CEO's vision. The brand development sounded exciting, but Jamie was surprised by the amount of time and resources that were being devoted to the creation of the brand. She was, however, extremely interested in finding out exactly what this branding campaign was and to have her questions answered by Rita. Also, Jamie was very concerned about having the employees in on the development of the brand. She felt their involvement was crucial because they would be representing the brand.

STARTING OFF ON THE WRONG FOOT

When Jamie arranged to meet with Rita, she was surprised by her abruptness. Rita said that she was very busy but was willing to spare a few minutes to fill Jamie in on the brand development. Jamie was puzzled by Rita's chilly treatment especially when she compared it to the friendliness of the other executive members.

At their meeting, Jamie was further taken aback by Rita's take-charge manner. The 15-minute meeting did not go as Jamie had envisioned. Not only had Jamie wanted a longer, more in-depth meeting, but she also had hoped that the two of them could discuss where their roles fell in the organization and how they could work together to make the branding campaign a success. Jamie knew that the employees would need a stake in the campaign in order for them to buy into it. She hoped that by including them in the brand development process, this would slowly initiate an organizational culture change and foster employee buy-in.

Jamie was astonished when Rita promptly told her that the marketing department was going to execute the brand development without any help from the rest of SHP. Rita argued that the brand research was confidential and she didn't see the need for employee involvement. She wanted to perfect the brand to meet the CEO's vision not the employees' and therefore did not want employee input. Rita believed that employee buy-in would be the easiest part. If she were successful at creating a distinct, high-quality brand, no employee would argue against its implementation. In fact, Rita argued they would feel privileged to represent SHP's new brand and automatically be motivated to reinforce the brand's high quality.

Jamie was astounded by Rita's logic. She tried to reason with Rita and explained to her that in order for the branding campaign to be successful at reinventing the company's image, Rita would need SHP employee buy-in. Many of the employees had been with the organization when it was a small, grassroots oriented senior services organization. If they did not get involved with these changes, they would surely resist the change.

Rita would not budge. She said her past experiences with brand development had taught her that the process should exclude employee involvement. Rita pointed out that she would fully involve the employees during the unveiling of the new brand. She explained that her department was already planning an unveiling ceremony where all of the employees would be introduced to the new brand.

WORKING INDEPENDENTLY

After that encounter, Jamie felt that her hands were tied. How could she manage the changing organization if Rita wasn't even going to include her in the brand development? Jamie viewed her participation in the branding campaign as a critical part of being the VP of Human Resources. She approached the CEO for guidance but backed down when he told her that Rita was highly experienced and knew what she was doing. Again, Jamie saw how important the brand was to him. He seemed so impressed by Rita's progress that he couldn't see past anything else.

Jamie set off to reorganize her department and the company structure so that it would be in alignment with what she perceived to be the new emerging corporate culture. Her department was very supportive of her. They jointly decided to create a way to open the communication lines between the employees and administration. Jamie viewed communication as one of SHP's current major weaknesses. Thus, she implemented a new medium for communication called the CEO's MessageBoard, created a policy that encouraged employees to eat lunch in the lunchroom instead of at their desks, and revamped the dress code to fit SHP's new corporate image. Her department also worked in conjunction with the executive team to revamp SHP's organizational structure. She thought that these changes should have been implemented long ago.

The CEO's MessageBoard was a hit with the employees. They loved the fact that they could anonymously submit messages to the CEO and have them answered on the company's on-line server. They felt comfortable voicing their concerns and the CEO gave his own input and answers to the questions. It was also available for the rest of the organization to view on-line. Jamie thought that the MessageBoard had helped to create a firm sense of partnership between management and staff while enhancing opportunities for employee growth and development.

The lunchroom policy did not receive rave reviews. Employees felt as if the HR department was telling them how to use their lunch time and felt that it was infringing on employee individualism. Yet, Jamie did not alter the policy. She felt that it was important to encourage employees to interact with each other away from their desks.

Jamie also felt that the organizational structure changes were greatly needed because of the high levels of duplication and geographic problems. Now that SHP had taken residence in their Newport Beach building, Jamie began working with the facilities director to reorganize the employees' workstations. She had wanted to arrange them all in appropriate work units. The employees, however, resented the cubicle changes and thought that HR was imposing a major inconvenience on them. Furthermore, 3 months after the cubicle swapping, the CEO announced that SHP would be relocating to a larger building with more space the following year. This added to the employees' annoyances with Jamie's department.

INTERDEPARTMENTAL CONFLICTS

Problems with marketing and interdepartmental organization made Jamie's job even more difficult. As Jamie and her department set out to make further changes, such as revamping the company newsletter and creating a newsletter for the consumers, she noticed that Rita was stepping into her territory.

During one pivotal executive meeting, Jamie unveiled the newsletters that she and her staff had spent weeks developing. Right there in front of the CEO, Rita expressed her disapproval and pointed out that they would not fit in with the consistency of the brand. Rita explained to the CEO and the executive team that in the future, any internal and external communication documents should be evaluated and approved by her department first. This was because the documents could wear away the brand integrity. Rita said, "Unfortunately good brand management does not always allow for individual creativity. We need to present a consistent image not just externally but internally as well."

Jamie left the meeting fuming. She could not believe what had just happened. Not only had Rita made her look foolish in front of the entire executive team, but she also implied that Jamie didn't know how to do her job correctly. She approached the CEO afterward with her concerns about Rita's infringement on her departmental duties. But Jamie knew he would be no help when she saw the look on his face as she mentioned the brand. He asked her if she had seen the final draft of the brand. She shook her head. His eyes lit up as he described how phenomenal it was. Rita had produced exactly what he had envisioned over the last 20 years. He said he was astounded and could not believe how excited he was. When Jamie voiced her concerns, he reiterated what Rita said regarding the importance of maintaining the brand integrity. He also mentioned that they were preparing to copyright certain terms that would be used to refer to their case managers as "Healthy Care Managers" and the senior services department as "Living with Independence." This would prevent other Medicare HMOs from stealing or copying the services that were unique to SHP.

Jamie was speechless. It was obvious that she could no longer depend on the CEO for support. Rita had him wrapped around her finger.

UNVEILING THE NEW BRAND

Two months later, the marketing department was set to release its new brand for SHP. They had organized a huge unveiling ceremony for the brand and asked Jamie's department for help. Jamie, although still upset from her encounters with Rita, decided that it would be in her best interest to cooperate with marketing. She had hoped that there would still be an opportunity for them to establish good interdepartmental relations.

She had agreed to lend her staff and HR would be in charge of spreading the word about the unveiling ceremony. Jamie began to feel more positive about the ceremony, especially since it now would appear to the employees that HR had played a big part in the brand development. Everyone was given the morning off to attend the ceremony at corporate headquarters.

The only glitch was that marketing had ordered polo shirts, caps, and lunch boxes with the new brand for employees. Because of the budget limits, however, they didn't have enough items to distribute to all of SHP's employees. Thus, Rita made the decision to only distribute items to permanent employees who had been with SHP for over a year.

Jamie objected to that proposal and pointed out that it could create animosity among the employees and temporary workers. Yet, Rita argued that it was too late to do anything about it and that it made sense to only offer long-standing employees the branded items. Jamie backed down and gave in. She had enough to worry about with the planning of the ceremony. She was scheduled to speak after the CEO and wanted to project the right image. The recent changes that she had made at SHP hadn't gone as smoothly as she had wanted, and Jamie knew that the ceremony was the perfect opportunity to redeem herself.

As Jamie had predicted, however, the employees were not only upset about the inequitable distribution of shirts, caps, and lunch boxes, but they were also resentful toward the new brand. Although they enjoyed having the morning off to attend the ceremony, they didn't understand exactly why SHP was revamping its external image. Many commented that SHP had sold out its grassroots heritage for a more corporate, snobby image. To make matters worse, they directed their anger toward the HR department. The employees had assumed that because HR had publicized the event, they were the major movers behind the brand development.

SIX MONTHS LATER

Six months after the unveiling ceremony, the situation between the HR department and SHP's staff had only worsened. While the marketing department had developed a whole new set of rules and regulations that accompanied the use of the new brand and the trademarked terms (Healthy Care Manager and Living with Independence), the executive team had given Jamie the job of enforcing the standards.

At first, Jamie had welcomed the chance to be in control of this area. She had thought that it would provide her with more control to mold SHP's employees and regain their trust. The employees, however, viewed the brand rules as a huge nuisance and resented the fact that they had to follow them. They felt that Jamie and her department were forcing SHP's staff to adjust to a new corporate image. They accused the HR department of eliminating the pioneering spirit of SHP by implementing a barrage of rules that accompanied the brand and the new culture.

Jamie was appalled by the situation. The employees were misinter-preting her actions. She, more than anyone else, wanted to maintain SHP's grassroots, pioneering spirit. It seemed that the only people who did not oppose her changes, however, were members of the executive team. They appeared to adjust well to the new emerging corporate culture. She finally realized that they were beginning to feel comfortable at SHP, because it was now so similar to the other HMOs they had left.

The executive team was troubled by the reactions of their employees. They did not understand why they were so against the changes. To make matters worse, the popular MessageBoard had evolved into a company therapy board. Departments used it as a medium to promote name-calling while others griped about the morale at SHP, whined about parking fees, and complained about dress codes. Even more disturbing to Jamie was that all of SHP's dirty laundry was being aired throughout the company. Instead of promoting good communication, the MessageBoard had turned into a disaster. Yet she was afraid of eliminating the MessageBoard because so many employees felt it was the only venue they could use to communi-cate their concerns.

LOOKING AHEAD

As Jamie turned off the television, she realized that the situation at SHP had reached a critical state. Already, she had droves of employees quitting their jobs, others were interviewing with SHP's competitors, and low employee morale was beginning to affect the quality of customer service. While the marketing department's branding campaign had been so suc-cessful at projecting a positive public image, the employees who upheld SHP's reputation were not supporting it. The way the cards had stacked up against her, Jamie knew that the executive team would blame her for the situation. Thus, Jamie would have to choose her next move very care-fully. The only problem was that she didn't know which way to turn.

26

Autumn Park

Cara Thomason
Park Terrace Senior Living, Rancho Santa Margarita,
California

Robert C. Myrtle
University of Southern California, Los Angeles,
California

Brad Douglas, the Executive Director of Autumn Park, was so tired and frustrated as he once again looked over the resident file of Mildred Puce. Brad was preparing for the afternoon meeting with Mildred and Hannah Meeks, a registered nurse and Director of Assisted Living of Autumn Park. Brad firmly believed in the company's principles, values, and beliefs (PVBs) on how to deal with resident issues and problems, yet everything he is doing with Mildred is going against those PVBs (see Exhibit 1).

THE HISTORY OF AUTUMN PARK

Autumn Park is one of the thirteen properties owned and managed by Abbot Retirement Communities (ARC), which owns and manages high-quality, full-service rental retirement communities nationwide, offering independent, assisted, and dementia care. ARC is passionate about enhancing the lives of seniors and is committed to delivering exemplary service with integrity, dignity, and compassion.

Statement of Principles, Values, and Beliefs

We are committed to exemplary service delivered with integrity, dignity, and compassion. Our communities for seniors are distinguished by warm, secure, and friendly environments.

We will enhance each resident's lifestyle by:
• Responding immediately to resident's needs and concerns.
• Offering high-quality, creatively designed programs.
• Encouraging independence.
• Promoting a sense of community and friendship.

We the staff are committed to:
• Teamwork
• Being professional
• Open communication
• Fostering a learning environment
• Continuous improvement
• Profitability

We live by a standard of conduct that encompasses honesty, accountability, personal development, and a passion for excellence.

Exhibit 1. These principles, values, and beliefs are referred to whenever important decisions are made at Autumn Park.

ARC is a family-owned company that was founded in 1990. The President and CEO of ARC, Anthony Abbot, was given a retirement property by his family as an investment. The original plan was to manage the property and improve its appearance and services, and then resell it for a profit. Abbot became so interested in managing the property that he decided to keep it and expand the business.

Abbot had a vision to grow ARC as a unique and enduring company dedicated to meeting the changing needs of the residents and their families. He wanted to create working environments where associates were appreciated and inspired to develop as individuals and where strengths and abilities were nurtured and rewarded. He wanted to own a company of high-quality retirement communities and services delivered with a warm and friendly feeling. He was committed to responsible growth, operational excellence, and superior financial results. He did not want the largest company in the industry; he just wanted the best.

In 1996, Abbot and his executive team wanted to develop a property from the ground up. Abbot wanted to build a high-end retirement community. The properties he had acquired previously were all middle- to upper-end properties, in appearance and price. Abbot was able to meet with the County Development Planning Department for a new city in Southern California. They found a center location for the property and bought the land. Also during this time, ARC moved their corporate office from North Carolina to Southern California.

ARC broke ground for Autumn Park in 1999, with an anticipated opening in March of 2000. Autumn Park was a community for independent and assisted living residents, with an additional neighborhood for dementia care. The goal for Autumn Park was to have no more than 40% of its residents on assisted living.

BACKGROUND OF MILDRED PUCE

In September of 1999, Mildred Puce visited the trailer that was advertising for Autumn Park while it was being built. After several visits with the marketing team about what Autumn Park could provide her, she gave her deposit in November of that year. Mildred already lived at another continuing care retirement community (CCRC), yet she was attracted to Autumn Park's centralized location; it was near shops, restaurants, churches, and grocery stores. Autumn Park offered what she had before, plus more services.

Autumn Park's marketing team was looking to fill up their new property as soon as possible. They were taking deposits and applications from anyone who was interested and seemed appropriate; but Mildred was different. Although she was already living in another CCRC, Mildred was in a motorized wheelchair, younger than 60, had multiple sclerosis, and the use of only her head and left arm. Autumn Park accepted her deposit based on the criteria that they had to have an exception letter from the state because she was under the age requirement to live in a CCRC, had special needs, and required a Vera body lift.

Due to unforeseen circumstances, Autumn Park's opening was postponed till July of 2000. In March, Autumn Park received doctor's orders that Mildred needed a Vera lift to get in and out of bed and to the toilet. The orders also indicated that she was able to operate the lift with little assistance. She also needed a motorized chair due to her disability and therefore needed a handicapped-access apartment. The Life Enrichment Assistant Coordinator of the CCRC in which she lived also wrote a letter to Autumn Park saying how wonderful a resident Mildred was and how sorry they are that she is leaving them.

In May of 2000, Autumn Park received another order from Mildred's doctor that stated Mildred could self-administer her own beta injections. The marketing department collected all of her information but did not share the information with the clinical staff to assess at that time. The physician disclosed all of her disabilities for the clinical staff to examine and consider in their assessment.

The assessment is done prior to the resident's moving in, and if the clinical staff does not feel that Autumn Park can take care of the needs of that person then the move-in is denied. The assessment is based on observation and conversation with the resident, along with a physician assessment of the resident's medications, diagnoses, disabilities, and abilities (see Exhibit 2). ARC policy states that after the initial assessment, the resident must be reassessed 30 days after the move-in date.

If the assessment indicates that the resident needs to be on assisted living, the resident is charged an additional $400 a month to go into assisted living, Level I, and another $300 for each additional level of assisted living care.

The original assessment given to Mildred, prior to her moving in, put her at a Level I for assisted living. Mildred was assessed at 10 minutes for bathing and showering, 15 minutes for grooming, and 15 minutes for assistance in transfers. Mildred also indicated in her assessment that she is fully capable of taking care of her two cats.

Autumn Park opened its doors July 1, 2000. During the first month of operation, the Executive Director resigned and the Director of Assisted Living was let go. In the interim of hiring replacements, the corporate staff brought in regional directors to fill in. By the end of August, Brad Douglas was hired as the new Executive Director of Autumn Park and Hannah Meeks was Autumn Park's new Director of Assisted Living.

Meeks reassessed Mildred at the end of August, 2 months after her move-in date, at a Level III. Mildred was taking 45 minutes of the caregivers' time for her showers, which were given three times per week. Mildred was also having the caregivers spend 20 minutes each day helping her with her oral care. It was also discovered that the caregivers were spending an extra 15–30 minutes with Mildred each time she had to use the restroom. Much of that time was spent helping her in and out of her Vera lift. It also took caregivers 20 minutes to transfer Mildred in and out of her bed, which they did once in the morning to get her out of bed and once at night to get her back into bed.

Each apartment at Autumn Park has two emergency call cords (e-cords), one in the bedroom and one in the bathroom. The e-cords are to be pulled only in case of emergencies. Once the e-cord is pulled, it shows up on a computer at the front desk, where the receptionist radios a caregiver to go to that specific room. If a resident wants a caregiver's help that is not an emergency the resident calls the front desk. After the receptionist receives that call, he or she radios a caregiver to go to that room for assistance. Since the e-calls are considered emergencies, they are put in top priority over the phone calls. It was discovered that Mildred was pulling her e-cord every 30 minutes to get the caregivers to help her with minor things, such as taking out the trash, turning on her lights, or feeding her cats.

Instructions for Level of Care Assessment

Bathing/Showering:
- 20 minutes—Resident requires daily bathing/showering due to incontinence
- 10 minutes—Requires total assistance, substantial assistance, or standby assistance during bathing/showering including help in and out, supervision/assistance with washing, shampooing, toweling, dressing, and so forth; bath/shower 3X/week; assist with dressing daily
- 5 minutes—Resident requires verbal reminders, clothes laid out, bathing items prepared, some assistance with buttons, zipper, and so forth
- 2 minutes—Resident requires minimal assistance, including reminders and follow-up
  Staff member does not need to be present during bathing and dressing
- 0 minutes—Independent

Oral Care:
- 10 minutes—Total assistance or standby assistance with and/or reminders for oral care including care of dentures, partials, and so forth
- 5 minutes—Reminder and setup only
- 2 minutes—Reminders only and follow-up check daily
- 0 minutes—Independent

Grooming: (includes hair care, shaving, and make-up application)
- 15 minutes—Total assistance or standby assistance daily
- 7 minutes—Reminders, setup, and follow-up only
- 0 minutes—Independent

Toileting/Incontinence:
- 50 minutes—Assistance and/or reminders to resident to use the bathroom every 2–3 hours; assistance with protective undergarments, assistance with removing and/or re-applying clothing; changing bed as needed
- 25 minutes—Reminders and directing only and/or frequent accidents (more than 1X/week)
- 10 minutes—Assist with cleanup of occasional accidents
- 0 minutes—Independent

Medication Management:
- 20 minutes—Total medication administration (4 plus X a day/dosing or more than 6 medications a day)
- 15 minutes—Supervision of medication administration (3X a day/dosing or 3–6 different medications a day)
- 10 minutes—Supervision of medication administration (2X a day/dosing or less than 3 medications per day)
- 5 minutes—Weekly medications setup only, or supervision of medication administration for P.R.N.s only
- 0 minutes—Independent

Mental Status/Behaviors:
- 60 minutes—Disoriented, requires 24-hour supervision and monitoring; occasional redirection

(continued)

Exhibit 2.   Level of care assessment criteria at Autumn Park.

(continued)

- 30 minutes—Disoriented, frequent reminders needed, but some direction or redirection required or depression requiring constant encouragement and frequent individual socialization
- 20 minutes—Mild disorientation, occasional behavior problems, needs reminders daily or depression requiring daily encouragement
- 10 minutes—Mild disorientation, no behavior problems, follows routines or some depression requiring occasional encouragement
- 0 minutes—Independent

Transfers/Ambulation:
- 10 minutes—Always assist with transfers; pushing wheelchair to meals, activities, or standby assistance for ambulation with walker
- 5 minutes—Occasional assistance for wheelchair transport to meals, activities, or standby assistance for ambulation with walker
- 0 minutes—Independent

Other Treatments:
- Other treatments, including follow-up of therapies, dressing changes, customary care, Unna boots, whirlpool treatments, application of ointments, blood sugar, frequent vital signs, or treatment. Record estimated/actual time per day to perform treatment. This includes weights or vital signs, more than once a month, daily bed change due to incontinence, and so forth.

Legend:

0–45   Minutes of care per day is   Level I

46–90   Minutes of care per day is   Level II

91–135   Minutes of care per day is   Level III

Greater than 130 minutes per day might require Alzheimer's care or nursing care. Each additional 40 minutes will be billed as an additional level.

Douglas, Autumn Park's new executive director, and Meeks also noted that Mildred was abusing her privileges with Autumn Park's scheduled transportation. Autumn Park owns a bus that is wheelchair accessible, and has a capacity for 20 people. The bus is normally used for scheduled outings and activities for the residents. Autumn Park also owns a Town Car that is used for doctor's visits and unscheduled errands. One hundred and forty residents must share these two vehicles. Although Mildred was aware of her restrictions on transportation since she could only use the bus, she still demanded that the bus take her to her doctor's visits on her schedule. She was not concerned that the bus was being used for another scheduled activity.

Mildred was constantly complaining that the caregivers don't understand her lift and don't understand English. She was continually pulling the e-cord. Once her present rent increased due to the time spent on her, she came back to Autumn Park with her attorney claiming discrimination under the Americans with Disabilities Act saying that Autumn Park only raised her rate, and no other resident's rate.

Every time Autumn Park showed her the minutes, she insisted that they were not right. She then dictated to Meeks which caregivers she wanted to care for her. Such a request was considered private duty in Autumn Park, which constituted a rate increase. Mildred once again claimed that Autumn Park was discriminating against her and threatened to sue.

In November of 2000, Meeks discovered that Autumn Park did not have any of the exception letters on Mildred's conditions to the state—injections, age, lift, and disability. Douglas and Meeks hoped that after they filed the exception letters, the state would no longer allow Mildred to live at Autumn Park. Yet, the exception letters came back approved by the state.

Also in November, Autumn Park gave Mildred a 30-day period to evaluate the minutes spent on her care. She was to keep a record and the caregivers were to keep a separate record of the minutes they spent with her. Yet, it was soon discovered that she manipulated the caregivers when to document the minutes and when to stop. Mildred denied any accusations that she manipulated the caregivers in their documentation of her care. Due to the dispute on how to record and how the minutes reflected the care, Mildred and Autumn Park redid the evaluation in January 2001.

Also, in January, a letter was sent to all residents at Autumn Park that there was a change in the price structure of assisted living. Instead of $400 for Level I, and $300 for Levels II and III, it will now be $500 for each level of care.

In March of 2001, a second evaluation of the minutes of care for Mildred was conducted. Mildred still didn't feel that the minutes documented a true reflection of the care she was given. Once again it was discovered that Mildred was manipulating the caregivers, because many came forward to talk about it with Meeks. Also, several of the caregivers wanted to quit because they no longer wanted to care for Mildred. They claimed she was verbally abusive and yelled at them. Mildred denied that she ever raised her voice to a caregiver or spoke to them in a derogatory way. She said that the caregivers must have interpreted her orders incorrectly. Also, in the span of 5 months, three caregivers were receiving workers compensation because they hurt their backs trying to care for her. Mildred still demanded only certain caregivers to care for her, and now she wanted no male caregivers giving her showers.

By this time, Douglas and Meeks were very frustrated with Mildred. They wanted her out of the property but didn't know how to dismiss her without getting sued or causing negative publicity. Douglas decided to visit the Executive Director of the CCRC Mildred lived in prior to Autumn

Park. The Executive Director agreed with Douglas about how difficult and manipulative Mildred was. She also told Brad that, "once we got her 30-day move-out notice we were jumping up and down in the halls. We wrote glowing letters about her just to make certain that Autumn Park would take her." Douglas was completely at a loss on what to do about Mildred Puce.

In May of 2001, Autumn Park talked to the ombudsman about the difficulties they were having with caring for Mildred. The demands she was putting on Autumn Park and the caregivers were causing a great deal of stress. The ombudsman agreed with Autumn Park that Mildred Puce had been a difficult resident.

In June, Mildred complained to the same ombudsman that her personal rights were being violated since Autumn Park was still allowing a male caregiver to give her a shower. The ombudsman then called the state licensing agent, who came out to Autumn Park and talked to Douglas and Meeks about the difficulty they had in caring for Mildred. Autumn Park provided the agent with all the information they had on Mildred including documentation of what skill level they provide for her in care and how Mildred needed more.

By this time, Mildred had developed severe edema in her legs due to poor circulation. This swelling in her legs has caused them to weigh around 50 pounds each. This increased the risk of caregivers injuring themselves when they lift one of her legs to reposition them in her wheelchair or her lift. If this edema persisted, her skin would break down, causing open, weeping wounds. If this happened, she would be immediately sent to the hospital.

Under the California state regulations, Title 22, a residential care facility for the elderly is obligated to give a resident a 30-day notice to move out if the facility feels that they can no longer provide the care a resident needs. Yet, if Autumn Park gives Mildred a 30-day notice, she will sue Autumn Park on the basis of the Americans with Disabilities Act. Mildred also threatened that she will call the local media about Autumn Park's treatment of a handicapped resident. Therefore, Douglas had made certain that he told the state licensing agent that Autumn Park can care for Mildred but not to her specifications.

Also, under these state regulations, a facility can refuse to permit a resident to return to the facility after a resident has been hospitalized, if the facility believes that they can no longer care for the resident. The regulations state that a resident in such a facility must have skilled health professionals take care of any open wound, skin tears, and/or pressure ulcers. In such cases, hospitalization may be necessary to receive such care or the facility will have an approved exception from the state that a home health nurse will care for the resident until their wound has healed.

As Douglas looked over Mildred's file, he felt that his hands were tied. Mildred needed custodial care not skilled nursing care. Yet, Mildred was a victim of her own circumstances since she could not afford the one-to-one care due to her insurance. Community care licensing agents had even evaluated Mildred, and they all agreed that Mildred Puce was not appropriate for a CCRC and needed a different level of care.

Douglas also thought about what the ARC corporate staff told him. They stated that anything is better than negative public press about Autumn Park or ARC. "Do what it takes to provide her care; avoid a lawsuit and negative publicity at all costs."

At the meeting with Mildred, Brad will offer her three legal options: (1) to get care from another agency that meets licensing requirements, (2) to move to another facility with more skilled care, or (3) to offer 12 hours of one-to-one care that will cost Mildred $7,000 a month.

27

Appalachian Home Health Services

Kathryn H. Dansky

Pennsylvania State University, University Park, Pennsylvania

Frances Matthews, the director of clinical services at Appalachian Home Health Services, Inc. (AHHS), was concerned. AHHS needed to hire a nurse quickly. One of the staff nurses had just handed in her resignation because her husband was being transferred out of state. The nurse who was leaving gave AHHS 2 weeks' notice, which complied with the agency policy; however, it still left the agency in a bind. Matthews knew that recruiting and interviewing home health nurses was a time-consuming process, and, even after a nurse was hired, several weeks of orientation were usually required before the nurse could perform independently. She knew that all of the regular staff nurses were working to capacity and that the loss of even one nurse would have major implications. She walked over to Kate Hennessey's office to discuss the situation. Hennessey was the director of administrative services. Matthews and Hennessey had started AHHS 4 years ago. Together, they made all final hiring decisions.

Matthews knocked on the door, saw that Hennessey was sitting at her desk, and walked in. "Sue is leaving. She sure picked a bad time to move!" She laughed halfheartedly, and said, "We need to replace her quickly. Do you have any brilliant ideas?"

From Dansky, K.H. (1991). Appalachian Home Health Services. In G.E. Stevens (Ed.), *Cases and exercises in human resource management* (5th ed., pp. 246–251). Homewood, IL: Richard D. Irwin, Inc.; used by permission of the author.

Hennessey sighed, and responded, more in the form of a statement than a question, "We don't have any decent applications on file, do we?"

"Nope."

"Great. Well, let's get our ad into the paper today; maybe something will turn up."

BACKGROUND

AHHS is a private, not-for-profit home health agency, located in a rural area of a midwestern state. The stated purpose of AHHS is to provide health care services at home to elderly individuals, persons with disabilities, and persons with short-term, specific health care needs that could be handled at home.

AHHS is a "fee-for-service" health care organization; it provides in-home services, then bills for the services, either to a public or private insurance carrier (e.g., Medicare, Medicaid, Blue Cross/Blue Shield), or to the patient directly. AHHS receives all (100%) of its revenue from billed services. As a private organization, it does not receive government subsidies or tax support.

Competition in the home health field is intense, particularly in rural areas, where the need for services fluctuates. Because services are expensive to provide, it is critical for agencies to generate a volume of visits sufficient to cover fixed expenses plus make a small profit. Competition for AHHS comes primarily from Care One, Inc., a multicounty operation that has been established in the area for well over 10 years. AHHS surpassed Care One in total number of visits after its second year of operation and has been steadily growing. Many of the physicians in the area, however, continue to use Care One, and Care One receives more referrals from nonlocal hospitals than does AHHS.

AHHS currently has 32 employees, including 15 registered nurses (full time and part time), 8 nursing aides, 1 physical therapist, 1 speech-language therapist, and 7 administrative staff. All but two employees at AHHS are female.

REFERRALS FOR SERVICE

Most of the business generated for AHHS is in the form of referrals. Hospitals (social workers, discharge planners) account for more than 70% of patient referrals; of this total, approximately 85% are from the two local hospitals and 15% are from out-of-town hospitals. The second most frequent source of referrals is the general public; former patients, potential patients, family members, clergy, and the like may request services directly. Approximately 20% of referrals come from this source. A small number of referrals come directly from physicians. Although this source is less than 10% of the total, it is important to AHHS, because of the power and status that physicians have in the community.

PATIENTS WHO RECEIVE HOME HEALTH SERVICES

Most of the individuals who receive in-home care are elderly. They usually have a chronic illness that requires monitoring or have a need for rehabilitation therapy following an acute episode, such as a stroke or hip fracture. Some patients have disabilities and require ongoing therapy at home. Some are convalescing from a hospital stay, and need short-term care (e.g., dressing changes). Others have a special type of medical need that does not require hospitalization, such as intravenous antibiotics or chemotherapy.

Most of the patients cared for by AHHS are indigenous to the area, live in rural areas, and are religious. Although not all patients fit this description, it is fairly safe to say that the patient population is elderly, traditional, and conservative.

THE ROLE OF THE HOME HEALTH NURSE

The registered nurse is the central caregiver in the home health field. The nurse must be able to function independently and comfortably in the patient's home, and must be capable of performing a wide variety of clinical procedures (e.g., giving injections, inserting catheters, obtaining specimens). Furthermore, the R.N. is considered both a "case manager" and a "gatekeeper" in coordinating medical, health, and social services (see Table 1). This position requires high-level skills in nursing and communications. Nurses with a bachelor of science in nursing (B.S.N.) and experience in home health or community nursing are usually sought for these positions.

ANSWERS TO THE AHHS ADVERTISEMENT

After Matthews left, Hennessey asked the office manager to run off a copy of their standard classified ad for a home health nurse (see Exhibit 1) and take it to the local newspaper's office. The next day, the newspaper carried the ad in the classified section. The ad ran for 3 consecutive days.

Table 1. Job description for home health agency registered nurse

Definition

The registered nurse administers skilled nursing services to a patient in accordance with a written plan of treatment established by the patient's physician. The incumbent is directly responsible to the Nursing Supervisor and ultimately to the Director of Patient Services.

Qualifications

1. Graduate of an approved school of professional nursing
2. Current license to practice as a registered nurse in this state

Responsibilities

1. Conduct initial patient assessment and evaluation
2. Evaluate the ongoing needs of patients on a regular basis
3. Initiate the patient's plan of treatment and any necessary revisions
4. Provide those services that require substantial specialized nursing skills
5. Initiate appropriate preventive and rehabilitative nursing procedures
6. Prepare and maintain clinical notes
7. Coordinate care with allied health professionals
8. Inform the physician and other personnel of changes in the patient's condition
9. Counsel the patient and family in meeting nursing and related health needs
10. Participate in in-service and continuing education programs
11. Supervise and teach other nursing personnel

Applicants were requested to call the office, or to send a résumé to the director of clinical services.

AHHS received two responses to the ad. One was a résumé from a student at a nearby technical college. The college had a 2-year (associate degree) registered nurse program, and the applicant was in the last quarter of her second year. Matthews read over the résumé. She knew, from past experience, that R.N.s from 2-year programs lacked many of the skills for this type of work. She decided not to interview this applicant.

The other applicant, Margaret Jenkins, called to express interest in this position; the conversation was pleasant and informal because the women knew each other. Jenkins had lived in the area all of her life, had family there, and was well known for her community activities.

Jenkins is a registered nurse, with a B.S.N. from the local university. She had most recently worked for 8 years for Dr. Edward Smith, a general practitioner in town. Prior to that time, she had worked at the state men-

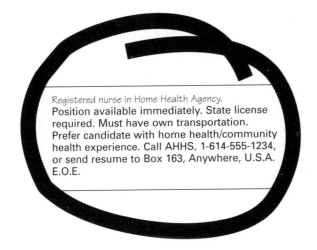

Registered nurse in Home Health Agency.
Position available immediately. State license
required. Must have own transportation.
Prefer candidate with home health/community
health experience. Call AHHS, 1-614-555-1234,
or send resume to Box 163, Anywhere, U.S.A.
E.O.E.

Exhibit 1.   Sample classified ad for a home health nursing position.

tal health center. References from both employers indicated that she was
hard working, responsible, and professional and got along well with
patients, staff, and physicians.

Eighteen months ago, Jenkins was involved in a domestic violence
situation in her home. During an argument with her husband, according to the press, Jenkins was physically attacked and the argument
ended in the death of her husband. Jenkins was charged with murder.
During the course of the trial, most of the details were made public.
Episodes of violence had occurred previously, resulting in a separation
of Jenkins and her husband, with a restraining order against the husband. Jenkins testified that on the night of the fatal argument, she was
home with her two children when he appeared and threatened all three
of them. While her husband was beating her, she managed to pick up a
kitchen knife and kill him. The court convicted her of involuntary
manslaughter and sentenced her to 10 years in prison. While she was in
prison, her attorney petitioned for early release, based on her standing
in the community and the fact that she was the sole support of two
young children. Also during this time, several concerned friends led a
successful campaign to have her nursing license reinstated. (The state
board of nursing had revoked her license to practice nursing, a standard
practice for convicted felons.)

Jenkins' immediate concern was finding employment. Dr. Smith, her
former employer, was semi-retired and not able to rehire her. When she
saw the AHHS ad in the paper, she thought it was her answer. Now that
she had her license back, she could begin working immediately.

THE INTERVIEWS

Because of Jenkins' good work record and because no other suitable applicants were available, Matthews asked Jenkins to come in for an interview, and set up an appointment for that afternoon. The procedure at AHHS was for all R.N. applicants to be interviewed first by the nursing supervisor, then by the two directors, Matthews and Hennessey.

Jenkins walked in to the AHHS offices and greeted everyone warmly. A Caucasian woman of average height and weight, she appeared to be in her mid-thirties. She was on time, was dressed appropriately, and looked a little nervous. Barbara Jones, the nursing supervisor, introduced herself and led Jenkins into the conference room. A half-hour later, Jones brought Jenkins to Hennessey's office, where the second interview would take place. Jones went in first and briefly summarized her interview. Although she had a positive overall impression, she was concerned about Jenkins' lack of experience with home health procedures, particularly interviewing and assessment skills. Because this part of the job was so important to the overall plan of care, it was essential that R.N.s have experience in this area. She then left the office and Jenkins went in.

Jenkins sat down with Hennessey and Matthews. The three women discussed AHHS policies and general personnel issues, including benefits. It was clear that Jenkins had the abilities and skills needed, she knew the geographical area well, and could communicate effectively with area physicians. Her only weakness was that she did not have home health experience. Her personal life was not discussed, but she did remark at one point, "You know, I really need this job." At the end of the interview, Matthews thanked her for coming, and said, "You do meet many of the qualifications, but I'm not sure if you're the right person for this job." Jenkins smiled grimly and said, "I wouldn't blame you if you don't want to hire me." With that, she picked up her things and walked quietly from the office.

Matthews and Hennessey looked at each other. "I don't know," Hennessey said. "I don't know either!" responded Matthews. They usually based their hiring decisions on qualifications plus "intuition," and usually agreed on an applicant's suitability. This case was different, however, and neither was sure whether they should hire Margaret Jenkins.

28

Suburban
Health Center

Bruce D. Evans
University of Dallas, Irving, Texas

George S. Cooley
Long Green Associates, Inc., Long Green, Maryland

The situation gave Helen Lawson good reason to pause. She had been supervisor of Metro City Health Department's Suburban Health Center for only 2 months and reflected that things had been going well. Yet, Lawson had one problem that, unfortunately, threatened to overshadow all of the good things, and she was not sure how to avoid trouble.

Dr. Morgan had just left her office, and he had merely added fuel to the fire. He was the staff doctor for a state-funded health project. He had come to plead that Dorothy Wilson be fired. Wilson, it seems, was the problem. As one of Lawson's staff nurses and one of only three in the office with a bachelor's degree in nursing, Wilson had been with the Suburban Center for 3 years. When Lawson was first hired, she had planned to rely heavily on Wilson, but so far she had not been able to do so.

Lawson knew, of course, that she did not have the authority to dismiss Wilson, because they were all municipal employees. She had had trouble convincing Morgan of this. He had been adamant. He had tried previously to have Wilson discharged because his people were unable to work with her. His staff had said her attitude conveyed that they were intruding in her domain and that she resented them. Wilson's actions did appear to reflect this attitude.

Morgan had related several incidents indicating that Wilson was a very weak communicator and that both her resentment and inability to communicate resulted in almost no coordination. Because coordination in community health services is very important, Morgan believed it was essential to replace Wilson with someone more mature who could work effectively with the state agency. Lawson had listened. Although reiterating the limitations of her authority, she promised to look into it further.

Appointments and lunch gave Lawson a brief respite from Morgan's comments. On her return, however, she felt compelled to carry through on her promise quickly. The first step was to review Wilson's personnel file carefully. To do so, Lawson called for her clerk to bring in the file. In passing she said, "Billie, why don't you go to lunch now. Ms. Wilson will be here to cover the phones." Billie replied excitedly, "Oh, no, Ms. Lawson! I'll just wait for the others to get back. Wilson can't handle them. I can never make out messages that she leaves after answering."

With the exchange ended, Lawson turned to the file. She had glanced casually at all the personnel files previously, but she had not looked thoroughly to see what they might reveal. Wilson's job application reflected that she had held eight assorted jobs in the 8 years preceding her application for this job. Lawson wondered what caused these job changes.

Pertaining to her education, Wilson's file reflected that her degree had been earned only after course work from five colleges and universities. Also, her excessive tardiness had delayed her attaining full employment status. Finally, her most recent performance report had been downgraded to "satisfactory" from her previous "excellent" ratings.

Armed with this, Lawson decided to meet with Lila Moran, the previous supervisor who had left to take a part-time position closer to her home. At her office, Moran added further information. "I confess I wasn't able to handle Wilson," she said. "I was afraid of her and did not want to confront her. After all, she is really a big woman and can be intimidating. Certainly her ratings were inflated, but I only did so to avoid trouble. Ms. Wilson's work—especially her reports—was often substandard. She often refused to do things, but the others covered for her in the office, so I let it go."

WILSON'S BEHAVIOR

The past 2 days' input weighed heavily on Lawson. Throughout all her subsequent findings, she recognized that Wilson's performance was continually unsatisfactory. As a result, Lawson felt compelled to begin to maintain a file on Wilson's performance. Despite incidents that had been related to her, Lawson found no specific deviations committed to writing. The depth of the problem was highlighted by the fact that it took less than 2 weeks to accumulate several memos in Lawson's file. Wilson's less-than-satisfactory performance, it seems, was hardly a rare occurrence.

One thing Lawson noted again and again was that Wilson consistently failed to leave word with anyone when she left the office. Not only did she fail to sign out, but also she failed to even mention where she was going or when she would return. This happened even at peak workload times when the entire staff was needed. Wilson seemed oblivious to these needs and went about tasks that could as easily have been scheduled for slower periods.

Lawson also noticed that Wilson always took 2 hours for lunch on Fridays. The staff jokingly seemed to know what she was doing and had covered for her often. Although Lawson did not object to occasional long lunch hours, the regularity and seeming secrecy bothered her.

In one specific incident, Wilson was gone for more than an hour one afternoon. When she returned, Lawson asked where she had been. "I went to get gas," she said. "I only use this one brand, and there is no station on my way home." Lawson asked her why she could not go out of her way after work. Rather than answering, Wilson appeared hurt and just stared away. Reacting to an awkward situation, she went off to sulk and was moody for the rest of the day.

Lawson next reviewed Wilson's time sheets and written reports. All employees were required to account for how their time was spent and report on the families for whom they were responsible. These reports resulted from periodic visits to the families' homes. Lawson noted that Wilson's sheet reflected consistently longer transportation and visit times than did those of the other staff nurses. Furthermore, Wilson's reports were poorly organized and provided scant information to justify the time spent. The reports did not reflect why she made the visit, what problems if any were noted, and what actions she planned to take to correct them. Rather, she gave a hazy narrative paragraph to show the visit was made.

When Lawson asked her about this, Wilson again seemed hurt, but she also indicated in a rather hostile manner that many of these problems were not her fault. "My district is the most spread out. I also find many families not at home. That's why my transportation time is higher. I can't help that." She also laid much blame on the coordinating agencies. "It's often the agencies' fault. They don't coordinate properly. I can't do it all myself." She said further that she often failed to get proper and adequate information because someone else slipped up.

LAWSON'S PROBLEM

Lawson considered this information for a few days and decided to discuss the situation with Betsy Graham—her immediate superior at the health department—in the hope that she could provide some useful guidance. Graham began by saying, "Yes, I was aware that Moran was having a personnel problem at Suburban, but it never officially got up to me, so I took no action. My main contact with Wilson came when Moran decided to leave. Wilson was senior there, and could have taken over your supervisory position, but she expressed no interest in it. She apparently had no desire to move up or accept more responsibility. The job remained essentially vacant until you arrived. Everyone pretty much looked after themselves."

Graham was unable to give Lawson any more first-hand information, nor did she seem to have any concrete advice for Lawson. Lawson puzzled over the facts as she drove back to the office. She realized there was sufficient information before her to solve the problem, but what she had not been able to do was put it together properly to come to the right conclusion. As she reached the office, she tried to sort out the issues, identify the causes of the problem, and decide what to do.

PART VI

Ethics Incidents

29

Ethics Incidents

Kurt Darr
The George Washington University, Washington, D.C.

ADMINISTRATIVE ETHICS

Incident 1: Borrowed Time

Annabeth Jackson is director for ancillary departments at Healing Hands Rehabilitation, a 120-bed acute rehabilitation center located in the Northwest. Jackson's departments include food and nutrition services (F&NS). Two years ago, she hired Frank Anderson as supervisor for F&NS, a department with 37 full-time employees (FTEs). Initially, Jackson was very pleased with Anderson's performance. However, problems have arisen over the past 8 months, including being tardy, taking numerous sick days, missing deadlines for employee performance evaluations, socializing (and partying) excessively with members of his staff, and addressing and engaging with staff in ways that are too familiar and casual. Some staff members have told Jackson that they are uncomfortable with Anderson's informality and overly friendly behavior. Jackson has verbally cautioned Anderson several times, noted these problems in his performance review, and even written a step one disciplinary memorandum, a copy of which was given to Anderson as well as put in his employment file. Actions to change Anderson's behavior have achieved no observable effect.

Healing Hands' human resources (HR) policies do not specify the appropriate relationship between supervisors and managers and staff. It is clear, however, that supervisors are expected to treat all staff with respect and maintain a certain distance between themselves and those for whom they are responsible. For example, HR policies specifically prohibit managers from borrowing money from those they supervise. This is to avoid placing a staff member in an untenable position if he or she refuses to lend money, or has to make efforts for repayment if money is lent.

Anderson's use of sick days causes him to use his paid time off (PTO) as quickly as he accumulates it. Employees earn 20 hours per month (240 hours per year) of combined sick leave, vacation, personal days, and bereavement time. Last week Anderson sent an e-mail to Jackson stating that he needed to take an extended medical leave due to the stress of his work. Under the federal Family and Medical Leave Act, Anderson is enti-tled to take the medical leave (with physician verification of his condition); however, he would need to use PTO hours to continue to be paid. Knowing that Anderson had only a few hours of PTO left for the year, Jackson wondered how he could maintain his level of income.

This morning Jackson learned that Anderson had sent an e-mail to three of his staff in F&NS asking them to donate some of their PTO to him. HR policies allow employees to voluntarily donate PTO hours to other staff. Jackson was angry; she saw this as a breach of the appropriate relationship between managers and staff. The situation raised several issues for Jackson. She pondered what course of action was necessary.

Incident 2: Emergency Department Repeat Admissions—A Question of Resource Use

Matt Losinski finished reading an article that provided grim details of a study of the overuse of emergency services in hospitals in central Texas. He smiled that sardonic half smile that meant there was a strong possibil-ity that County General Hospital (CGH) might have the same problem. As chief executive officer (CEO), Losinski always saw the problems of other hospitals as potential problems at CGH, a 300-bed, acute care hos-pital in a mixed urban and suburban service area in the south central United States. CGH was established as a county-owned hospital; however, 10 years ago the county wanted to get out of the hospital business and the assets were donated to a not-for-profit hospital system. The new owner has continued a strong public service orientation, even though CGH no longer receives the tax subsidy it did when it was county owned; it must look to itself for fiscal health.

The study data showed that nine residents of a central Texas commu-nity had been seen in emergency departments (ED) a total of 2,678 times over 6 years. One resident had been seen in an ED 100 times each year for the past 4 years. Given that an ED visit can cost $1,000 or more, the nine residents had consumed $2.7 million in resources. These high users were middle age, spoke English, and were split between male and female. To

Losinski, the problem seemed like a manifestation of Wilfredo Pareto's classic 80/20 rule.

Losinski forwarded the article on a priority basis to Mary Scott, his chief financial officer (CFO), and asked her to see him after she read it. Scott stopped by Losinski's office late the next day and began the conversation by asking him why he thought the article was a priority. Scott reminded Losinski that Medicaid paid 75% of *costs* for eligible ED users and that the cross subsidy from privately insured and self-pay ED admissions covered most of the unpaid additional costs. Losinski had a good working relationship with Scott, but he was a bit annoyed by her rather indifferent response.

Losinski wanted details on the use of the ED at CGH. He asked the administrative resident, Aniysha Patel, to gather data that would identify use rates for persons repeatedly admitted to the ED. The findings that Patel gave to Losinski two weeks later were not as extreme as those reported from central Texas; however, they did show that a few persons were repeatedly admitted to the ED and accounted for hundreds of visits in the past year. The clinical details were not immediately available, but a superficial review of the admitting diagnoses suggested that most of the admissions involved persons with minor, nonspecific medical problems— persons commonly known as the "worried well." Although Scott was correct that Medicaid covered the majority of costs, the fact remained that over $200,000 each year was not reimbursed to CGH. Were that money available, it could go directly to the bottom line and be used for several needed enhancements to health initiatives for the community. In addition, repeated admissions to the ED contributed to crowding, treatment delays, and general dissatisfaction for other patients.

Losinski presented the data to his executive committee, which includes all vice presidents, the director of development, and the elected president of the medical staff. The responses ran the gamut from "So what?" to "Wow, this is worse than I would have imagined." Losinski was bemused by the disparity of views. He had thought that there would have been an almost immediate consensus that this was a problem in need of a solution. The financial margins for CGH were already very thin, and the future for adequate reimbursement was not bright. A concern echoed by several at the meeting was the requirement of the federal Emergency Medical Treatment and Active Labor Act (EMTALA) that all persons who present at an ED that receives federal reimbursement for services must be treated and stabilized.

Losinski asked his senior management team for recommendations on addressing this problem.

Incident 3: The Administrative Institutional Ethics Committee[1]

The CEO of Community Health Plan (CHP), a small not-for-profit HMO, has been approached by a group from "north of the river." This area of the city is economically depressed and has lost many of its health services organizations (HSOs) and physicians to the suburbs during the last decade. It seems to be in a downward vortex with no apparent bottom. An increasing number of uninsured patients means that HSOs are less and less able to continue serving the area. The city-owned hospital has made several ill-fated attempts to serve "north of the river" with a clinic system, but its efforts have been scandal-ridden. The system is a political football with little credibility in the community.

The representatives from "north of the river" are community leaders, none of whom appear to have any political ambitions. They seem genuinely willing to do whatever they can to assist in delivering high-quality health services in the community. They proposed that CHP establish and staff three store-front clinics in the area. The community leaders stated they would get volunteers to remodel the facilities and work in clerical capacities.

The CEO described the proposed activity to the administrative institutional ethics committee (IEC), which included members of governance, managers, and physicians and others from clinical areas. In making the presentation, the CEO stressed the plan's historical role in providing health services to those in need, its not-for-profit status, and its continuing modest surplus. The members listened patiently, but the minute the CEO finished all of them seemed to speak at once. Several were opposed and made the following points about the suggested venture:

1. "North of the river" is the city's responsibility. Providing care to the needy is not something a small, not-for-profit health plan should attempt.

2. They have a primary obligation to enhance benefits for their enrollees, rather than get involved in new schemes. Several of their physicians and many plan members have requested additional services.

3. The modest surplus that the plan has accumulated over several years could easily be consumed. The chief financial officer noted that they are expecting an increase in reinsurance premiums in the next quarter.

4. If the plan pulls the city's political chestnuts out of the fire by providing even stop-gap assistance, the city will never get its house in order and develop the system needed "north of the river."

Several spoke in favor of working "north of the river":

1. Helping the "north of the river" community is the right thing to do. The people there deserve health services. It was noted that CHP's own start had come about when several physicians in the community fought the prevailing attitude among their peers about prepaid practice.

2. Those opposed are putting dollars ahead of people's health. They must be willing to assist those less fortunate.

3. Plan members will support such an initiative if it is properly explained to them.

4. The positive publicity will further plan interests by increasing the number of enrollees.

It seems to the CEO that this is a no-win situation. The organizational philosophy is not well developed, and the proposal is a major step. Something should be done to assist the "north of the river" community. The IEC members are raising valid points that merit further discussion.

Incident 4: Bits and Pieces[2]

John Henry Williams really liked his new job in the department of radiology at Affiliated Nursing Homes and Rehabilitation Center. He had recently been appointed acting head when his predecessor, Mary Beth Jacobson, went on maternity leave. As acting head of radiology, John Henry is responsible for two and a half full-time equivalent (FTE) technicians, an appointments clerk, and more than $250,000 worth of equipment. He has authority to purchase radiographic supplies, including certain types of film. The total value of these purchases is approximately $90,000 per year. Most are obtained from three vendors, companies with which the organization has done business for many years.

When Mary Beth oriented John Henry to the demands and responsibilities of the job, she told him that some of the best parts were the meetings with the sales representatives from the three vendors. She said that most of these meetings were held at nice restaurants in the suburban area around the center. Some were held in her office. When that was the case, she said, the sales representatives invariably brought along a "little something." When John Henry asked what that meant, Mary Beth gave examples: perfume, a bottle of French brandy, and a pen set in a nice case. John Henry remembered thinking that his wife might like the perfume.

He asked Mary Beth whether there was a policy concerning accepting gifts from vendors. Mary Beth was a little put out by the question, because it seemed to suggest something might be wrong with the practice. She responded somewhat curtly that the center's senior management trusted its managers and allowed them discretion in such matters.

Personally, John Henry was more interested in the lunches, because it seemed to be a chance for him to leave the facility occasionally and get away from the dreary cafeteria as well as his routine sack lunches. Mary Beth described the lunches as nothing especially fancy. She estimated their cost to the sales representative as about the same as small gifts—the $40–$50 range.

John Henry asked whether the action might not suggest to some members of the staff that her decisions were being influenced by the pecuniary relationship with the sales representatives. Mary Beth's anger flashed. She quickly gave four reasons in justification to John Henry:

1. Taking clients to lunch or providing small gifts was common in business relationships.

2. There was no cost to the center because the vendors paid for everything and they could charge it against their expense account, or get reimbursed by the company.

3. At least one of the sales representatives had become a friend over the years and she enjoyed his company on a social level as well.

4. There was absolutely no possibility her judgment could be influenced for the small amounts of money involved.

Somewhat heatedly, Mary Beth added, "I know you're thinking that somehow this whole thing doesn't look right. But that isn't fair at all. I work long hours as a manager and get paid very little extra. It also takes more effort and time to do the ordering and keep the inventory of supplies at a proper level. If anything goes wrong, it's my neck that's in a noose. These gratuities from vendors are a little something to help compensate me for those activities. My work for the center has been very effective. I'd be happy to talk to anyone who thinks otherwise!"

Incident 5: A Potentially Shocking Revelation

Geraldene Jones had been a nurse before she earned her master of health services administration degree and began her trek to the top of the corporate ladder, a trek that sometimes seemed agonizingly slow. Her love of long-term care and improving the way it is provided fuels her goal to become the chief executive officer of a large nursing facility. Currently, Jones is the vice president for support services at a large nursing facility. It is part of a for-profit chain that owns more than 100 facilities; most of them are large and have more than 200 residents. The facility has an excellent reputation, and there is a waiting list for admission.

Jones's facility is undergoing a major expansion of its physical plant, one that will almost double the square footage. The new space will house rehabilitation services and will add a new respite care program and about 50 new private residents' rooms. Jones volunteered to be responsible for the building program, and some of her other duties were reassigned. She volunteered because she believed success in getting the building program completed on time and under budget would bring her to the attention of corporate headquarters and would make her more promotable.

One day as Jones walked through the half-completed structure, she overheard a heated conversation between the foreman for the electrical contractor and the county electrical inspector. The inspector was pointing out a long list of discrepancies, which ranged from the number of amperes of overall electrical service to the location and number of outlets. The contractor stated repeatedly that the inspector was being overly aggressive in applying the county electrical code. After the inspector left, Jones approached the electrical contractor and asked him whether there were any problems that she should know about. The electrical contractor rubbed two of his fingers and thumb together and said, "Nothing that a little 'grease' won't take care of." It was obvious that the contractor was talking about bribing the inspector. Jones expressed shock and was rebuked by the contractor. "Obviously, you're new to the construction game. Payoffs are common, and I've dealt with this kind of thing before. I know what to do and it's what we'll have to do if you want this building completed on time. I have an account for just such a contingency, but you may have to add to it if the electrical inspector isn't reasonable."

Jones was stunned. She had no idea what to say or what to do.

CLINICAL ETHICS

Incident 6: Protecting the Community[3]

University Hospital has a unique role. It is not only a tertiary referral hospital for the region but also a major source of service to the community. In 1977, it experienced an outbreak of *Legionella* (the bacteria causing Legionnaires' disease). A number of patients were affected; several died.

Legionella is a bacterial infection of the respiratory tract and lungs that may result in death if not diagnosed and treated early. It is especially dangerous for elderly people and those with medical problems that weaken their general resistance. A factor requiring even greater caution on the part of hospital management is that, at the time of the outbreak, the process for identifying the organism in the laboratory took several days. Thus, patients were at great risk until a confirmatory diagnosis was obtained. Epidemiological studies showed a relationship between air conditioning cooling towers and the fine mist they give off and spread of the disease through the aerosol. Workers exposed directly to the aerosol have contracted severe cases of *Legionella*. Chlorinating the water in the cooling towers eliminates the organism.

Although a cooling tower was implicated in the 1977 outbreak at University Hospital, the relationship was never confirmed. The infection control committee of the hospital did not develop any standing orders or policies after the first outbreak. In May 1982, there was evidence of another outbreak of *Legionella*. Chlorination was immediately undertaken and the number of new cases dropped dramatically. An undetected failure in the chlorination system, however, brought a second outbreak in early June.

When the first cases were detected in May 1982, the administrator was notified. He met with various staff members, including physicians on the attending staff. It was decided that information about the outbreak should be kept from the community, lest there be a panic and a sudden drop in census, as well as loss of public confidence. A confidential letter was sent to staff physicians advising them of the problem and asking that they keep in mind the *potential* for infection when making admissions decisions. Admissions were not limited to emergencies, however, and there was no prospective review of elective admissions to determine whether patients at risk for pulmonary infections such as *Legionella* should be sent elsewhere. Nor was there any review of indications for, and necessity of, admission. The medical staff developed a protocol (standing order) stating that unexplained acute-onset pneumonias were to be treated immediately with a very potent antibiotic shown to be effective against *Legionella*. No provision was made, however, for effective review to determine that the protocol was actually followed on a concurrent basis.

Incident 7: Decisions[4]

Mrs. Nickleby is in her mid-forties and has severe multiple sclerosis, a chronic disease that impairs muscular control. She has been a resident of Hightower Nursing Home for almost 3 years. Her two teenage daughters live with her sister in a nearby subdivision and visit her often. Mr. Nickleby, a middle-management executive with a local firm, divorced her 5 years ago.

Mrs. Nickleby has frequent acute attacks of asthma. To date they have been caught in time by the nursing staff; on a couple of occasions she has had to be rushed to the emergency room of the local community hospital. Her physician, who treats her at Hightower Nursing Home, has ordered "no code" if Nickleby has a cardiac arrest during an acute asthma episode at the nursing home—that is, she will not be resuscitated. (Skilled nursing facilities [and acute care hospitals] have different signals, or codes, that are used to call a resuscitation team over the loud-speaker system to respond to a cardiac arrest without alarming other patients and visitors.)

As far as the nurses know, Nickleby's physician made his decision without having discussed it with the patient or her family. One of the nurses is very upset because the decision conflicts with her professional values, although she admits in private that, if she were Nickleby, she would find the situation intolerable and that she would not want to continue living in those circumstances. None of the nurses has heard Nickleby express the same opinion about her condition, even though she has become increasingly depressed, especially after each episode. The nurses have asked the administrative director of the unit for advice.

Incident 8: The Missing Needle Protector[5]

E.L. Straight is director of clinical services at Hopewell Hospital. As in most hospitals, a few physicians deliver care that is acceptable but not of very high quality; they tend to make more mistakes than the others and have a higher incidence of patients going "sour." Since Straight took the position 2 years ago, new programs have been developed and things seem to be getting better.

Dr. Cutrite has practiced at Hopewell for longer than anyone can remember. Although once a brilliant surgeon, he has slipped physically and mentally over the years, and Straight is contemplating steps to recommend a reduction in his privileges. However, the process is not yet complete, and Cutrite continues to perform a full range of procedures.

The operating room supervisor appeared at Straight's office one Monday afternoon. "We've got a problem," she said, somewhat nonchalantly, but with a hint of disgust. "I'm almost sure we left a plastic needle protector from a disposable syringe in a patient's belly, a Mrs. Jameson. You know, the protectors with the red-pink color. They'd be almost impossible to see if they were in a wound."

"Where did it come from?" asked Straight.

"I'm not absolutely sure," answered the supervisor. "All I know is that the syringe was in a used surgical pack when we did the count." She went on to describe the safeguards of counts and records. The discrepancy was noted when the records were reconciled at the end of the week. A surgical pack was shown as having a syringe that was not supposed to be there. When the scrub nurse working with Cutrite was questioned, she remembered that he had used a syringe, but, when it was included in the count at the conclusion of surgery, she didn't think about the protective sheath, which must certainly have been on it.

"Let's get Mrs. Jameson back into surgery," said Straight. "We'll tell her it's necessary to check her incision and deep sutures. She'll never know that we're really looking for the needle cover."

"Too late," responded the supervisor, "she went home the day before yesterday."

Damn, thought Straight. Now what to do? "Have you talked to Dr. Cutrite?"

The supervisor nodded affirmatively. "He won't consider telling Mrs. Jameson that there might be a problem and calling her back to the hospital," she said. "And he warned us not to do anything, either," she added. "Dr. Cutrite claims it cannot possibly hurt her. Except for a little discomfort, she'll never know it's there."

Straight called the chief of surgery and asked a hypothetical question about the consequences of leaving a small plastic cap in a patient's belly. The chief knew something was up but didn't pursue it. He simply replied that there would likely be occasional discomfort, but probably no life-threatening consequences from leaving it in. "Although," he added, "one can never be sure."

Straight liked working at Hopewell Hospital and didn't relish crossing swords with Cutrite, who, although declining professionally, was politically very powerful. Straight had refrained from fingernail biting for years, but that old habit was suddenly overwhelming.

Incident 9: Demarketing to Avoid Bankruptcy[6]

Chris Hines had finally gotten down far enough in the stack of papers on her desk to get to last month's emergency department (ED) activity report. She had already digested the grim news about the continued financial hemorrhage affecting Community Hospital. The current deficit was $500,000— and it was only the fourth month of the fiscal year. Because Community served a largely inner-city population, many of whom were uninsured or whose care was paid by a chronically underfunded Medicaid program, there seemed to be little hope of the financial situation improving.

Hines knew that more than 40% of Community's inpatient admissions came through the ED, and that about half of those admissions arrived by taxi, by private automobile, or on foot. The other half was brought in by the ambulance service run by the city government. Hines had tried to implement a plan to increase the number of elective admissions (and thus improve the payer mix) by encouraging physicians to bring their private patients to Community. This effort failed, however, largely because of the difficulty physicians had in getting their patients admitted—ED admissions were taking too many beds. Hines then tried to work with city officials to implement a new ambulance routing system that would give Community a chance to improve its financial condition. This effort also failed because city officials were unsympathetic.

Hines knew that Community's endowment would carry the hospital about 3 years, but that it would be forced to close if it were not breaking even by then. Because there was nothing that could be done with the city, Hines concluded that the key to survival lay with reducing the number of uninsured and Medicaid admissions through the ED.

Hines spoke with several marketing consultants, one of whom offered to do *pro bono* work for Community. He seized on the idea of "demarketing" the ED. He reasoned that it was the fine reputation Community's ED had in its service area that was largely responsible for the 50% of ED patients who came in other than by city ambulance. He then set out to identify ways in which ED could be made less attractive to potential patients. The plan he developed included reducing ED staffing to the very minimum; closing the parking lot near the ED; reducing housekeeping services so that the physical plant would be dirty and unkempt; deferring indefinitely all non–safety-related maintenance; changing the triage policies, procedures, and staffing so as to increase waiting time for nonemergency patients; using staff who were most likely to be rude and inconsiderate; and encouraging rumors that the closure of the ED was imminent.

The consultant knew there might be repercussions beyond the ED, but Community Hospital was desperate, and he believed there was no choice but to take extreme action.

Incident 10: Something Must Be Done, But What?[7]

Stunned, Carolyn Aubrey, the CEO of Metropolitan Hospital, sank into her chair and stared out the window for a very long time. She realized when Dr. Midmore's wife had angrily insisted on seeing the CEO that something was afoot. Even in her worst nightmares, however, Aubrey could never have imagined that Mrs. Midmore would tell Aubrey that she was suing her husband, an orthopedic surgeon, for divorce because he had given her AIDS. As Mrs. Midmore left Aubrey's office, she had turned back and said, "I was sure you'd want to know—surely you'll want to do something."

Fleetingly, Aubrey thought Mrs. Midmore's remarks might be nothing more than the ravings of an angry, vindictive wife, but that was not likely. As she considered what she had just learned, she recalled an incident several years ago involving Dr. Midmore and a male orderly. In retrospect, it now suggested that he might be bisexual. Aubrey thought, too, about the department of surgery meeting last year when there had been a long discussion about the desirability of knowing the HIV status of all surgical patients. The special risks of torn gloves and cuts during orthopedic surgery had been described in detail.

Now it seemed that Dr. Midmore's patients were at special risk. Aubrey called operating room scheduling and learned that Dr. Midmore was maintaining a full surgical load. Aubrey asked her secretary to call the hospital attorney and the medical director and set up an emergency meeting for 7:00 A.M. the following morning. *Mrs. Midmore might have been telling the truth*, thought Aubrey. *We will have to do something, but what?*

ENDNOTES

1. From Darr, K. (2005). *Ethics in health services management* (4th ed., pp. 100–101). Baltimore: Health Professions Press; reprinted by permission.
2. From Darr, K. (2005). *Ethics in health services management* (4th ed., pp. 132–133). Baltimore: Health Professions Press; reprinted by permission.
3. From Darr, K. (2005). *Ethics in health services management* (4th ed., pp. 200–201). Baltimore: Health Professions Press; reprinted by permission.
4. Adapted from Aroskar, M. (1977, August). Case No. 461, Case studies in bioethics. *Hastings Center Report*, p. 17; used by permission.
5. From Longest, Jr., B. B., Rakich, J. S., & Darr, K. (2000). *Managing health services organizations and systems* (4th ed., pp. 725–726). Baltimore: Health Professions Press; reprinted by permission.
6. From Darr, K. (2005). *Ethics in health services management* (4th ed., pp. 287–288). Baltimore: Health Professions Press; reprinted by permission.
7. From Darr, K. (2005). *Ethics in health services management* (4th ed., p. 199). Baltimore: Health Professions Press; reprinted by permission.